Community Oral Health

Community Oral Health

Edited by

Cynthia M. Pine BDS PhD
Senior Lecturer, Honorary Consultant in Dental Public Health, University of Dundee Dental School

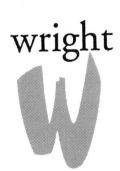
wright

Wright
An imprint of Butterworth-Heinemann
Linacre House, Jordan Hill, Oxford OX2 8DP
A division of Reed Educational & Professional Publishing Ltd

A member of the Reed Elsevier plc group

OXFORD   BOSTON   JOHANNESBURG
MELBOURNE   NEW DELHI   SINGAPORE

First published 1997

British Library Cataloguing in Publication Data
A catalogue record for this book is available from the
British Library

Library of Congress Cataloguing in Publication Data
A catalogue record for this book is available from the
Library of Congress

ISBN 07236 1095 9

Printed and bound in Great Britain by the Bath Press

Contents

Contributors

Ronald M. Andersen, PhD
Wasserman Professor and Chair, School of Public Health, University of California, Los Angeles, USA

Alexia Antzcak-Bouckoms DMD, ScD, MPH
Assistant Professor of Medicine, New England Medical Center, Boston, Massachusetts, USA

F. M. Andreasen
Research Associate, Pedodontic Department, Gothenburg Dental School, Copenhagen, Denmark

J. O. Andreasen DrOdontHC
Associate Director, Department of Oral and Maxillofacial Surgery, Gothenburg Dental School, Copenhagen, Denmark

Hamilton, T. Bellini PhD
Professor, Jundiai, Brazil

Gillian Bradnock PhD, BA
School of Dentistry, Birmingham, UK

Ewald Bronkhorst PhD, MSc
Department of Cariology and Endodontology, Nijmegen, Netherlands

Brian A. Burt BDS, MPH, PhD
School of Public Health, University of Michigan, Ann Arbor, Michigan, USA

Meei-shia Chen PhD, MPH
Research Associate (Associate Professor), Center for Health Administration Studies, University of Chicago, USA

Terry W. Cutress BDS, PhD, FRACDS
Director, Dental Research Unit, Wellington School of Medicine, New Zealand

Murray Dickson DDS, DPaed, MPH
Community and Health Facilitator, College of Dentistry, Saskatoon, Saskatchewan, Canada

Martin C. Downer DDS, PhD, DDPH
Head of Department of Dental Health Policy, Eastman Dental Institute for Oral and Dental Health Care Sciences, London, UK

Stephen A. Eklund DDS, DrPH
Associate Professor of Dental Public Health, University of Michigan, School of Public Health, Ann Arbor, Michigan, USA

Sabrina Fuller MSc, LDS, RCS(Edin)
Senior Dental Officer (Dental Health Promotion) for Tameside and Glossop Community and Priority Services NHS Trust and Oldham NHS Trust; Honorary Lecturer in Oral Health Promotion, University of Manchester, UK

Helen G. Gift PhD
Chief, Disease Prevention and Health Promotion Branch, National Institute of Dental Research, Bethesda, Maryland, USA

Martin H. Hobdell PhD, BDS, LDSRCD (Eng.)
Head, WHO Collaborating Centre for Oral Health, and Dean, Faculty of Dentistry, University of the Western Cape, Cape Town, South Africa

Dorthe Holst DDS, MPH
Professor (Community Dentistry), Institute of Community Dentistry, Oslo, Norway

Sheila Jones MPH
Department of Clinical Dental Sciences, University of Liverpool School of Dentistry, Liverpool, UK

Albert Kingman PhD
Chief Statistician NIDR, Bethesda, Maryland, USA

Michael A. Lennon MDS, FDSCRS(Ed), DPD
Department of Clinical Dental Sciences, University of Liverpool School of Dentistry, Liverpool, UK

David Locker BDS, PhD
Professor, Department of Community Dentistry, Faculty of Dentistry, University of Toronto, Ontario, Canada

Walter Mautsch DR med dent, MSc (Dental Public Health), Klinik für Zahnaerztliche Prothetik, Aachen, Germany

Pauline Mc Goldrick MSc
Clinical Psychologist, Lecturer in Behavioral Sciences in Relation to Dentistry, Dundee Dental School, Dundee, UK

John J. Murray BChD, MChD, PhD, FDSRCS, MCCD
Dental School, Newcastle upon Tyne, UK

Denis M. O'Mullane BDS, PhD, FDS, FFD
Head of University Dental School and Hospital, Professor of Preventive and Paediatric Dentistry, Cork, Eire

Poul Erik Petersen DDS, DrOdontSci, BA, MSc (Sociology)
Professor, Head of Department for Community Dentistry, University of Copenhagen, Denmark

Taco Pilot
Professor, WHO Collaborating Centre for Oral Health Services Research, Groningen, Netherlands

Cynthia M. Pine BDS, PhD
Senior Lecture/Honorary Consultant in Dental Public Health, Department of Dental Health Dental School, University of Dundee, UK

Victor Gomes Pinto PhD
Former Chief of the National Dental Services, Brasilia, Brazil

Nigel B. Pitts BDS, PhD, FDS, RCD Eng, FDS RCS Eng
Director of the Dental Health Services Research Unit and Head of the Department of Dental Health, University of Dundee, UK

Andrew J. Rugg-Gunn RD, DSc, PhD, BDS, FDS
Professor of Preventive Dentistry, and Head of the Department of Child Dental Health, University of Newcastle upon Tyne, UK

Flemming Scheutz DrPH, Dr odont
Senior Associate Professor, Royal Dental College, Aarhus, Denmark

Lone Schou BDS, PhD (Cph), PhD (Edin)
Associate Director, Division of Dental Auxiliary Education, Copenhagen, Denmark

William C. Shaw PhD, MScD, BDS, FDS, D.Orth RCSEng, DDORCPSG1as,
Professor of Orthodontics and Dentofacial Development Dean, University Hospital of Manchester, UK

Aubrey Sheiham BDS, PhD, DHC
Professor, Department of Epidemiology and Public Health, University College London, UK

John Spencer PhD
Professor of Social and Preventive Dentistry, University of Adelaide, Australia

Grace W. Suckling FDSRCSEng, DDSc
Dental Research Unit, Wellington, New Zealand

Gert-Jan Truin PhD
Professor, Department of Cariology and Endodontology, University of Nijmegen, Netherlands

Richard G. Watt BDS, MSc
Lecturer, Dental Public Health, University College London, UK

Helen P. Whelton BDS, PhD
Deputy Director, Oral Health Services Research College, Lecturer in Preventive Dentistry and Public Dental Health, Cork, Eire

B. Alex White DDS, DrPH, MS
Senior Investigator, Center for Health Research, Portland, Oregon, USA

Preface

This textbook is designed for dental under-graduates, postgraduates and health profession-als with an interest in understanding and promoting oral health within communities. The terms 'community oral health', 'community dentistry' and 'dental public health' are essentially synonymous and may be defined as the science and art of preventing oral disease, prolonging oral health and improving the quality of life through the organized efforts of society. The study of community oral health will involve an appreciation of aspects of several disciplines, including sociology, psychology and health-related behaviour, epidemiology and statistics, health economics, health promotion and health service organizational methods. Although community oral health is concerned with the health of populations rather than individual patient care, an appreciation of the health of the broader community, their needs and expectations is essential to the provision of high quality treatment services. The principal diseases of the mouth, caries, periodontal disease, and increasingly in some communities, oral cancer are chronic diseases that are lifestyle-dependent. Choices favourable to the maintenance of oral health include a diet low in refined sugars, regular effective oral hygiene, fluoride enhancement, avoidance of tobacco and moderation in alcohol consumption. Many within affluent societies faced with excess, consumerism and conflicting messages develop, and are encouraged to maintain, the least healthy option. As disease levels have improved, those most vulnerable in society are carrying a greater burden of disease and the gap between the health of the rich and poor has widened. In developing countries, acute conditions are still common. Increasing commercialism alongside the debts from aid are combining to increase oral disease and favour inappropriate health service provision. The chapters in this textbook tackle all of these issues and many more and provide a rich source of information and examples from many countries. This textbook deliberately takes a broader, international perspective. The problems to be tackled in promoting oral health will benefit from co-operation across countries. Furthermore, optimal solutions for health service provision are often hard won and many can benefit from the lessons of others. Those who have contributed to this textbook have expert knowledge of their specialist area, care deeply about the subject and are pre-eminent in their field. This book is commended to student and teacher alike and health professionals who seek to understand and promote oral health within communities large and small.

Acknowledgements

As always, in creating such a valuable resource many people have been involved. My thanks are due to each contributor. They agreed to take part with only minimal persuasion, kept to time and made editing an absorbing process. Mary Seager at Butterworth-Heinemann, as Development Editor, gently guided the book from the outline to the finished product. My personal thanks to Anne Byres, my secretary, who helped me in the preparation of the manuscript and to Heidi Goodship for assistance with proof-reading. Finally, thanks to my family who lived with 'the book' for two years and are still waiting for the video and T-shirt.

This textbook is dedicated to my late father, Frederick Freeman who believed that education opened all doors and to my husband, Geoffrey Pine who shares my philosophy.

1

Introduction, principles and practice of public health

Cynthia M. Pine

Introduction

Public health was defined in the Acheson report (1988) as 'the science and art of preventing disease, prolonging life and promoting health through the organised efforts of society'. This has been adapted in dental public health to become 'the science and art of preventing oral disease, promoting oral health and improving the quality of life through the organised efforts of society' (Downer *et al.*, 1994). Dental public health is the name of the specialty in the UK, but elsewhere a more familiar term would be community dentistry. Dental health is much wider than a consideration of the dental tissues alone. It encompasses all oral conditions, and is an important part of general health. The use of the term oral rather than dental is gaining prominence, therefore the more internationally recognized term community oral health is used in this book.

The aim of public health is to enhance the health of *populations* (Last, 1994). It is clear from these aims and definitions that the study of oral health in the community will require an appreciation of other disciplines, for example sociology, psychology and health-related behaviour, epidemiology, health economics, health promotion and health service organizational methods. All these aspects are covered in detail in the chapters that follow. Since each chapter gives examples in the oral field, it seems pertinent as an introduction to take a broader perspective of public health. This chapter begins with a brief historical overview, leading to the up-to-date view of public health. The next section considers lifestyle influences on health, continuing with the concept of population approaches to preventing disease and a brief evaluation of the practice of public health. The final sections discuss tackling social inequalities in health, concluding with implications for teaching and research.

Historical overview of public health

There have been three phases of activity in public health and organized health care in Europe and North America since the middle of the 19th century and we are now part of the fourth phase (Ashton, 1993).

The *first phase*, 1840–1900, was characterized by industrialization and rapid urbanisation leading to desperate living conditions for the poor. Public health achievements were principally those of sanitary reform. This was the time when medical and epidemiological approaches were successful in detecting causal relationships involving malnutrition, unhygienic conditions and infectious diseases. John Snow's classic study of the cholera epidemic of 1854 is one of the best examples. He mapped the location of each of the over 500 deaths in Soho, London which occurred in a period of 10 days. From the map, he found a distribution with a central point thinning towards the periphery. The central point in Broad Street housed a pump from which the local people obtained their drinking water. At Snow's insistence the handle of the pump was removed and the epidemic immediately subsided (James and Beal, 1981). These types of battles still occur in developing countries. Infectious diseases, that we have largely forgotten, can still wreak havoc in the appalling conditions in which many people in the world have to live today.

The *second phase*, 1880–1930, saw advances in bacteriology and immunization bringing personal prevention on a population basis. This also saw the growth in maternal and child welfare. In the UK, for instance, school meals and school milk were introduced and partly compensated for malnutrition in the poor.

The *third*, therapeutic *phase*, from 1930 to 1974, was characterized by medical services shifting their principal focus to hospitals, increasing complexities of medical treatments and less emphasis on public health. This also coincided with the disappearance of the major infectious diseases.

The *fourth phase*, sometimes called the 'new public health' (Ashton, 1993), had its origins in the growing awareness of the limitations of therapy to tackle chronic lifestyle diseases and the spiralling costs of health care. This led to the publication of new perspectives on health (Lalonde, 1974), closely followed by the World Health Organization (WHO) Health for All concepts.

The 'new public health'

Over the last 20 years the focus of public health has been changing (Dean, 1994). The 1977 World Health Assembly resolution added impetus with the aim that by the year 2000 all citizens of the world would attain a level of health permitting them to live socially and economically productive lives. Several health policy documents followed giving specific health goals, internationally presented by WHO (1981, 1985). The next step was the national setting of targets by many governments, for example, within Europe, as Health for All by the Year 2000 policies and strategies. There have been health gains in this period, for example, major reductions in infant mortality and increasing life expectancy. However, one of the notable trends, common across the world, has been the increasing difference between the rich and poor in economic and social conditions

both within and between countries. Many studies have shown that this phenomenon underlies the growing disparity in health between these groups in society. This division has become accentuated because the occurrence of the most prevalent diseases, e.g. cancer, heart disease and dental caries, are determined by our lifestyle. One of the focuses in public health is to promote the establishment of healthy environments by working in settings such as cities or schools. The aim is to strengthen community action and develop personal skills for health protection. These approaches are discussed in further detail later in the book with the theoretical framework in Chapter 11 and the practical examples in oral health in Chapter 15.

In developed countries, public health is seen as a complex area in which social conditions such as poverty, the absence of hope for the future, a self-centred society and economic influences are increasingly important (Nijhuis and van der Maesen, 1994). At the same time modern medicine has retreated more and more into its own professional domain. *Quality of life* and not just *survival* has become a core issue for public health.

Lifestyle influences on health

In oral health, the two principal diseases are dental caries and periodontal disease with aetiological factors of sugars in the diet and bacterial dental plaque. Oral cancers afflict a minority, but the prevalence is increasing in some countries. The two major risk factors are smoking and alcohol consumption. Further details of aetiology, prevalence, incidence and trends are given in Chapters 6 and 8. Lifestyle influences, including diet, effective oral hygiene and smoking, are pivotal to the occurrence of oral diseases. This finding is in common with other chronic conditions affecting general health, for example coronary heart disease. Examining trends in these conditions can illuminate our approach to oral health and disease.

Much has changed since the days of Snow and the cholera epidemic. Today in the developed countries smoking is the greatest cause of preventable death. The Health Education Authority estimated that 110 000 deaths in the UK in 1988 were attributable to smoking, representing about 1 in 6 deaths. Differences in mortality between people classified according to their occupations were very marked. Between 1972 and 1992, the percentage of male smokers with professional occupations more than halved from 33% to 14%, but reduced by only one-third in men with unskilled manual occupations–from 64% to 42%. Occupation is a reflection of education which is closely linked to lifestyle. Lifestyle encompasses the likelihood of making healthy choices in relation to diet, smoking, hygiene and use of health services. In terms of perpetuating risk behaviour, the report also confirms the clear link between children's smoking habits and that of their parents (Social Trends, 1995). Occupation is a reflection of education which is closely linked to lifestyle. Lifestyle encompasses the likelihood of making healthy choices in relation to diet, smoking, hygiene and use of health services.

Despite some reductions over the last 20 years, heart disease is the largest single cause of death, with the main risk factors being virtually entirely lifestyle-related: cigarette smoking; raised cholesterol levels (directly linked to dietary fat); lack of physical activity. There has been a decline in deaths due to coronary heart disease (in those aged 40–69) of approximately 14% in men and 5% in women in England and Wales between 1970 and 1986 (Beaglehole, 1990). In contrast, in the USA the decline has been over 50% for both sexes. In all countries, the disease has been greatest in higher social class groups and this has led to widening in social inequalities in health within countries. Some reports have claimed that much of the reduction has been due to advances in medical care for coronary heart disease patients. However, although these advances have influenced the quality of life of those with the disease, there are few data to support claims of influencing the population mortality data. This is because of the natural history of the disease. Most deaths occur out of hospital in people without major clinical manifestations of the disease. An analysis of trends in population risk factors for coronary heart disease in the USA from the early 1970s to 1980s found smoking rates had declined by 10% in men and women aged 25–59; total cholesterol levels decreased by around 4%, and blood pressure levels improved (Beaglehole, 1990). Work examining the relationship between lifestyle factors and coronary heart disease found that in almost all countries with major falls or rises in mortality, there are corresponding decreases or increases in animal fat consumption. Therefore, the principal causes of the improvement in mortality rates are reductions in cigarette smoking and animal fat consumption.

Similarly, the reduction in dental caries in children in developed countries in the last 20 years has not occurred because of the undoubted advances in dental care but because of the widespread use of fluoridated toothpastes. For caries, improvements in dietary risk factors have been minor; indeed, total sugar consumption in children has little changed. The fact that children now drink more carbonated drinks may be contributing to a relatively new condition at the population–level, that of dental erosion (O'Brien, Hinds and Gregory, 1995).

There are other similarities between coronary heart disease and dental caries. Until recently, both caries and coronary heart disease were epidemic diseases only in western industrialized countries. There have been pronounced declines in mortality (and caries) in affluent countries, with mortality increasing in some less affluent industrialized countries, e.g. eastern Europe, with rapid growth in both conditions in some newly developed countries. As one social group changes its habits, other markets are searched for and pressure is exerted on other social groups to increase their consumption, e.g. in the USA and the UK, young women have become the focus of attention of the tobacco and alcohol industries. This pattern is repeated internationally, with multinational companies exploiting the huge markets in less developed countries. The effect of traditional health promotion campaigns on increasing social inequalities reflects their focus on individual patterns of behaviour, in particular consumption of food and tobacco. New health promotion approaches as expressed in the Ottawa Charter for Health Promotion (1987) may help to avoid this problem. They emphasize public policy and the creation of healthy environments, supporting the production and availability of healthy products, so facilitating healthy behavioural options (Beaglehole, 1990). The background to these initiatives is fully explored in Chapter 11.

One of the most firmly established patterns in social epidemiology is the relationship between socioeconomic status (SES) and health (Davey Smith *et al.*, 1990; and see Chapter 3). This relationship exists throughout the industrialized world and in developing countries. Concepts of differences in racial predisposition to disease have been thoroughly researched and discounted, except for a few relatively rare conditions like sickle cell, which more truly reflect protective adaptation to environmental effects (Williams *et al.*, 1994). Some of the largest studies have shown that migrants to new countries adopt the lifestyle of the host country, often within one generation, and in consequence acquire similar prevalences of diseases as the indigenous population, even though those diseases may have been rare in their community of origin. In studies finding differences in health between races, when racial disparities in health status are adjusted for SES appropriately, racial differences are substantially reduced or eliminated. However, even within the same SES group, life experiences can be markedly different across racial groups with, for example, deprivation being more profound because of inherent effects of racism on employment prospects and living conditions (Williams *et al.*, 1994). Any health intervention should take into account its target audience and select appropriate advice and appropriate vehicles to capture the attention of all vulnerable groups in society. These aspects are discussed further in Chapters 3, 11 and 15.

The average life span in developed countries is increasing by around 2 years every decade (Social Trends, 1995). In the UK, a boy born in 1996 can expect to live until he is 74; a girl, until she is nearly 80. In contrast, average life expectancy of a person in one of the least developed countries is 43 years (Subramian, 1995). Just over half of men in the UK and around two-fifths of women were overweight or obese in 1991–1992. This profile would be similar but somewhat higher in the USA One-fifth of the world is overeating and dealing with the problems of excessive food intake, while four-fifths of the world is malnourished.

Overall, there have been marked changes in the UK diet in the last 20 years comparing the early 70s to the early 90s. The consumption of breakfast cereals has increased dramatically; table sugar has fallen continually (Social Trends, 1995). However, this has been compensated by hidden dietary sugar, e.g. a very large increase in sweetened drink consumption (see Chapter 13). The energy content of food brought into the home had reduced to around 1800 calories per day in 1993 compared to 2600 in 1970.

However, the former figure excludes food eaten outside the home and confectionery and soft drinks, which are making an increasing contribution to our total energy consumption.

In concluding this section on lifestyle influences on health, it is salutary to remember that mental illness costs the National Health Service in the UK more than coronary heart disease. Suicide is three times more common in men than women and the rates for men aged 25–44 have risen steeply in the last 20 years. From government surveys, up to half of the increase can be accounted for by the increasing numbers of men remaining single or becoming divorced. Unemployment is undoubtedly one of the additional factors. Therefore, lifestyle is impacting on health across a wide range of parameters. The goals of public health include knowledge and understanding of health problems and their causes, technical capability to deal with the problems, a sense of values that the problems matter and political will. The last of these is the most important (Last, 1994). It is encouraging to remember that there are many examples where epidemiological knowledge has become part of general knowledge and popular culture, changing social norms. This has been the case since the early days of public health when the knowledge of spread of infection through lack of appropriate sanitation and clean drinking water led on to establishing prevention by personal and communal cleanliness. Later, regulations and laws were enacted reinforcing many of the new societal norms and helping establish them, for example, car seat belts; restrictions on alcohol when driving; mandatory immunizations before admission to primary school; conscientious dental hygiene; use of sunscreen barrier creams; no-smoking rules throughout hospitals and many workplaces. Therefore, although some habits seem to be immutable, we need to remember that change can filter through, resulting in new social norms.

Population strategies in prevention

In his seminal paper on 'Sick individuals and sick populations', Geoffrey Rose (1985) described two strategies in the control or prevention of illness. The first is the *'high-risk' approach* which seeks to identify and protect susceptible individuals. The second strategy is the *population approach* which seeks to control the occurrence of new disease in the population as a whole. One classical example is the prevention of coronary heart disease. In the high-risk approach, the aim would be to screen the population to detect those with risk factors to the disease, e.g. raised serum cholesterol levels or raised blood pressure. These people would then become *patients* and be treated medically for their blood pressure, advised to change their diet, stop smoking and exercise regularly. They would be monitored subsequently and the level of risk factors checked periodically for improvement.

Taking a population approach to the prevention of coronary heart disease would be to try to reduce the prevalence of risk factors for all. Therefore, smoking, diet and exercise would be the targets using health education and health promotion initiatives including legislation, community and industrial participation. Examples would be: a complete ban on cigarette advertising; restriction of smoking in work environments and public places; differential taxation; campaigns to reduce consumption of animal fats; and work with industry to make healthier products more available and affordable. In reality, both approaches are often followed at the same time, but there is increasing evidence that the population approach is the more powerful.

One of the philosophical objections to the *high-risk approach* is that apparently healthy people become patients, frequently put on long-term medication for 'prevention'. Some of the practical disadvantages of prevention by the high-risk strategy relate to problems of screening for diseases that have yet to develop or are in the preclinical phase with no signs or symptoms. The difficulties and costs of screening have been encountered both in general medicine and dentistry. Misclassifications of risk are a problem (misclassifications are described in Chapter 5). For example, although high serum cholesterol levels result in higher relative risk to coronary heart disease (Kannel *et al.*, 1971), there is still a high degree of overlap between those individuals with high levels who go on to develop disease and those who, despite them, remain healthy. Commonly, the best predictor of future major disease is the presence of existing minor disease (Rose, 1985). Thus, a high blood pressure today is the best predictor of its future rate of rise. Exactly the same has been found

from many studies designed to identify which subjects will go on to develop dental caries in the future. The presence of existing caries is the best predictor (Beck *et al.*, 1992). Similarly, children who have ever experienced toothache are the most likely to have high caries levels and teeth extracted by 5 years of age (Mitropoulos, 1994). Where disease is absent at the time of screening, our ability to predict future disease accurately for that individual is the poorest. The cost:benefit ratio (see Chapter 10) of screening procedures is often unfavourable and this is compounded by the sequelae of false-positive diagnoses. For example, the continuance of the UK breast cancer screening programme is being questioned. For every 1000 women screened, only 6 cases are detected but 54 are recalled for further investigation (Social Trends, 1995). False-positive diagnoses can cause considerable distress and anxiety and the vast majority of breast cancers are still self-diagnosed. Furthermore, it is commonly found with screening programmes that there are problems with uptake and those people who access them are often those least at risk of the disease. For example, more than 1.6 million women in the UK were invited for breast cancer screening in 1992–93 but 480 000 did not attend (Social Trends, 1995). Since many of the diseases of the developed world have major lifestyle components in their aetiology, those with unhealthy habits are less likely to present. Similar considerations are found surrounding oral cancer screening, where the two most important predictors are smoking and drinking alcohol. In 1992 in the UK, men in the unskilled manual group were three times more likely to smoke than those in the professional group (Social Trends, 1995). If we combine this knowledge with reported dental attendance of adults in the UK in 1988 (Todd and Lader, 1991), we find that those least likely to attend the dentist with any regularity are men in unskilled occupations, so reducing the possibility of effective opportunistic screening of oral cancer by general dental practitioners.

The *population approach* attempts to control the determinants of incidence, to shift the whole distribution in a favourable direction. In the population strategy we are trying to remove the underlying causes that make the disease common. A small reduction for all would have a dramatic effect. Smoking is a classic example. Smoking cessation clinics begun in many doctors' surgeries in the late 70s and early 80s proved to be very labour-intensive with a few hard-won cases that were successful. However, health promotion on smoking cessation backed up with local restrictions, e.g. in the number of public places smoking is allowed, is beginning to make non-smoking the social norm for considerably more people. Once the new social norm of behaviour has become accepted and supply industries have adapted, as has happened with some dietary changes, e.g. extensive ranges and widespread availability of lower-fat milks, then maintaining the new pattern is no longer an effort. A population approach to improving periodontal health through effective oral hygiene is discussed in Chapter 6.

In a population strategy two approaches can be distinguished. The first might be described as the restoration of biological normality by removing abnormal exposure. Examples here would be stopping smoking, cleaner air and water, reducing some of our dietary indiscretions like excessive fat, sugar and salt in the diet. The second approach leaves intact the underlying cause of incidence of disease and seeks to prevent occurrence by giving some protective intervention. Examples here would be immunization and water fluoridation. Then, Rose (1985) argues, it is up to those proposing the intervention to demonstrate safety. This is discussed in detail in Chapter 14 on fluoridation. Population strategies to reduce the incidence of disease are the classical public health approach. Traditionally, this has involved mass environmental methods: clean water, clean food, maternal and child welfare screening, immunization, water fluoridation. Its modern form is attempting, much less successfully, to alter relevant society norms of behaviour. The skills required to encourage behaviour change have been unfamiliar in most clinical training; many practitioners feel on uncertain ground. Even more difficult is the ability to see health as a population issue and not simply a problem for individuals (Rose, 1985). This is changing and has been formally recognized in the requirement to teach behavioural sciences in the undergraduate curriculum (General Dental Council, 1990).

Some would argue that with the polarization of caries in children, a high-risk approach may be appropriate. This aspect is discussed in greater detail in Chapter 8. There are advantages and disadvantages. The principal advantage is that resources, which are increasingly limited, could be directed towards those who are likely to experience the disease. The disadvantage is that to date our screening techniques are most successful when disease is present, so that our targeting would be for treatment of existing disease as well as prevention of future disease. The second disadvantage is that caries is a multifactorial disease with incidence determined by social and lifestyle factors. Therefore, without tackling the broader problems, the next generation would present with the same problems. The resource may be better spent looking for a change in the established norms of that societal group. A consideration of the practical issues in health promotion initiatives is described more fully in Chapter 15.

Evaluating the practice of public health

Objectives for the year 2000 were set in the USA as national health objectives. One of the targets was for 90% of the population to be served by a local health department effectively carrying out the core functions of public health (Public Health Service, 1990). The three core functions of public health were defined as assessment, policy development and assurance. Assessment covers three areas: *assess* the prevailing status and health needs of the community; *investigate* adverse events and health hazards; *analyse* the determinants and contributing factors of disease locally and the adequacy of existing health resources. Policy development is similarly defined in three stages: *advocacy*, which requires establishing networks of support and communication with health-related organizations, the media and the general public; *prioritizing* needs from community needs assessment; *planning* in terms of an action plan for the community, with a long-range strategic plan reflecting wide participation. Assurance practices describe management plans; *implementation* and *evaluation* of mandated programmes and services; and finally *informing* and *educating* the public about current health status, health care needs, positive health behaviours and health care policy issues (Turnock *et al.*, 1994). A nationally representative survey of US local health departments was undertaken to determine how effective they were in meeting these performance indicators. Interestingly, 83%

felt they were complying with their requirements to assess health needs, but only 56% felt they fulfilled their advocacy role. This finding would not be dissimilar to dental public health purchasing in the UK. Many local commissioning authorities have achieved their target of health needs assessment particularly for children in undertaking centrally coordinated local surveys of dental health (Pitts and Palmer, 1995). However, many would feel less confident about their success in advocacy or implementation of locally appropriate health promotion initiatives. We have a stronger historical framework for counting cases of sickness than we have of advocating for health.

Implications for teaching and research

Recommendations are being made to define the curriculum needs more clearly and identify the need for skills training. This will need the teaching of behavioural sciences to extend from the preclinical part of the undergraduate course, which is the case in some dental schools, to bring it into the clinical course, thus making it directly relevant to individual patient care, for the clinical dentist, and to appropriate health promotion for the public health dentist. This latter point in particular can best be achieved by providing some integration of dental public health teaching with the behavioural sciences (McGoldrick and Pine, 1996). It is only half the story to teach the theoretical basis of lifestyle choices and health behaviour without teaching the tools (skills) the dentist will need to support individual patients and groups to make healthy choices. Both these aspects are considered in Chapter 11 and 12 of this book.

The organization of health services is increasingly market-based with a purchaser/provider model that is being required to become sensitive to consumer expectations. Those in public health need to be aware of health needs assessment on an individual patient basis and on a community or health service planning basis. From an individual clinician's point of view, treatment planning, although often led by normative need (conditions defined as disease by the profession), invariably has had to consider other factors. At the simplest level—willingness and ability to pay are present at the point of delivery of dental care in the majority

of oral health care systems for adults (see Chapters 16 and 17). Presenting symptoms and ability to accept care options are factors together with an assessment of the patients' ability to sustain the planned outcome. These aspects of treatment planning may not have been taught in the past and were sometimes hard-won from clinical experience in general practice. However, undergraduates are increasingly taught to consider psychosocial factors, for example, what the patient is looking for from the visit and the reality of patients' expectations of outcomes of treatment. The concept of negotiation of treatment plans is being taught in some dental schools and is found in standard texts (Jacob and Plamping, 1989; Locker, 1989). Undoubtedly, some clinicians have been let down by classical dental teaching which provides a standard prescriptive treatment for a specific normative need despite the day-to-day reality in oral health care of one person's mild impairment being another's profound handicap (see Chapter 4). Assessment is the key to successful treatment planning and normative need is only one part of the assessment. The social, psychological and lifestyle profiles are integral when dealing with oral conditions since these are largely preventable.

From a public health perspective, planners need to be able to prioritize effectively and allocate resources based on need (normative, felt and expressed) and on the reality of the type and extent of services they can provide within their current oral health care system. We need to be aware that sometimes care is sought for conditions for which the efficacy of treatment is doubtful – classically, minor orthodontic anomalies. One mechanism already in place in some purchasing policies prioritizes which patients will be treated first by using the Index of Orthodontic Treatment Need. This has a normative and aesthetic component of need. However, the aesthetic component is often measured by the clinician, who marks deviations from the norm much more severely than the patient. At the least, we should encourage these to be child/parent-led assessments of aesthetic need. In the face of limited resources, we have to consider the balance between patient/public demands for orthodontic treatment which can lead to inequity of uptake.

Health needs assessment is at the commencement of the planning cycle. We need to move forward from these being largely based on normative need for the treatment of diseases to incorporating measures of health, patient/public desires from the health care system and effectively measuring these to evaluate the outcome of our planned interventions. Clearly we still have a long way to go in health needs assessment and progress in this field is detailed in Chapter 4. These broader measures of need will help in treatment planning for the increasing numbers of adults retaining their teeth into old age. Perceptions of dental health are changing with the expectation of a dentition for life. The discipline of health needs assessment will become central to planners faced with the economic realities of finding effective and equitable systems for rationing health care from the potential of increasing patient demand.

A new focus in research is needed when looking at causation of the modern multi-factorial diseases. The constraint in early epidemiological studies was the inability to examine all the relevant variables at one time. It is essential that we study interrelationships rather than controlling for 'confounding' influences; the use of multivariate analyses and modelling is emphasized to help us understand the moderating multiple influences that constitute true causation (Dean, 1994). All these factors are considered in Chapter 5, presenting the principles of oral epidemiology and Chapter 9, appropriate statistical techniques. New approaches to public health policy and practices focus action on the causes of ill health in *communities* (Dean, 1994). A recent study conducted in the north-west of England provides an example of this approach (Gratrix and Holloway, 1994). This study sought to identify indicators in community profiles which make them more at risk of their children having increased experience of dental caries. This approach contrasts with individual risk behaviour studies which have provided disappointing results. In this population study, two communities were investigated, one in which the young children (5-year-olds) suffered from high levels of dental caries and one with children with excellent dental health. The study employed both quantitative and qualitative approaches. Fifteen potential indicators were identified; most were surrogates for deprivation and poverty (Gratrix and Holloway, 1994). The communities with children with high caries activity had fewer normal-birth-weight babies, lower uptake of

vaccinations, more children born to single parents, lower percentage with cars or private housing, more children in receipt of clothing allowances and free school meals because of household poverty and their children were less likely to attend school regularly. From an infant feeding perspective, the babies were more likely to have been bottle-fed, weaned earlier, used feeding bottles longer, given baby fruit juices more often and, as schoolchildren, have a greater consumption of confectionery after school. One of the more salutary conclusions from this work was that the lifestyles that influence different risks to disease are so fundamental and ingrained that change will only come with difficulty and over long periods.

The qualitative data in the above study were collected by interviewing people involved in health and education within the community with special knowledge of the primary school children. Qualitative approaches will often be a powerful tool in this type of research, since qualitative methods take a holistic approach which preserves the complexity of human behaviour (Strong, 1992). Qualitative methods have their own rigour and have the capacity to reveal what is the background or perceptual concepts without attempting to measure frequency or association, which would be more the realm of epidemiological approaches of causation described in this book in Chapter 5. Qualitative methods enhance quantitative methods. One of the most powerful potentials in qualitative research is the enhanced ability to validate information on reported behaviour. As described, much of ill health in developed countries is based on unhealthy lifestyle practices. These practices often persist in the presence of knowledge about their effect. For example, few people could claim nowadays to be unaware of the link between cigarette smoking and lung cancer. Smoking prevalence has reduced, as has its social acceptance. Traditional quantitative studies are likely to lead to underreporting with people giving the socially correct answer. The same is true in reporting frequency of dental attendance (Nuttall and Davies, 1991). Qualitative approaches allow a subject to be explored face-to-face in greater depth, providing a more open discussion around lifestyle practices that lead to ill health. Research should be conducted with scientific rigour and the most appropriate tools to answer the research question should be used which will lead to an increasing role for qualitative techniques (Black, 1994).

Tackling social inequalities in the future

From the review of the evidence it is clear that social inequalities lead to inequity in health, what can be done about that? A report by the King's Fund contains a strong agenda for action (Benzeval *et al.*, 1995). The aim is 'to outline a number of practical and affordable ways in which the situation could be substantially improved, if the political will existed to recognize that tackling inequalities in health is a fundamental requirement for social justice for all citizens'. This is familiar to those who have followed the application of the primary health care approach described in Chapter 2. The report takes four key areas for intervention (with an example in each): the physical environment (housing); social and economic factors (income maintenance); barriers to adopting a healthier personal lifestyle (smoking); and access to appropriate and effective health and social services (access to health care). Although a recent review welcomed the report, a note of caution was made (Mackenbach, 1995) in that only interventions of established efficacy in reducing these inequalities should be pursued. Evidence-based interventions, like evidence-based medical procedures (Peckham, 1991), for example, 'natural' experiments, in which favourable changes occur for reasons other than to reduce inequalities in health should be sought. Mackenbach (1995) suggests that these would include 'changes in employment opportunities, housing or the price of cigarettes'. In oral health, the classical natural experiment that led to removing inequity in health is fluoridated water supplies, the history of which is fully explored in Chapter 14. Unfortunately, water fluoridation has reached an impasse in many developed countries and increasingly the use of other vehicles for fluoride needs to be explored (see Chapter 7). The marked decline in dental caries in these countries has been ascribed to the use of fluoride toothpastes and methods of increasing the use of toothpastes is seen as one approach to achieving the national targets set for improved dental health (Davis *et al.*, 1995).

In summary, health improvements in the future are most likely to be gained from enhancing healthy lifestyles choices.

The next chapters provide an excellent exposition of community oral health. The knowledge reviewed and questions raised provide a rich source for student, teacher and public health professional.

References

Acheson, D. (1988) *Public Health in England: Report of the Committee of Inquiry in the Future Development of the Public Health Function*. HMSO, London.

Ashton, J. (1993) Institutes of public health and medical schools: grasping defeat from the jaws of victory? *Journal of Epidemiology and Community Health* **47**: 165–168.

Beaglehole, R. (1990) International trends in coronary heart disease mortality, morbidity and risk factors. *Epidemiologic Reviews* **12**: 1–15.

Beck, J.D., Weintraub, J.A., Disney, J.A., Graves, R.C., Stamm, J.W., Kaste, L.M. and Bohannan, H.M. (1992) University of North Carolina caries risk study: comparisons of high risk prediction, any risk prediction, and any risk etiologic models. *Community Dentistry and Oral Epidemiology* **20**: 313–321.

Benzeval, M., Judge, K. and Whitehead, M (eds) *Tackling Inequalities in health; An Agenda for Action*. King's Fund London.

Black, N. (1994) Why we need qualitative research. *Journal of Epidemiology and Community Health* **48**: 425–426.

Davey Smith, G., Bartley, M. and Blane, D. (1990) The Black report on socioeconomic inequalities in health 10 years on. *British Medical Journal* **301**: 373–377.

Davies, R.M., Holloway, P.J. and Ellwood, R.P. (1995) The role of fluoride dentifrices in a national strategy for the oral health of children. *British Dental Journal* **179**: 84–87.

Dean, K. (1994) Editorial: Creating a new knowledge base for the new public health. *Journal of Epidemiology and Community Health* **48**: 217–219.

Downer, M.C., Gelbier, S. and Gibbons, D.E. (1994) *Introduction to Dental Public Health*. FDI World Press, London.

General Dental Council (1990) *Guidance on the Teaching of Behavioural Sciences. Report of the Working Party on the Behavioural Sciences*. General Dental Council, Wimpole Street, London.

Gratrix, D. and Holloway, P.J. (1994) Factors of deprivation associated with dental caries in young children. *Community Dental Health* **11**: 66–70.

Hinds, K. and Gregory, J.R. (1995) *National Diet and Nutrition Survey: Children aged 1½ and 4½ years. Volume 2: Report of the Dental Survey*. HMSO, London.

Jacob, M.C. and Plamping, D. (1989) *The Practice of Primary Dental Care*. Wright/Butterworth, Oxford.

James, P.M.C. and Beal, J.F. (1981) Dental epidemiology and survey procedures. In: *Dental Public Health. An Introduction to Community Dental Health*. John Wright, Bristol.

Kannel, W.B., Garcia, M.J. and McNamara, P.M. (1971) Serum lipid precursors of coronary heart disease. *Human Pathology* **2**: 129–51.

Lalonde, M. (1974) *A New Perspective on the Health of Canadians*. Minister of Supply and Services, Canada.

Last, J. (1994) New pathways in an age of ecological and ethical concerns. *International Journal of Epidemiology* **23**: 1–4.

Locker, D. (1989) *An introduction to Behavioural Science and Densitry*. Tavistock/Routledge, London.

McGoldrick, P. and Pine, C.M. (1995) *Report into the Teaching of Behavioural Sciences in the United Kingdom Dental Undergraduate Courses*. University of Dundee, Dundee.

Mackenbach, J.P. (1995) Tackling inequalities in health. *British Medical Journal* **310**: 1152–1153.

Mitropoulos, C. (1994) The contrast in dental caries experience amongst children in the north-west of England. *Community Dental Health* **10**: (suppl. 2) 9–18.

Nijhuis, H.G.J. and van der Maesen, L.J.G. (1994) The philosophical foundations of public health: an invitation to debate. *Journal of Epidemiology and Community Health* **48**: 1–3.

Nuttall, N.M. and Davies, J.A. (1991) The frequency of dental attendance of Scottish dentate adults between 1978 and 1988. *British Dental Journal* **171**: 161–165.

O'Brian, M. (1994) *Children's Dental health in the United Kingdom* 1993. HMSO, London.

Ottawa Charter for Health Promotion (1987) *Health Promotion* **1**: iii–v.

Peckham, M. (1991) Research and development for the National Health Service. *Lancet* **338**: 367–371.

Pitts, N.B. and Palmer, J.D (1995). The dental caries experience of 5-year-old children in Great Britain. Surveys coordinated by the British Association for the Study of Community Dentistry in 1993/94. *Community Dental Health* **12**: 52–58.

Public Health Service (1990) *Healthy People 2000: National Health and Promotion and Disease Prevention Objectives*. DHHS publication no. (PHS) 91-50212. US Government Printing Office, Washington, DC.

Rose, G. (1985) Sick individuals and sick populations. *International Journal of Epidemiology* **14**: 32–38.

The Smoking Epidemic: Counting the Cost in England (1991) Health Education Authority, London.

Social Trends (1995) *Social Trends 1995*. Central Statistical Office, HMSO, London.

Strong, P.M. 1992. The case for qualitative research. *International Journal of Pharmacy Practice* **1**: 185–186.

Subramian, M. (1995) The World Health report 1995: bridging the gaps. *World Health* **2**: 4–5.

Todd, J.E. and Lader, D. (1991) *Adult Dental Health 1988. United Kingdom*. HMSO, London.

Turnock, B.J., Handler, A., Hall, W., Potsic, S., Nalluri, R. and Vaughn, E.H. (1994) Local health department effectiveness in addressing the core functions of public health. Public health reports. *Journal of the US Public Health Service* **109**: 653–658.

WHO (1981) *Global Strategy for health for All by the Year 2000*. World Health Organization. Global.

WHO (1985) *Targets for health for all: Targets in Support of the European Regional Strategy for health for ALL*. World Health Organization, Copenhagen.

Williams, D.R., Lavizzo-Mourey, R. and Warren, R.C. (1994). The concept of race and health status in America. *Journal of the US Public Health Service* **109**: 26–41.

2

The primary health care approach

Walter Mautsch and Murray Dickson

Primary health care (PHC) is essential health care based on practical, scientifically sound and socially acceptable methods and technology, made universally accessible to individuals and families in the community through their full participation and at a cost that the community and country can afford to maintain at every stage of their development in the spirit of self-reliance and self-determination (WHO/UNICEF, 1978). PHC remains a viable strategy for improving health in both industrialized and Third World countries. This chapter will provide an overview of PHC, adapt it to become primary oral health care (POHC) and propose certain implications, for to pursue POHC is to pursue equity in dental care and to promote holistic views about oral health.

In the 1970s, disillusion grew with prevailing biomedical models of health care with their focus on symptoms and diseases, individuals and professional expertise and treatments and cure, all of which incurred substantial costs. Not sufficiently considered, it was argued, were the social, political, economic, educational and psychological determinants of health and social equity (Navarro, 1974, 1977; Illich, 1976, McKeown, 1978, 1979; Doyal, 1979; Doyal and Doyal, 1984). A convergence of factors, including critical theories linking health with development, led to an international conference in Alma Ata, in the former Soviet Union, in 1978, and the Declaration of Alma Ata (WHO/UNICEF, 1978) which affirmed the now famous goal of 'Health for all by the year 2000'. PHC was featured within the declaration as the critical strategy for

achieving better health for more of the world's population. Commissions and panels have since met throughout the world, always coming away with the same recommendations: health care systems should be reoriented away from an emphasis on curative interventions to an emphasis on disease prevention and health promotion; and services should be moved from institutions to the community.

Concept of primary health care

The Alma Ata Declaration was a radical break with conventional thinking. For the first time issues like dependence and poverty were linked with health status in an official statement signed by countries and international organizations. Challenges were made for the health sector to supplement individualistic approaches (both in curative and preventive aspects) with wider analyses about health and disease. People's interpretation of PHC ranged from services at a primary level of care, to a set of health-related activities, to a philosophy out of which will arise socially progressive actions.

PHC as a level of care

PHC was seen by many to be merely 'the first level of contact by individuals, the family and community with the national health system thus bringing health care as closely as possible to where people live and work' (WHO/UNICEF, 1978). Unfortunately, many industrialized countries equated primary care with PHC and so concluded that PHC was not necessary for them.

PHC as a set of activities

PHC was also seen to be pursuing a number of activities simultaneously as part of a whole, such as:

- education about prevailing health problems and the methods for preventing and controlling them;
- promotion of food supply and proper nutrition;
- adequate supply of safe water and basic sanitation;
- maternal and child health care, including family planning;
- immunization against the major infectious diseases;
- prevention and control of locally endemic diseases;
- appropriate treatment of common diseases and injuries;
- provision of essential drugs.

PHC as a philosophy

A key philosophical basis for the Alma Ata Declaration and PHC was the belief that social, economic and environmental determinants are more important for the health of the people than is medical care. A PHC approach moved people beyond biomedical actions and paternalistic systems of care to considerations about social justice and equity, empowerment of people and acceptance of more holistic views about health (Walt and Vaughan, 1981).

A legitimate worry was always that, although the vocabulary and even the technology may change, it is not necessarily intended that anything else will. The danger in presenting an alternative ideology like PHC is that, in the hands of the same people of influence, a new set of ideas becomes as dominating as the old set (Elliott, 1979). Indeed, many health programmes remained separate or vertical in nature rather than integrated or horizontal (Rifkin and Walt, 1986). This was, in part, rationalized by the need for 'selective primary health care' (Walsh and Warren, 1979), which advocates focusing on programmes that are more economically and organizationally feasible – an approach favoured by many donor agencies as it guarantees

professional support and provides measurable results. And so, fluoride mouthrinse programmes are presented in public schools with little consideration of the surrounding poverty.

In fact, PHC is all of these interpretations: a philosophical commitment to equity, empowerment, and holism; a full range of health-promoting activities; and services close to where people live and work. The framework is the five PHC principles: equitable distribution, community involvement, focus on prevention, appropriate technology, and a multi-sectoral approach (Walt and Vaughan, 1981).

Oral health in the light of PHC principles

Imperative for change

In his seminal paper on primary health care, Mahler (1981) clearly lays out the imperative for changing the health care system. He cites too few resources, poor allocation of existing resources, the drain of doctors from poor to rich countries, little control by ordinary people over their own health, and an inherent mistrust by health professionals of people being able to make good decisions about health matters. His arguments apply equally well to dentistry, for in every country of the world there are significant numbers of people who have no permanent access to dental services. They live in distant locations, in the slums around large cities of the world, in inner cities. They are not always unemployed, for struggling working-class families are also dentally neglected. Oral health for them will remain a dream as long as it continues to be understood in purely technical terms–fillings, extractions, dentists, clinics, equipment.

If the dream of oral health for more people is to become a reality, dental interventions as we know them have to be transformed because they are beset with problems. First, resources for programmes are few and those that now exist are likely to be reduced even further as a result of economic adjustment processes that have been put in place in both 'developed' and 'developing' countries. Second, purposes have been inverted. Achieving oral health, which should be the overriding goal, has been replaced by oral treatment, which really should be one of its strategies. Dental models that focus on services and treatment continue to predominate. This, in turn, ensures that there is better care for a few, a dependence on professionals, an emphasis on curative care, a dependence on sophisticated technologies, and little intersectoral work–the very opposite of WHO's PHC principles. Third, the determinants of oral health are far too narrowly defined. Research suggests that contributions to an individual's health status are apportioned in the following manner: health care system–25%; biological endowment–10%; physical endowment–15%; social environment–50% (Saskatchewan Public Health Association, 1994). Fourth, prolonged conditioning has disabled professionals in that they do not know how to engage people who need them most. Instead, their attention is directed at those with whom they have most in common–the less poor and largely middle-class. As well, professional training nurtures a certain arrogance in which scientific knowledge is considered superior to what people know and understand and believe–what is often called 'popular knowledge' (Chambers, 1983). This is consistent with Mahler's (1981) premise that health care professionals essentially distrust public involvement in decision-making about health care matters.

We have to swing away from the kind of paternalistic thinking that leads to doling out things and creating dependence. Besides, clinic-based, capital-intensive approaches to improved health are unrealistic given the excessive costs and continued inadequacies in coverage. With growing concerns over escalating costs associated with providing dental care, it is time to ask challenging questions about who are appropriate providers of care; how services are delivered; and how costs are apportioned between curative, preventive and health promotion activities (Robinson, 1990).

Primary oral health care

PHC remains as valid today as when it was first articulated in 1978 but, as Elliott (1979) once advised about PHC, an overly naïve espousal of primary oral health care (POHC) without a readiness to face deeper issues is likely to result in bitter disappointment. The five principles of PHC lead us directly toward acknowledging and confronting the kind of issues with which he was concerned and which continue to face dentistry.

Equitable distribution

Inequity refers to differences that are unnecessary and unavoidable, and that are also unfair and unjust. In order to describe a situation as being inequitable, one examines underlying causes and then decides if a situation is right given what is happening with the rest of society. Admittedly, we can never achieve a situation where everyone has the same level of oral health or suffers the same degree of disease, but the crucial test is whether people choose that situation or whether it was mainly out of their control. Equity is then concerned with creating equal opportunities for health and bringing health differentials down to the lowest possible levels (Whitehead, 1991).

It would seem logical that disadvantaged people have poorer oral health because they have fewer healthy alternatives and fewer opportunities for care. Sadly, what is termed the 'inverse care law' is all too prevalent in dentistry: deprived communities that suffer the most and so have the most need receive the fewest resources (Tudor Hart, 1971). Even sadder is the fact that so many dental institutions essentially ignore this reality and effectively encourage the status quo to continue. Recent studies in the USA show repeatedly that people who are poor and with limited education, minorities and older people who live in difficult circumstances all continue to be dentally neglected (Allukian, 1993; Harmon, 1993; Clark, 1994). A study of Canadian aboriginal children clearly demonstrates that the general decline in caries is not occurring among aboriginal children. And yet, three-quarters of aboriginal children had a dental visit in the past year (Leake, 1992). This has to be food for thought for dentists who continue to formulate dental programmes for others. Even in a rich country like Germany, which has a dental insurance system that covers more than 90% of the population, extreme differences in oral health can be found. As seen in Table 2.1, a small percentage of people account for the majority of decayed and filled teeth (Duenninger and Pieper, 1991).

One of the most important innovations of the PHC movement has been the preparation of community dental workers who provide basic preventive, promotive and treatment services and who become a referral link to the nearest dental clinic. Originally called auxiliaries and seen as substitutes for dentists, accumulated experience has revealed their value in ways not previously apparent. As POHC workers, they make equity a realistic goal because they provide equal access to available programmes according to need. In Peru, health workers in remote rural

Table 2.1 Distribution of DMF-T and dmf-t in Germany

8/9 years	13/14 years	35/54 years
22% have 46% of dmft		
43% have 90% of DMFT	41% have 68% of DMFT	40% have 5% of DMFT
23% have 82% of DT	23% have 66% of DT	27% have 7% of DT
35% have 100% of FT	35% have 67% of FT	37% have 5% of FT
		41% have 8% of MT

dmft = Decayed, missing, filled deciduous teeth;
DMFT = decayed, missing, filled teeth; DT = decayed teeth;
FT = filled teeth.

From Duenninger, P. and Pieper, K. (1991), with permission.

health centres were trained to carry out simple dental measures. They established links with the primary schools in their catchment areas and started small-scale oral health programmes. Integrated fully into the health system, they are supported by public health dentists (Mautsch *et al.*, 1995). With relevant skills, confidence and ongoing support, community dental workers have many advantages: if they are women, they become role models for other women; they are an entry point for more holistic community analysis and development work; they are accountable to community members and so offer a means for both sustainability and advocacy about oral health issues; and they can make quality dental services available to all (Robinson, 1990).

Community involvement

A fundamental element of PHC was always seen to be input by non-professional community members. As seen in the accompanying graphic used by Fletcher (1995) to teach the PHC concept (Fig. 2.1), all the components of the bicycle can be in place but, without the participation of people at the community level driving it forward and energizing it, nothing will happen.

Failing to involve communities in ways that are based on their own cultures, values and experiences has doomed many a logical health initiative (Airhihenbuwa, 1994). The critical discussion revolves around the meaning of participation. To ordinary people, a phrase like 'decentralizing power and decision-making and encouraging people to participate in the policy-making process', which appears so frequently in oral health plans, all too often means 'getting people to cooperate so that

official plans can work' (Whitehead, 1991). Elliot (1979) is quite correct when he observes that community involvement in decision-making can easily become a charade in which decisions are minimized and managed and so patterns of domination continue. Community participation means more than establishing a dental committee or involving community leaders.

In Porto Alegre, Brazil, a community in a local health district is actively involved in the analysis of its own oral health problems and in the search for realistic solutions. It is demonstrating that people living in deprived communities are able to link oral health with their struggle for human rights, and that an organized community can effectively pressure policy-makers (Baldisserotto, 1995). For programmes to be appreciated and used, they have to be relevant, and the road to relevancy begins by building on what people understand and feel is important about the world they know. It is more effective to begin work in a community dealing with issues community members have identified as important, rather than beginning with predetermined services. This community development approach initiates a problem-solving process which may become a permanent feature of community life.

Focus on prevention and health promotion

While we recognize in the literature the value of prevention, it remains in practice, as Elliott (1979) once said, 'the slumland of the medical (and dental) townscape'. Increasingly, the meaning of prevention has become compressed to be another service like placing a sealant, applying fluoride and providing dental education. Not surprisingly, a provider–recipient dynamic is established which ends up disabling the empowerment purpose of health promotion–

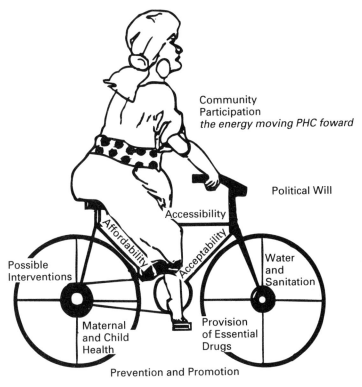

Fig. 2.1 The primary health care (PHC) bicycle. From Fletcher (1995), with permission.

the sister component of prevention. The term health promotion captures what was never sufficiently part of prevention. It focuses on personal and community growth in the sense that information can be power and, if it is supplemented with resources and provided in ways that create in people a critical awareness, they will use that awareness to challenge the unhealthy context that surrounds them (Minkler and Cox, 1980).

At the heart of health promotion is empowerment, which is achieved when people are enabled to set their priorities, make decisions and plan and implement their own strategies for achieving better health. Empowerment may be an outcome when participation deliberately nurtures personal confidence and an ability to analyse one's own contextual reality. Not being in control is recognized as a risk factor for disease, whereas being in control–empowerment–has been shown to be an important promoter of health (Wallerstein, 1992). The proposition is that personal and community

empowerment is what is needed for real oral health changes to occur.

One road to empowerment is through community development which, in turn, is the process of working with people to generate 'grassroots' support for desired change. Community development is an educational process and is not simply better roads, better latrines, having toothbrushes; it is something of the spirit, not just something material. It is found and tapped by reaching into the deep social values of people. Without these, it matters little whether the road is paved or not, whether you go to the woods or to a latrine, whether a community is materially rich. When we build on values, physical solutions follow and in their proper order–including oral hygiene. Teachers of the dental *agente* (therapist) course in Mozambique are exploring community development and participatory action research in order better to practise and teach oral health promotion. Course development arose out of the teachers' own analysis of country realities (Rosenbloom *et al.*, 1995). Using their own version of problem-based learning, they are successfully provoking their students, beyond acquiring skills, to think critically and care about people.

Werner (1985) is quite correct that health work is never apolitical. Either it is done in ways that help people take greater control over factors that affect their health or it tries to keep people under control and dependent on over-professionalized yet inadequate services. There is a choice–primary oral health care can be people-empowering or it can be people-disempowering. Further considerations of health promotion principles are given in Chapter 11, with practical applications in Chapter 15.

Appropriate technology

The singular treatment strategies emphasized in the dental schools of the world require equipment that are often worth thousands of dollars. It is no wonder that students upon graduation feel obliged to set up similar practices that cater only to people who pay. They feel like a fish out of water when having to function with no equipment close at hand. A resulting ethical dilemma for educators is teaching skills that require materials which, in turn, need to be imported at considerable cost to the government or to those who have to pay through higher fees. Meanwhile, an unmodified transfer of science and technology to poorer societies burdens their systems with an unbearable inflow of materials that are difficult to control and maintain. A classic example is the donation of old dental units and other equipment items which then require training and further complementary technologies (Pereira, 1995). The net effects are to work against the principles of equity and empowerment.

Research on the processes of oral disease and on improved filling materials has led to the development of the atraumatic restorative treatment (ART) technique (Frencken, 1995). ART offers a less threatening treatment for caries at an early stage and at low cost, for it can be provided where electricity is not available or where electricity exists but it is not possible to afford and maintain expensive dental equipment. The challenge is to treat oral diseases appropriately but at a cost that individuals and communities can afford. The objective is not the production and use of cheap, second-class materials and equipment. Rather it is helping dental workers cope with economic and technological constraints and so become more self-sufficient. At question is the paradigm that only high-tech is able to provide good oral health care.

In a community-based project in Mexico, oral health promoters make their own explorers, mouth mirrors, scalers, curettes and suction devices. The project has developed folding dental chairs and a portable dental unit with a dual energy supply: electric and using solar panels. Toothbrushes are made from local materials as well as low-cost toothpaste. And research is occurring in the use of herbs and plants for treatment of oral diseases (Yaschine, 1995).

Multisectoral approach

A major reason for the lack of success of many oral health programmes is the fact that they operate in isolation, separate from the general health care structure (WHO, 1989). As Sheiham (1988) points out, oral health could be better integrated into general health programmes by tackling common causes, by including oral health in general health education, and by adopting population strategies. This approach is powerful in tackling causes that are common to a number of chronic diseases. Adopting a common risk/health factor approach can impact on several diseases at a lower cost than disease-specific approaches by controlling certain risk factors while, at the same time, promoting health factors. For instance, unhealthy diets affect the incidence of heart disease and cancer as well as oral disease, and so reducing intake of sugars, fat and salt together with increasing intake of complex carbohydrates and fruits, vegetables and cereal products is healthier–and more likely to succeed–than simply stressing control of sugars for caries reduction. Similarly, since tobacco smoking affects heart disease, respiratory diseases and oral diseases, it makes sense for dental workers actively to support programmes aimed at reducing tobacco smoking (Mautsch and Sheiham, 1995).

Oral hygiene should be included in general hygiene teaching and actions carried out by parents, teachers and health workers. Brushing of teeth then becomes less of an isolated practice and more an important part of grooming and body cleanliness. Links can be readily made with such important issues as the need for uncontaminated water and food source, sewage and latrines and other forms of waste disposal, including in a dental clinic. Adopt a population rather than a high-risk group strategy. Individual care is important but, if oral health is to improve, more attention must be given to the population as a whole through policies and strategies that require multisectoral cooperation and action: increasing the availability of fluoride; promoting sugar-reduced products; and establishing codes of practice for advertising (Mautsch, 1995).

By describing oral health only in individual terms, people's social context remains hidden and yet it contains significant oral health determinants. If a person's emotional poverty is also considered as a risk factor for oral disease, then dental professionals need to learn how to participate with colleagues in community actions that aim to improve the well-being of women; literacy; and feelings of self-esteem, dignity, and being in control (Dickson, 1993). A shift from narrow, vertical programming to an integrated and horizontal approach expands the scope for dealing with oral disease (WHO, 1990; Daly *et al.*, 1991) and promoting oral health. In a case study described by Mautsch *et al.* (1995), oral health was located within a social context of nutrition, agriculture, sanitation and community health. School curricula were adapted, and both schoolteachers and community workers learned how to incorporate oral health education into their own activities. Oral health was part of health-promotional activities which included the building of water pipelines, latrines, the improvement of indigenous crops and the nutrition of the families. If lasting solutions to oral health problems are to be realized, collaboration and programme cooperation have to be instituted. Working together provides the most sustainable possibilities for continued services and a wider distribution of oral health.

Implications

To pursue primary oral health care as both a philosophy and strategy for action, four implications are proposed, recognizing that there will be others to work through as well.

Pursue partnerships

Equity cannot be achieved by dentists and related personnel in isolation. Linkages are needed with sectors that influence oral health determinants like education, nutrition and food security, environment, social welfare, small business and community development. For dental personnel really to pursue POHC, they need to 'partner with people' and so contribute to the overall development of their communities. Dental programmes, whether to improve primary care or teaching, need to acknowledge that people's oral health cannot be achieved by dental providers; make an explicit philosophical commitment to pursue equity in dental care; and work with institutions and groups that have a spirit of social equity, community participation and activism.

Evaluation and research

Evaluating and researching with local people helps to ensure that important questions are asked and that visible actions occur as a result of information gained (Dickson, 1995). This helps ensure that dental personnel remain accountable to their communities. The realities of life and work require front-line personnel who can think and problem-solve because they have options upon which to draw. To work on their own and accept responsibilities, they must be able to evaluate progress being made, ask critical questions about underlying causes and make wise decisions which may include changing course.

Reform existing pedagogy

We have to move away from the idea that oral health is something to be delivered. It is not; it is something to be achieved. In PHC work, it is often said that changes in attitude and ways of doing things are accomplished ever so slowly and patience is required. Usually such a statement is made in reference to lay people, especially those considered to be uneducated. But those having community experience will testify that the attitudes and approaches most difficult to modify are not those of the public but of professionals. The training of professionals does not prepare them to adapt easily or work with local people. In fact, their training actively conditions them against it. If dental personnel are to practise POHC, their preparation has to be radically different. A reaffirmation of goal, revised content and a different set of values are required. To be relevant, community dental workers need to be able to assess changing circumstances, plan programmes and evaluate progress being made as a result of their efforts. Values to be nurtured include caring for people and being humble enough to recognize that local people have more expertise than professionals do about their local realities. As Chambers (1983) points out, professionals do not feel, and therefore really know, the realities of other people; even more worrisome is when they do not know that they do not know.

Begin with self

To formulate an effective strategy for improving health and survival, we must first re-examine the causes that lead to the present high levels of sickness and death–especially among vulnerable groups. We must follow the chain of causes all the way to its source, even if its final link frames a mirror in which we begin to rediscover ourselves (Werner, 1989). Time, temperament and trust are the ingredients for both initiating and sustaining community work. Time is needed for community empowerment. Necessary also is an orientation that one can learn from community people, and that power-to-the-people is desirable. Trust in this case is believing that, over time and with support, people are capable of analysing their own situations and deciding what is best for them (McFarlane and Fehir, 1994). If we really want to pursue equity and promote oral health in our communities, a new kind of professional is required. As Bea Shawanda, a Canadian aboriginal teacher said, 'we talk a lot about others and their culture but what of our own culture? If our culture-talk says that we care for the suffering and the unfortunates, then we have to do those things. We must be responsible. We must live those things we talk about' (Shawanda, 1990). The first step is always the one I can take myself.

References

Airhihenbuwa, C.O. (1994) Health promotion and the discourse on culture: implications for empowerment. *Health Education Quarterly* 21: 345–353.

Allukian, M. (1993) Introduction. Symposium: Oral disease: the neglected epidemic–what can be done? *Journal of Public Health Dentistry* 53: 45.

Baldisserotto, J (1995) Community participation in a decision making process in a local health council in Porto Alegre city, Brazil. In: *Promoting Oral Health in Deprived Communities* (W. Mautsch, A. Sheiham, eds), pp. 253–263, Berlin, German Foundation for International Development (DSE).

Chambers, R. (1983) *Rural Development: Putting the Last First*, Essex, Longman.

Clark, W.B. (1994) Access to oral health and health care reform–inside the President's task force. *Journal of Dental Education, 58*: 291–294.

Daly, B., Hobdell, M.H., Sadlier, D. and Jennings, N. (1991) The Kilkenny integrated oral health project. *Irish Journal of Medical Science* 160, (suppl. 9): 50–54.

Dickson, M. (1993) Oral health promotion in developing countries. In: *Oral Health Promotion* (L. Schou, A. Blinkhorn, eds), pp. 233–247, Oxford, Oxford University Press.

Dickson, M. (1995) Community-based research in dentistry. In: *Promoting Oral Health in Deprived Communities* (W. Mautsch, A. Sheiham, eds), pp. 229–237. Berlin, German Foundation for International Development (DSE).

Doyal, L. (1979) *The Political Economy of Health*. London, Pluto.

Doyal, L. and Doyal, L. (1984) *More than the Sum of Parts*. London, Pluto.

Duenninger, P. and Pieper, K. (1991) Ergebnisse zur Praevalenz von Karies und Dentalfluorose. In: *Mundgesundheitszustand und -verhalten in der Bundesrepublik Deutschland. Ergebnisse des nationalen IDZ-Survey 1989* (W. Micheelis, J. Bauch, eds), pp. 205–260. Koeln, Deutscher Aertze-Verlag.

Elliott, C. (1979) *Is Primary Health Care the New Priority? Yes, but... In The Principles and Practice of Primary Health* Care (Contact special series No. 7), pp 67–72. World Council of Churches.

Fletcher, D. (1995) Participation, poverty and politics: working in international health into the 21st Century. *Pearson Notes* 8: 4–8.

Frencken, J. (1995) A new atraumatic technique (ART) for treating tooth decay. In: *Promoting Oral Health in Deprived Communities* (W. Mautsch, A. Sheiham, eds) pp. 401–402, Berlin, German Foundation for International Development (DSE).

Harmon, R.G. (1993) Oral health care for the underserved in the 1990s: the HRSA perspective. Symposium: Oral disease: the neglected epidemic–what can be done? *Journal of Public Health Dentistry* 53: 46–49.

Illich, I. (1976) *Limits to Medicine*. Marion Boyars.

Leake, J.L. (1992) *Oral Health Survey of Canada's Aboriginal children aged 6 and 12*. Department of Community Dentistry, University of Toronto, Canada.

McFarlane, J. and Fehir, J. (1994) De Madres a Madres: a community primary health care program based on empowerment. *Health Education Quarterly* 21: 381–394.

McKeown, T. (1978) Determinants of health. *Human Nature* April issue, 61–67.

McKeown, T. (1979) *The Role of Medicine: Dream, Mirage or Nemesis?* Oxford, Basil Blackwell.

Mahler, H. (1981) The meaning of 'health for all by the year 2000'. *World Health Forum, 1*: 5–22.

Mautsch, W. (1995) Oral health in a multisectoral approach. In: *Promoting Oral Health in Deprived Communities* (W. Mautsch, A. Sheiham, eds), pp. 267–282. Berlin, German Foundation for International Development (DSE).

Mautsch, W. and Sheiham, A. (1995) Editorial. In: *Promoting Oral Health in Deprived Communities* (W. Mautsch, A. Sheiham, eds), pp. 29–42. Berlin, German Foundation for International Development (DSE).

Mautsch, W., Paniagua Gamarra, M. and Sobrino Mora, E. (1995) Integrating oral health: a project in Peru. In: *Promoting Oral Health in Deprived Communities* (W. Mautsch, A. Sheiham, eds), pp. 283–299. Berlin, German Foundation for International Development (DSE).

Minkler, M. and Cox, K. (1980) Creating critical consciousness in health: applications of Freire's philosophy and methods to the health care setting. *International Journal of Health Services* **10**: 311–322.

Navarro, V. (1974) The underdevelopment of health or the health of underdevelopment: an analysis of the distribution of human health resources in Latin America. *International Journal of Health Services* **4**: 5–27.

Navarro, V. (1977) Justice, social policy, and the public's health. *Medical Care* **XV**: 363–370.

Pereira, S. (1995) Appropriate technology for health. Dependence–self-determination–technical cooperation. In: *Promoting Oral Health in Deprived Communities* (W. Mautsch, A. Sheiham, eds) pp. 413–426. Berlin, German Foundation for International Development (DSE).

Rifkin, S.B. and Walt, G. (1986) Why health improves: defining the issues concerning 'comprehensive primary health care' and 'selective primary health care'. *Social Science and Medicine* **23**: 559–566.

Robinson, S.A. (1990) Primary health care experience in the developing world: lessons for Canada? *Canadian Family Physician* **36**: 95–100.

Rosenbloom, J., Dickson, M. and Tanda, A. (1995) Researching deficiencies: a first step in curriculum restructuring in Mozambique. *Journal of the Institute of Health Education* **33**: 16–19.

Saskatchewan Public Health Association (SPHA) (1994) *The Determinants of Health*. Canada.

Shawanda, B. (1990) Reclaiming health: who is responsible for what? *The Four Worlds Exchange* **2**: 9–11.

Sheiham, A. (1988) Integrating strategies for improving oral health and general health. *World Health* October, 28–29.

Tudor Hart, J. (1971) The inverse care law. *Lancet* **1**: 405–412.

Wallerstein, N. (1992) Powerlessness, empowerment, and health: implications for health promotion programs. *American Journal of Health Promotion* **6**: 197–205.

Walsh, J.A. and Warren, K.S. (1979) Selective primary health care. An interim strategy for disease control in developing countries. *New England Journal of Medicine* **301**: 967–974.

Walt, G. and Vaughan, P. (1981) *An Introduction to the Primary Health Care Approach in Developing Countries*. Ross Institute of Tropical Hygiene No.13. School of Hygiene and Tropical Medicine, London.

Werner, D. (1985) *Public Health, Poverty, and Empowerment–A Challenge*. Convocation address at Johns Hopkins School of Public Health. Paper available from the Hesperian Foundation, Palo Alto, California, USA.

Werner, D. (1989) *Health for No One by the Year 2000: The High Cost of Placing 'National Security' Before Global Justice*. Presentation to the National Council for International Health. Paper available from the Hesperian Foundation, Palo Alto, California, USA.

Whitehead, M. (1991) The concepts and principles of equity and health. *Health Promotion International* **6**(3), 217–228.

WHO (1989) *Research and Action for the Promotion of Oral Health within Primary Health Care*. Basel, WHO/Ciba/Geigy.

WHO (1990) *Oral Health in Community Health Programmes*. Copenhagen, WHO/Regional Office for Europe.

WHO/UNICEF (1978) *Primary Health Care, Alma Ata 1978*. 'Health for All' series no. 1. Geneva, World Health Organization.

Yaschine, A. (1995) Community-based programme for training, care, and self-reliance in dentistry (PROCAO). In: *Promoting Oral Health in Deprived Communities* (W. Mautsch, A. Sheiham, eds), pp. 391–400. Berlin, German Foundation for International Development (DSE).

3

Society and oral health

Poul Erik Petersen

Introduction

During recent years dramatic changing patterns of oral diseases have been observed at a global level. While dental caries seems to be rapidly declining as a problem of public health concern in the advanced industrial societies, caries may now take on the dimensions of a major 'epidemic' in the Third World countries. These two divergent trends present quite contrasting problems for dentistry in the future. However, these two quite different trends have one thing in common, which is that neither is susceptible to a traditional technical solution provided by clinical dentistry. In fact, the point is underlined that modern dentistry has to reach beyond the conventional clinical disciplines. The future challenges to dentistry and public health care planning are confined to areas of expertise that relate to the non-clinical dimensions of dental practice–health promotion, community-based preventive care and outreach activities.

A proper understanding of the social context of oral health and illness is a prerequisite to the provision of such care by the dental profession and its participation in public health action programmes. The social sciences are the academic disciplines that offer the theoretical and practical foundations in this respect, and in particular, the discipline of sociology. It is sometimes difficult for dental professionals with a background in the natural sciences to come to an understanding of the relevance of sociology which, after all, focuses on the impact of social

factors. While anatomy, biochemistry and physiology deal with apparently objective, demonstrable and measurable phenomena, sociological concepts by contrast seem to be both more subjective and more abstract. Furthermore, there often appears to be much more controversy among sociologists about how to study social phenomena than there is among those working in the natural sciences about how to study their particular areas of interest. This appearance of subjectivity and controversy, however, should not be allowed to deter dental professionals or public oral health planners. Much of the sociological contribution to dentistry is not controversial. Moreover, the problem of subjectivity is not really a problem peculiar to sociology since subjectivity is inherent in making social judgements and evaluations of any kind.

The social construction of reality

Reality is socially construed and formed through the membership of social or human groups (Berger and Luckman, 1967). In making sense of the world, most people are what philosophers call 'naïve realists', i.e. they assume that what they 'see' and 'believe to be there' about the world around them is indeed how things are. For the sociologist, however, concepts about reality are drawn from social processes of definition. In a sense, reality, is 'in the eye of the beholder' and therefore what people see and understand about the world around them is shaped by their social or cultural experience. It follows, for example, that the view of the world and of its opportunities is very different depending on whether you happen to be a factory worker or, say, a medical or dental practitioner.

This perspective on 'reality' has great relevance for dentistry as well. For the dental professional there is a common understanding of what constitutes oral disease and related disorders and anomalies of the mouth, and the jaws. This common understanding is based on certain biological criteria that help define what is, and what is not, oral pathology and hence in need of treatment. But for the sociologist oral health and illness is a social concept. Virtually everybody suffers to some extent from caries or periodontal disease. However, for only a minority is the interference with normal social activities such that disease-related signs and symptoms prompt a visit to the dentist. Furthermore, the way in which these signs and symptoms are filtered is again a social process: oral discomfort, bad breath, packing of food–these are likely to be the cues for action rather than any 'objective' assessment of the underlying biological condition.

Moreover, there is another sense in which oral health is a social concept. Much of the usual round of human activity that is related to oral health is *not* concerned with health as conventionally understood. Except for a few cases of extreme oral pain, dental problems do not normally threaten a person with sickness or social incapacity. Instead, the great public interest in oral health seems to originate more from a concern to conform with certain cultural ideals of body image, especially in the symbolically important area of the mouth. The shape and configuration of the teeth, mouth and jaws are obvious cases. Appearance rather than 'health' is important here. But more than this, standards of oral hygiene, cleanliness and health of the dentition and gums, absence of discomfort and embarrassing blemishes are all related to central cultural ideals of body image, health and vitality.

It follows from what has been noted so far that, for the sociologist, social factors can be seen to impinge on every aspect of oral health and 'illness'. Perhaps the best-researched area in the social context of oral health is that of aetiology. This is the area in oral health science known as social epidemiology. Much of the research here has been designed to document social variations in the two principal oral diseases of dental caries and periodontal disease, in particular, with respect to the effect on oral health status across social classes.

The sociological perspective

Sociology is the study of human groups. The discipline focuses on two interrelated areas of study: social factors and recurrent relationships among people. Sociology is not concerned with behaviour unique to individuals or with particular situations. These lie outside the boundaries of the sociological perspective since sociologists are interested in patterned human relationships rather than individual behaviour. This approach assumes that the behaviour of a group or people's behaviour within a group is not primarily determined by the characteristics of its individual members. The sum of a group is not equal to its parts. Something new is created when individuals come together as a collective, originally emphasized in 1895 by one of the classic sociologists, Emile Durkheim (Durkheim, 1966). Individualistic explanations of group behaviour are inadequate because all human activities are influenced by social forces that individuals have not created themselves and cannot control. We live in groups ranging in size from a family to an entire society, but they all encourage conformity. Thus, people who belong to similar groups tend to think, feel and behave in similar ways. Such patterns may form the basis of culture, norms and traditions. This is clearly demonstrated by the fact that European, American, African and Chinese citizens have distinctive eating habits, types of dress, religious beliefs and attitudes toward family life.

Conformity within a group occurs partly because most of its members believe that their group's ways of thinking, feeling and behaving are the best; they have been successfully taught to value their group's ways of living. Group members also tend to conform even when their personal preferences are not the same as their group's. This is due to social or peer pressures. Whether it is because members value their group's ways or because they yield to the social pressures of the moment, behaviour within a group is not usually predictable from knowledge about its individual members.

Sociological schools of thought

The perspective you take influences what you see. One perspective emphasizes certain aspects of an event while another perspective puts the accent on different aspects of the same event. Moreover, when a perspective highlights certain parts of something, it necessarily places other parts in the background. Sociology provides several perspectives for looking at human or group behaviour: functionalism or consensus theory, conflict theory and interactionism (Giddens, 1982). Each of these perspectives provides a slant on human behaviour in groups. Exclusive use of any one perspective prevents seeing other aspects of group life. All perspectives together, however, allow us to see most of the important dimensions of social life. This holistic approach holds true also for the analysis of oral health and health related-behaviour.

Functionalism or *consensus theory* emphasizes the contributions (functions) that each part of a society makes to it. It focuses on social integration, stability, order and cooperation. Accordingly, the parts of a society are organized into an integrated whole. Consequently, a change in one part of a society (e.g. the economy) leads to changes in other parts (e.g. the family or the health care system). Most aspects of a society have evolved to perform certain necessary functions. It is for this reason that all complex societies have economies, families, religions, health care systems and governments. If these elements did not contribute to a society's well-being they would not survive. Consensus theory assumes that most members of a society agree on what is desirable to have and to achieve–in other words, that there is a consensus on values and interests. The high degree of consensus on democracy and social welfare accounts for the great degree of cooperation found in any society. This is applicable to the health care system as well. Consensus on the value of health and oral health, goal-setting and priorities, and organization of work by health professionals and health workers provides for cooperation and ultimately for improved oral health of the population.

On the other hand, *conflict theory* emphasizes competition, change and constraint within a society. The roots of this theoretical perspective go back as far as functionalism. Karl Marx (1818–1883) contended that the nature of a society is based upon its economy, and that

inequalities and class conflicts are inevitable in all capitalistic economies (Marx, 1967). Modern conflict theorists do not limit themselves to economic determinism and class conflict (Giddens, 1982). They broaden Marx's insights to include conflict among any aspects or segments of a society. Conflicts may exist, for example, between living conditions of people, the structure of the health care system, and the standard of health of people. Thus, conflict theorists focus on the inevitable disagreements among people in groups, and individuals and groups compete (conflict) with one another as they attempt to preserve and promote their own special values and interests. Such conflicts also are often seen among health professionals or between health professionals and health politicians or administrators.

Briefly, society experiences inconsistency and conflict at every moment everywhere, a society is continually subjected to change, elements of a society tend to contribute and, due to power, a society rests on the constraint of some of its members by others.

Interactionists are concerned with how people interpret the social situations they are participating in. Both consensus and conflict theory deal with large social units and broad social processes. *Interactionism* attempts to understand social life from the viewpoint of the individuals involved. Accordingly, groups can only exist because their members influence one another's behaviour. Three basic assumptions are outlined (Mead, 1934). First, we act according to our interpretation of reality; second, subjective interpretations are based on the meanings we learn from others and, third, we are constantly interpreting our own behaviour as well as the behaviour of others in terms of the symbols and meanings we have learned.

Although the assumptions of these three theoretical perspectives are often contradictory, we learn more by using all three than we would by limiting ourselves to any one of them alone. This will become evident also from applying the perspectives to health-related behaviour and oral health as social phenomena.

Social classes and society

Social structure is found in all human groups and refers to the patterned relationships among individuals and groups. Such relationships are present in smaller groups like the family (*microsociology*) and larger groups as in the society (*macrosociology*). A society is the largest and closest to self-sufficient group in existence. A society is theoretically independent of all its outside groups. It contains smaller social structures–family, economy, government, religion or health service system–to fulfil all the needs of its members. Societies have been classified by anthropologists and sociologists in various ways. One important classification system is based on the way the problem of subsistence is solved. Historically, societies have become larger and more complex as the means for solving the subsistence problem have improved. The major types of societies are hunting and gathering, horticultural, agricultural and industrial. The emergence of postindustrial societies is now foreseen.

Social inequality or social stratification appears to be a nearly universal characteristic of social life. Significant contributions to the study of social stratification and classes have been made by the functionalist tradition as well as by sociologists of the conflict school of thought. For conflict sociologists, the economic factor has been considered an independent variable explaining the existence of social classes. Originally, Karl Marx recognized the existence of several social classes in the industrial society but predicted that capitalist societies would ultimately be reduced to two social classes. Those who owned capital (the bourgeoisie) would be the rulers; those without ownership of the means of production (the proletariat) would be the ruled. Consequently, the capitalists controlled all social institutions. They could structure the legal system, educational system and government to suit their own interests. Whereas conflict theory focused on the relationship to the means of production as the cause of social stratification, functionalist or consensus theory examined the consequences of people's relationship to the economic institution. These consequences have been termed life chances: the likelihood of securing the good things of life such as housing, education, health and food. An important dimension of social stratification is the prestige, or social recognition, respect, and admiration from others. Prestige is always a cultural and social matter. In the first place, favourable social evaluations are based on the norms and values within a group. Occupational prestige scores vary according to compensation, education

required, skills and ability needed, power associated with the occupation, the importance of an occupation to a society and the nature of the work (mental or white-collar work versus manual or blue-collar work).

Three basic and practical approaches have been developed for the identification of social classes at the community and societal levels–reputational, self-location and objective. The reputational methods imply a strategy in which knowledgeable people are asked to rank individuals and families in terms of their place in the community's stratification structure. The self-location method requires members of a community to identify the social class to which they think they belong. For example, people may be asked to place themselves within a set of social classes presented to them by the researcher. A commonly used set of social classes includes lower class, working class, middle class and upper class. The objective method involves ranking individuals or families/households on such standard criteria as income, occupation and education. Objectivity is increased because the researcher does the ranking on predetermined scales which provides some consistency in placing people in social classes. Eventually, an index of social position or status may be constructed from several criteria.

Such principles are widely used in the UK as well as in Scandinavia enabling, to some extent, cross-country comparisons of stratification or class structures. The UK Registrar General's categories are as follows:

- Social class I: Professional (e.g. accountant, doctor, lawyer; 5%).
- Social class II: Intermediate (e.g. manager, nurse, schoolteacher; 18%).
- Social class III NM: Skilled non-manual (e.g. clerical worker, secretary, shop assistant; 12%).
- Social class III M: Skilled manual (e.g. bus driver, butcher, carpenter, coal-face worker; 38%).
- Social class IV: Partly skilled (e.g. agricultural worker, bus conductor, postman; 18%)
- Social class V: Unskilled (e.g. cleaner, dock worker, labourer, 9%).

Consequences of stratification

Three umbrella-like dimensions of class-related social repercussions are life chances, lifestyle and

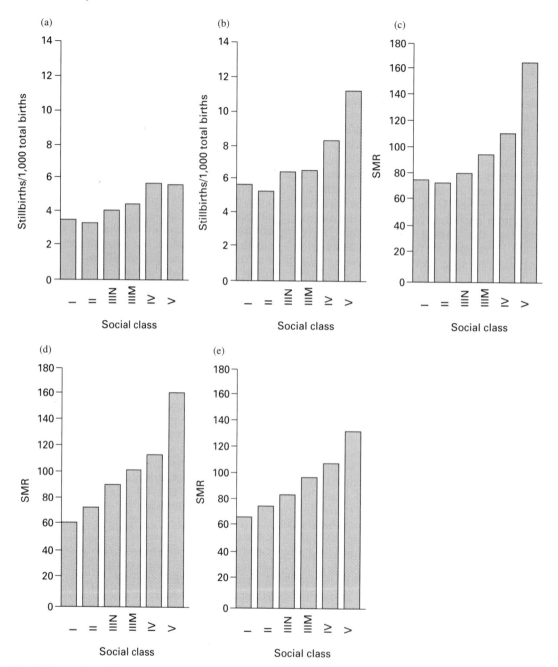

Fig. 3.1 Occupational class and mortality in infants, children and adults. England and Wales: (a) stillbirths, 1990; (b) infants, 1990; (c) children aged 1–15, 1979–83. UK: (d) men aged 20–64, 1979–1983; (e) women aged 20–59, 1979–1983. SMR = Standardized mortality rate. Modified from Whitehead (1992).

personality. Life chances refer to the likelihood of possessing the good things in life. Such living conditions include health, happiness, education, wealth and legal protection. The probability of acquiring and maintaining the material and non-material rewards increases with social class level, whereas the probability of possessing life itself declines with social class level.

Whether measured by the death rate or by life expectancy, the likelihood of a longer life is enhanced as people move up the stratification structure (Fig. 3.1; Whitehead, 1992). This disparity in the most fundamental life chance may be due to differences in living conditions, the value placed on medical attention, concern with proper nutrition, attention to personal hygiene and the ability to afford what these things cost. In the light of this, it is not surprising that physical health is affected by social class level (Whitehead, 1992). Those lower in a stratification structure are more likely to be sick or disabled and to receive poorer medical treatment once they are ill. It is no different for mental health. People in lower-class groups have a higher probability of becoming mentally disturbed and are less likely to receive therapeutic help, adequate or otherwise.

Life chances are often linked to the economics of social class. Since life chances can be improved with access to wealth, they can be changed quickly. Lifestyle, on the other hand, changes less easily because this is related to culture. Research has shown that the rich and the poor really are separated by much more than money. Social class differences have been observed in many areas of life, including language, marital and family relations, child rearing, political attitudes and behaviour, religious affiliation and participation in social activities. Just as life chances and life styles are correlates of stratification structure, social class is associated with different personality characteristics. This occurs because the patterns of socialization vary from social class to social class. This is not to say that all members of a social class share a given personality trait. It does mean that, as a whole, members of one social class exhibit a given characteristic more than members of another class do.

Social stratification and oral health

The research literature is rich with evidence of social factors impacting on oral disease and illness (Beal, 1989). For the UK, the oral health impact of social classes as well as the broader societal changes over time have been documented in the most recent *Adult Dental Health Survey in the United Kingdom 1988* (Todd and Lader, 1991). The purpose of the study was to establish the state of dental health of adults and to compare the 1988 results with similar studies carried out in the 1960s and the 1970s. A national representative sample of adults (non-institutionalized) was chosen. In all, 6825 adults were interviewed and 4331 were dentally examined.

Table 3.1 illustrates important trends for the changes in oral health conditions from a societal perspective. The reductions in total tooth loss in the UK for the period 1978–1988 were most dramatic among the three 10-year age groups 35–44, 45–54 and 55–64. Although the level of total tooth loss had fallen for both sexes, the proportion of women who were edentulous in 1988 was similar to that for men in 1978. The final factor considered was the social class of the head of the household in which the informant lived. The proportion of edentulous adults in each of the three grouped social classes had fallen since 1978, with a smaller decrease for people in social class III non-manual. However, the unskilled manual classes in 1988 had not yet achieved a reduction to the levels of edentulousness that the non-manual classes had achieved in 1978; 22% of adults with backgrounds dependent on non-manual occupations were edentulous in 1978, compared with 32% of adults in unskilled manual occupations in 1988.

Similar trends are found in Scandinavia. Table 3.2 presents results from two interview studies of adults in Denmark undertaken 10 years apart

Table 3.1 The percentages of adults with total tooth loss in the UK for different age, sex and social class groups for 1978 and 1988

	1978	1988
Age (years)		
16–24		
25–34	4	1
35–44	13	4
45–54	32	17
55–64	50	37
65 and over	79	67
All ages	30	21
Sex		
Male	25	16
Female	33	25
Both sexes	30	21
Social class of head of household		
I, II, III NM (skilled non-manual)	22	14
III M (skilled manual)	29	24
IV, V (unskilled)	38	32
All	30	21

From Todd and Lader (1991), with permission.

(Petersen, 1990). The proportions in different age groups and social groups who reported having few or no teeth left are shown. The participants were classified by social class according to the method described by the Danish National Institute for Social Research. The main criteria are level of education, occupational status and training, and number of subordinates. Groups I and II represent the highest social positions (upper-level salaried employees and large-business self-employed) while group V (unskilled manual workers) are the lowest positions. In all social classes the proportion of respondents with few or no teeth left decreased over time, in particular in the younger individuals, diminishing the social difference. However, the social inequality in dental health was found to be significant in the older groups.

For adults, the impact of social class on oral health status has also been documented through several oral epidemiological studies (for review; see Beal, 1989), especially with respect to dental caries and periodontal conditions. The disadvantaged social groups have a higher proportion of teeth or tooth surfaces with unmet need for treatment; number of teeth missing due to caries; lower numbers of filled/restored teeth, compared with the advantaged groups. This pattern of dental caries experience holds true for the child population as shown in the recent UK study of children's dental health (O'Brien, 1994; Table 3.3). For both ages 12 and 15, the proportion of children with any known decay was higher for those with a background of social classes IV or V. Similarly, in a Danish survey of

Table 3.2 Percentage of Danish adults who report having few or no teeth left in relation to age group, social group and year of investigation (1976 and 1986; sample *n* = 2008)

| | Age group | | | | | |
| | 35–44 years | | 45–54 years | | 55–64 years | |
	1976	1986	1976	1986	1976	1986
Social Group						
I	2	1	14	7	38	25
II	12	4	27	15	39	31
III	19	10	51	26	58	54
IV	30	9	48	37	64	57
V	52	24	73	56	86	80
Total	30	11	54	36	68	61

From Petersen (1990), with permission.

Table 3.3 The proportion of children with actively decayed, filled and missing teeth in the permanent dentition and the mean number of affected teeth by age and household social class in the UK in 1993

| *Tooth conditions and household social class* | *Age* | | | |
| | *12 years* | *15 years* | *12 years* | *15 years* |
	Percentage of children with condition		Mean number of teeth affected	
Actively decayed				
I, II, III non-manual	17	25	0.3	0.5
III manual	27	25	0.5	0.6
IV, V	32	36	0.6	0.9
Filled				
I, II, III non-manual	35	48	0.7	1.4
III manual	38	59	0.7	2.0
IV, V	50	59	1.1	2.2
Missing due to decay				
I, II, III non-manual	3	4	0.1	0.1
III manual	6	6	0.1	0.1
IV, V	15	19	0.3	0.3
Any known decay				
I, II, III non-manual	45	58	1.1	2.0
III manual	51	68	1.4	2.7
IV, V	68	72	2.0	3.4

From O'Brien (1994), with permission.

Table 3.4 Multiple dummy regression analysis of caries experience (defs = decayed, extracted, and filled surfaces and DMFS = decayed, missing due to caries, and filled surfaces) and logistic regression analysis of odds for dental caries among 6-year-old Danish children (*n* = 197)

Independent variable	Dummy variable	Regression coefficient	Odds ratio
Frequency of daily tooth-brushing	Three times or more often	0.22	1.42
	Twice	0.19	1.17
	Once		
Consumption of sweets	High	0.38*	2.08*
	Moderate	0.29	2.51**
	Low		
Pocket money for sweets	High	0.54*	1.55*
	Moderate	0.28	1.14
	Low		
Consumption of sugary drinks	High	0.44*	1.58
	Moderate	0.13	1.01
	Low		
Parent's education	Primary school		
	Grade 7–9	2.63*	2.46**
	Grade 10	1.46*	1.32
	Secondary school	−0.24	0.91
	High school		
Family income	<DKR 200 000	0.87*	2.14*
	DKR 200 000–299 999	0.06	1.28
	> DKR 300 000		

Dummy regression: intercept = 0.65.
*P < 0.05; **P < 0.01.
DKR = Danish kroner.
From Petersen (1992), with permission.

6-year-old children, multivariate analyses of dental caries experience outlined the existence of a social gradient (Table 3.4; Petersen, 1992). The relative risk of dental caries (odds ratio) as well as the total amount of dental caries were higher for children with family backgrounds of low education or poor family income. Moreover, the consequences of risk behaviour in terms of frequent consumption of sweets was demonstrated.

Health, illness, sickness and culture

Social factors are involved not just in the aetiology of oral problems; they are also implicated in the very processes by which those problems come to be defined and seen as socially significant. These are processes of definition at the level of the whole culture–what is seen to be the cultural ideal of body image and oral health–but they are also processes conducted at the interpersonal level, for example in response to highly visible aspects of the oral condition like

the shape of the mouth and jaws. The simple disease model of social epidemiology has to give way to one that draws more fully on the social construction perspective of sociology. In other words, people *define* their oral problems; they don't just experience them.

An important way in which social factors determine–rather than merely define–oral health is in patterns of active prevention and self-care. In oral health care, as in medicine, there is a range of clearly defined actions that people can carry out to maintain and enhance their health. The important difference is that in the case of oral care the procedures and the philosophy of conscious self-care and prevention seem to be much more widely diffused in the population. The classic case is, of course, that of tooth-brushing, which is almost a universal practice in the populations of the advanced industrial societies. Fluoride toothpaste, dental floss, disclosing solution and dietary control follow some distance behind. All these practices, however, vary strongly by social group and reflect powerful society-wide cultural influences

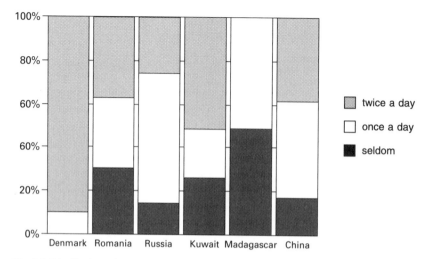

Fig. 3.2 Distribution of 6-year-old children (%) according to frequency of tooth-cleaning and by country. Data from Petersen, 1992; Petersen *et al.*, 1990, 1991, 1993, 1994, 1995.

that are frequently more closely linked to grooming behaviour and the cultivation of body image than they are to the maintenance of health. The extensive cross-cultural variation in oral self-care practices is illustrated in Figure 3.2. In these cross-cultural studies, the same basic questionnaire was used to collect information on tooth-cleaning habits in the different population groups of 6-year-olds and the impact of cultural factors would seem apparent (Petersen, 1992; Petersen *et al.*, 1990, 1991, 1993, 1995; Petersen and Escheng, 1994).

In modern health sociology, some basic terms have been introduced to the analysis of health related behaviour (Patrick and Scambler, 1982). *Health behaviour* is the broad concept implying actions undertaken by people which have positive or negative consequences to health. Effective tooth-cleaning practices are indicative of positive oral health behaviour whereas frequent consumption of sugary foods represents negative health behaviour (or risk behaviour). The concept encompasses conscious as well as non-conscious behaviour. The interpretation of symptoms or signs of illness–especially pain–and the search for relief is a social process drawing on past experience and involving interaction with others in defining a solution to an oral health problem. Sociologists have called this process *illness behaviour*. In the case of conditions that are visible and that affect the social identity or acceptability of a person, more

complex processes of decision-making are involved in the lay culture. In such instances, both the pressures from others and the will to accede to such pressures in the interests of social conformity are much greater. Sociologists have called this process of influence and response *labelling behaviour*. Finally, the social role of a sick person has been considered. To be ill is more than a medical condition. The patient has a customary part to play in relation to the health professional and to his or her family and to other members of society, and in turn they expect him or her to behave in certain prescribed ways–the *patient role*. Four aspects of the *sick role* have been emphasized. First, the sick person is exempted from normal social responsibilities, depending on the severity of the illness. Second, the sick person cannot help him or herself and must be cared for. Third, the sick role is regarded as a misfortune, so it is assumed that the sick person will want to get well, and is under obligation to do so. The fourth aspect is the obligation of the sick person to seek competent help, usually from the health professional, and to cooperate with him or her in the process of getting well. The typical sick role is temporary and society expects that most patients will get well. In conclusion, a conceptual model regarding health-related behaviour is presented in Figure 3.3 (Petersen, 1990). The distinct levels of relevance to the analysis of health and illness behaviour are outlined and the influences of

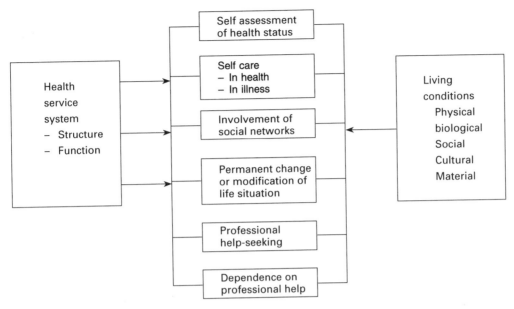

Fig. 3.3 A conceptual model for the analysis of health-related behaviour. From Petersen (1990).

living conditions as well as the structure and function of the health service system are stressed. Further considerations of health behaviour are given in Chapter 12 of this book.

Culture and health-related behaviour

Social research has demonstrated the association of distinct ways of thinking, feeling and behaving with social class level. In fact, this association among social class, attitudes and behaviour has led many sociologists to think of social classes as subcultures. Because of the difficulty in specifying all of the factors affecting class-related differences, it is more correct to think of these differences as being correlated with rather than caused by social class level. This does not down-grade the impact of social class on human behaviour, but it does mean that social class is one of several factors contributing to the variations observed in social life.

In a sociological perspective, culture consists of all humanly created physical objects and patterns for thinking, feeling and behaving that are passed from generation to generation among members of a society. In all societies, health cultures are found which influence how people tend to cope with health problems, either through contact with the formal health care system or by alternative lay health care practices.

The sociological standpoint is that human behaviour is learned. There are three broad dimensions to culture–material, cognitive and normative. *Material* culture is composed of the concrete, tangible aspects of the culture (e.g. houses, cars, money, dental instruments, dental office facilities). Material objects have meanings only when people assign meanings to them. *Beliefs*, the most important aspect of the cognitive dimension, are ideas about what is considered to be true. Whether or not they are actually true, beliefs have a great influence on members of a society or within a human group. The *normative* dimension of culture is composed of norms, sanctions and values. *Norms* are rules defining appropriate and inappropriate ways of behaving. There are several types of norms. Folkways are not considered vital to a group and may be violated without significant consequences. Norms of great moral significance are thought to be vital to the well-being of a society. In more advanced societies, laws are a third type of norm. Laws are norms that are formally defined by designated persons. In a society, the two latter types of norms emerge slowly and are often unconsciously created whereas laws are consciously defined and enforced. Since norms must be learned and accepted by individuals, conformity to them is not automatic. Groups must have some means for teaching norms and encouraging conformity to them. *Sanctions* are rewards and punishments used to encourage socially acceptable behaviour. Informal sanctions–which can be applied by most members of a group–may be positive or negative. Formal sanctions may be given only by officially designated persons, such as judges or health authorities.

Norms and values are not the same thing. *Values* are broad cultural principles defining what is good or desirable. For example, in most societies health and quality of life are desirable. Values are so general that they do not specify appropriate ways of thinking, feeling and behaving. Thus, it is possible for different societies or different groups within the same society to have quite different norms based on the same value. Cultural diversity exists in all societies in part because of the presence of social categories, i.e. persons who share a social characteristic such as age, sex or religion. Such differences are also demonstrated within oral health due to the fact that oral self-care practices as well as utilization of professional dental services tend to vary by sex and age. For example, the recent UK data (Todd and Lader, 1991) showed that dentate women were more likely than dentate men to say they had been to the dentist in the last 12 months (72% of women, 62% of men), and overall relatively more women claimed to go for regular check-ups or preventive reasons (Table 3.5). There was also a large variation in time since the last visit for people of different ages. In 16–24-year-olds, 69% said they last visited the dentist within the last year as compared with only 32% of the age group 65–74. This is partly explained by the higher proportion of edentulous people in old age and partly by lack of dental care traditions. Evidence is now available for the industrialized countries that for the coming generation of old age people, utilization of services is growing, indicating the shift in oral health culture (Petersen and Holst, 1995).

Cultural diversity is also promoted by occupation or social class. As indicated by the UK dental health survey (Todd and Lader, 1991), higher social classes more often reported dental visits compared with lower social classes. Table 3.5 presents the dental attendance rates in adults by social class of the head of the household. People with backgrounds dependent on non-manual occupations were significantly more likely to have said that they attend for a regular check-up, 51% of non-manuals compared with 23% of unskilled manuals. Conversely, people of unskilled manual occupations were more likely than those from non-manual backgrounds to say that they only go when having trouble with their teeth. Furthermore, in the advantaged social classes more people tend to believe that tooth loss is preventable than do so in the disadvantaged group.

Values and norms with respect to oral health

Table 3.5 Dental attendance patterns by social class of the head of household as defined by occupation and sex–all adults and dentate adults in the UK (1988)

Dental attendance pattern	Social class of head of household						All	
	I, II, IIINM		IIIM		IV, V			
	M (%)	F (%)	M (%)	F (%)	M (%)	F (%)	M (%)	F (%)
All adults								
Regular check-up	47	54	28	40	20	25	35	43
Occasional check-up	16	11	10	9	10	9	13	10
Only with trouble	27	18	40	24	47	27	35	22
Edentulous	10	18	22	26	23	40	16	26
Base	991	1066	747	677	366	480	2150	2335
Dentate adults								
Regular check-up	52	65	36	54	26	41	42	58
Occasional check-up	17	13	13	12	13	14	16	13
Only with trouble	30	22	51	33	61	45	42	29
Base	889	878	583	499	282	290	1795	1737

From Todd and Lader (1991), with permission.

Table 3.6 Percentages of Danish adults 25–44 years of age reporting having undertaken various kinds of dental health behaviour in relation to their level of education (n = 749)

	Education				
	Primary school (grades 7–8) (n = 310)	Primary school (grades 9–10) (n = 155)	Secondary school (n = 155)	High school (n = 129)	Total (n = 749)
Regular dental visits	75	92	95	94	86
Tooth-brushing at least twice a day	75	82	91	90	83
Tooth-brushing after breakfast	37	57	58	70	51
Regular use of toothpicks	38	42	53	49	45
Regular use of dental floss	9	27	31	33	22

From Petersen (1990), with permission.

Table 3.7 The percentages of parents with high levels of dental knowledge, positive attitude to prevention and dental health-related behaviours in relation to parent's level of education

	Education			
	Primary school grade 7–9	Primary school grade 10	Secondary school	High school
High level of knowledge about sugar and caries (score 6–7)	83	69	88	93
High level of knowledge about prevention of dental diseases (score 3)	52	66	71	88
Positive attitude to prevention (score 4)	56	69	73	80
Frequent consumption of sweets (score 12–13)	39	49	36	33
Frequent consumption of healthy foods (score 15–18)	24	46	54	63
Tooth-brushing at least three times a day	15	23	16	36
Parents brush the child's teeth every day	39	27	39	65

From Petersen (1992), with permission.

are reflected in knowledge, attitudes and self-care practices. Since oral health behaviour is conditioned by culture, the variations by education are often most prominent. Table 3.6 illustrates such findings from a national Danish study of 25–44-year-olds (Petersen, 1990). As supported also by Table 3.7, high scores on dental knowledge and attitudes to teeth and dental care tend to be more frequent in people (parents) with a background of high education (Petersen, 1992), and such parents also more often claimed to brush their child's teeth on a daily basis than parents of lower education. The evidence of a cultural basis of values and norms in oral health is also supported by a number of studies in the UK which focus on oral health in ethnic minorities. For example, oral health conditions of children have been shown to be poor in Bangladeshi, Vietnamese, African or Asian children compared with white UK children (Plamping et al., 1985; Laher, 1990; Martin and Smith, 1991; Williams et al., 1991). Poor living conditions are also often observed among ethnic-minority groups, suggesting that socio-economic status may be a critical determinant of oral health.

Family, socialization and health

So far we have seen that social life is patterned and orderly because of the existence of culture and social structure. Since we are not born with culture and social structure in our genes, a lot of learning is required before we can participate in group life. The process of socialization enables us to take part in group life and acquire many of the characteristics we think of as human.

Table 3.8 The percentage of parents who gave support to their child every day, in relation to the child's place in the family

	1 (first born)	2 (second born)	3 + (third or higher)
Parents brush the child's teeth every day	53	35	42
Parents check the child's teeth every day	67	47	38
Parents talk about tooth-brushing every day	31	28	23

From Petersen (1992), with permission.

Socialization takes place within groups. Early or primary socialization usually occurs exclusively within friendly, small intimate groups. The principal example of this type of group–known as the primary group–is the family. Later we enter groups that tend to be larger and more impersonal. The secondary groups, important in the process of secondary socialization, range from the kindergartens, and the schools we enter at age 5 or 6, to larger work-related groups, continuing to the old-age homes we may die in.

As mentioned previously, *interactionism* is the sociological position which stresses the importance of socialization to the study of social behaviour. We use groups to evaluate ourselves and to acquire attitudes, beliefs, values and norms. Groups used in this way are called *reference groups*. However, we need not be a member of a reference group. Those whose judgements are most important to our self-concept are called *significant others*. For a child, significant others are likely to include mother, father, grandparents, teachers and playmates. Teenagers place heavy reliance on their peers. The variety of significant others is greater for adults, ranging through parents, friends and neighbours.

The importance of family support in the development of appropriate oral health care habits of the child and the young has been shown in the literature. For example, a recent UK study demonstrated that dental care habits as well as dental health status of children improved when their mothers undertook regular dental care themselves (Gratrix *et al.*, 1990). Positive oral health attitudes in parents and emotional support to children are considered important to 'dental socialization'. However, equally important is the practical help from parents. In a study of parents of 6-year-old children the influence of family structure on parental support in oral health was shown (Petersen, 1992). As indicated in Table 3.8, support in tooth-brushing was relatively often given to the first-born child

of the family, while the younger children in larger families often enjoyed less assistance from parents. Recent studies in Norway provided further evidence to support the assumption that the family serves as a major influencing agent on health behaviours (Rossow, 1993). The potential for parental influence on adolescents' health behaviour was found to be larger if both parents were consistent in their behaviours and the influence of parents was present throughout the late period of adolescence. Moreover, the interrelationship between oral health conditions and social network activity is also documented for adults. In a study of old-age pensioners (Petersen and Nörtov, 1989), dental health status and dental health behaviour were poor among persons with weak social network relations (Table 3.9). A similar pattern of poor oral health was found for persons with a less active lifestyle (Table 3.10). Those old-age pensioners who infrequently participated in various social or cultural activities tended to have relatively poor scores on dental status and were less likely to be regular dental attenders.

Towards theoretical explanations of social inequalities in oral health

So far the societal aspects of oral health and health-related behaviour have been outlined. From a sociological point of view the associations between social class and health represent effects at the *macro level*. The interrelationships between health and social networks, lifestyles and culture are effects at the so-called *meso level*. In health sociology, efforts are undertaken to organize the extensive empirical evidence and, thereby, help us to understand the social context of health and health care. Also, theoretical models may guide further research in the field as well as the design of public health intervention programmes. How do we interpret the meaning of social differences

Table 3.9 Percentages of 67-year-old Danes who were edentulous, denture-wearers and reported dental symptoms and regular dental visits among people with *low positions* on social network activity. Each column represents only respondents with weak social network relations (*n* = 216)

Dental health variable	Weak social network				
	Family (n=51)	Friends (n=61)	Neighbours (n=113)	Single living (n=63)	All respondents (n=216)
Edentulous	47	41	57	46	38
Denture-wearer	70	65	67	65	59
Symptoms from teeth/gums within the last 12 months	11	28	24	18	23
Regular dental visits	45	36	44	38	46

Total sample: *n* = 216.
From Petersen and Nörtov (1989), with permission.

Table 3.10 Percentages of 67-year-old Danes who were edentulous, denture-wearers and reported dental symptoms and regular dental visits in relation to lifestyle activity (*n* = 201)

Dental health variable	Index of lifestyle activity				
	Very low (n=51)	Low (n=44)	Moderate (n=56)	High (n=50)	Total (n=201)
Edentulous	51	31	36	34	39
Denture-wearer	68	50	56	58	59
Symptoms from teeth/gums within the last 12 months	39	19	18	16	23
Regular dental visits	31	45	48	60	46

From Petersen and Nörtov (1989), with permission.

in oral health and the policy implications that flow from them? A number of approaches to an explanation of these fundamental questions have been proposed, though none until now has provided a wholly satisfactory answer. Theoretical explanations of the relationship between health and inequality may be roughly divided into four categories:

1 Artefact explanations;
2 Theories of natural or social selection;
3 Materialist or structuralist explanations;
4 Cultural/behavioural explanations.

In the following, each of these approaches will be described in general terms and then their relevance with respect to oral health is discussed.

Health inequality as an artefact

The artefact explanation argues that inequalities in health are not real but artificial. They are an effect produced in the attempt to measure something (health, social class) which is more complicated than the tools of measurement can appreciate. More an expression of scepticism than a theoretical explanation, this view is often held by statisticians who claim that the evidence of health inequality is so complicated by changes in classification of social class that it is impossible to tell whether things are getting better or worse. Furthermore, it is argued that changes in occupational structure are likely to combine with age to confound any attempt to measure inequality in health even at a point of time. The observed social gradient is thus really caused by a skewed age structure of the lower social class rather than by the poorer health of its members.

Natural and social selection

Explanations in terms of selection accept that social inequalities in health do indeed exist, but suggest that the differences are caused by a health selection process (functionalism). Occupational or social class is here relegated to the state of dependent variable and health acquires the greater degree of causal significance. According to this explanation, people in poor health would tend to move down the occupational scale and concentrate in the lower social classes, while people in good health would tend to move up into higher classes. In other words, the observed differences in health reflect a process of social mobility. The class structure is seen as a filter or sorter of human beings, and one of the major bases of selection is health, i.e. physical and mental strength. The gap between the health of higher and lower social classes would therefore be kept open indefinitely and would be inevitable whatever improvements in health occur over the entire population.

Materialist or structuralist explanations

The materialist explanation emphasizes the role of external environment–the conditions under which people live and work and the pressures on them to consume unhealthy products. Inequalities in health in this context would come about because lower social groups are exposed to a more unhealthy environment. They do more dangerous work, have poorer housing and have fewer resources (e.g. income) available to secure the necessities for health and to use the available health services. In other words, health inequality occurs as a result of material deprivation, i.e. a shortage of the material resources on which healthy human existence depends. The definition of deprivation is not absolute but always relative to social and economic norms. When living standards rise in general, rich and poor improve their life expectation and the gap in life chances is maintained. At a more general level, the whole structure of society is implicated. The materialist/structuralist approach reflects the conflict theories in sociology.

Cultural/behavioural explanation

This fourth approach stresses differences in the way individuals in different groups choose to lead their lives: the behaviour and voluntary lifestyles they adopt. Such explanations thereby focus on the individual as a unit of analysis, emphasizing unthinking, reckless or irresponsible behaviour or incautious lifestyle as the moving determinant of poor health status. Inequalities in health evolve because lower social

groups have adopted more dangerous and health-damaging behaviour than the higher groups, and may have less interest in protecting their children, by the excessive consumption of harmful commodities, refined foods, tobacco and alcohol, by lack of exercise, or by underutilization of preventive health care. Part of the culture of any social group is concerned with ideas and practices about health. Some would argue that the distinct pattern of behaviour, knowledge and health attitudes within certain social groups is a consequence only of lack of education. This perspective is also called the theory of cultural deprivation or cultural poverty.

Which of the theoretical approaches are then of great relevance to the explanation of inequalities in oral health?

The various explanations for health inequality differ in their assumptions. Artefact explanations tend to be favoured by statisticians and by those who reject the empirical data. However imperfect the measuring tools, there can be no doubt that inequalities in oral health exist. It should be stressed that, compared with general epidemiology, valid measures of the oral diseases may be obtained, i.e. number of teeth affected by dental decay or number of edentulous persons. Also, the health selection theory must be considered of minor importance to the explanation of inequalities in oral health. In a wider perspective it seems rather unlikely that oral health, even in terms of dental appearance, can determine subsequent social position and thereby be of relevance to social mobility.

The two last approaches have pure theoretical aims and are essentially sociological explanations. The argument that inequality in health reflects material or cultural deprivation is a sociological position. It states that health is a product of social forces whether these take a material (economic) or a cultural (normative) form. Health is assumed to be a property of social environment and the individual's relationship to it. The data on oral health presented in this chapter are more supportive of the materialist/structuralist and the cultural/behavioural explanations. Arguments for the first approach would be, for example, that oral health is so clearly influenced by both living and environmental working conditions. Furthermore, the reduction of tooth loss across all social classes and increased utilization of professional dental services in industrialized countries are likely to have occurred as a result of social and health policy initiatives, e.g. improved standards of living and the establishment of systematic oral health care systems. Arguments for a cultural/behavioural explanation would be that oral health status and treatment needs are so clearly related to individual health behaviour (e.g. sugar consumption, oral hygiene and dental visiting habits).

However, empirical data suggest that inequalities in oral health are not completely explained by social differences in oral health behaviour. Several commentators are beginning to question whether the distinction between the two approaches is artificial, as behaviour cannot be separated from its social context. Certain living and working conditions appear to impose severe restrictions on an individual's ability to choose a healthy lifestyle. The two models are therefore interrelated rather than mutually exclusive. This new perspective has also been suggested with respect to oral health. In a study of an industrial population (Petersen, 1990), a conflict model of dental visiting habits was proposed (Fig. 3.4). The model emphasizes that environmental factors (living and working conditions, structure and function of the dental health service system) dictate behaviour and, in turn, are conducive to the development of group-specific norms and values regarding dental health (i.e. dental health culture).

Health systems and society

In community oral health, three areas may benefit from the sociological perspective and approach (Petersen, 1986). The first area, *social epidemiology*, is concerned with the social causes of oral diseases. The epidemiological concept of multiple causality is central and sociological methods may be used to study how social and physical settings bring about diseases. The second area, which may be called *odontological social psychology*, deals with the reactions of individuals and groups to oral health and oral diseases. This means the cultural-based concepts, knowledge, attitudes and the behaviour of individuals with respect to oral health, the prevention and treatment of oral diseases. The last area of studies may be called *sociology of the oral health care system*. The structure and the function of oral health care service, the making of decisions, organizational positions and roles in society of the oral health personnel are central subjects. Such aspects call for the application of theories of social organization and systems analysis.

A formal organization is a group deliberately

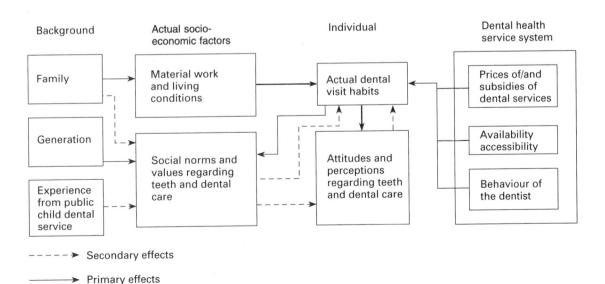

Fig. 3.4 Conflict model for the explanation of actual dental visit habits in adults. Model stresses the primary effect (arrows in bold) of structural factors and the secondary importance of normative factors.

created for the achievement of one or more goals. This is the case also for organizations or systems within the health care sector in a society. Organization involves deciding who has the authority and responsibility for what and formulating procedures for such aspects as communicating, making decisions, management, planning for the future, handling financial matters, and rewarding and punishing organizational members. Once established, organizations tend to assume a life of their own; they continue to exist despite changes in personnel. The stability and continuity of organizations are partially due to the fact that they are based on formal positions and duties rather than on intimate, personal relationships. For people working within an organization or system (including oral health systems), the social structure around them seems to have a certain solidity and permanence almost similar to that of a material structure like a building. Certainly this is how it seems if they try to make any major changes in the system or if they try to depart too radically from its established procedures.

Sociologists have classified organizations according to who benefits from them most. In mutual-benefit organizations (political parties, labour unions or professional associations) the prime beneficiary is the membership. These organizations exist to promote the interests of those who belong to them. Business organizations, on the other hand, are expected to serve the interests of their owners. Since these are profit-oriented organizations, their emphasis is on the achievement of maximum gain at the least cost. The prime beneficiary of a service organization is its clients. The goal of social-work agencies, schools, hospitals or oral health systems is to aid those who qualify for their professional services. These differences among organizations are important but so are the similarities. Similarities among modern organizations exist primarily because most of them are bureaucratic. Bureaucracy may occur within a formal organization but the informal side of bureaucracy should also be considered. The informal groups can either help or hinder the achievement of formal organizational goals and shall be taken into account by leaders or the management staff. This perspective is valuable also to understanding cooperation and conflicts within the oral health service systems.

For sociologists the interest therefore is in the social organization of oral health care; that is,

the way in which the provision of oral health services of one kind or another has become the centre of an elaborate structure of occupations with associated organizational and financial arrangements. These systems have evolved in the advanced industrial societies over the last century or so and reflect quite varied cultural and political environments. Beneath this apparent variety, however, oral health care systems perform certain core functions and show common organizational features. Of special interest to the sociologist–and to the dental professional–is the very particular occupational form that dentistry, like other professions, has taken. The organization of dentistry as a profession has implications for its relationship to other occupations in the medical field, quite aside from its unique internal arrangements which require, for example, an elaborate and extended induction period through dental school for the new recruit. These issues are related to the societal role of the dental professional.

The essential features of the principles of delivery of oral health care in a number of countries are discussed further in Chapters 16 and 17.

Research methods in social sciences and health sociology

In this chapter reference has been made to social research and empirical results of sociodental surveys. People tend to get information from non-scientific sources such as intuition, common sense and authority. Generally speaking, these sources are inadequate for obtaining knowledge about social life as well as the social aspects of oral health and illness. In an effort to obtain accurate knowledge, researchers use the scientific method which involves the application of several distinct steps to the problem. The steps include identifying a problem, construction of variables, formulating hypotheses, developing a research design, collecting data, analysing data and stating conclusions. Although nearly all researchers use the steps in the scientific method as a model, they do not all use the same methods for collecting data or strategies for testing hypotheses or theories. Physical and natural scientists depend on the controlled or laboratory experiment, as do many psychologists. Though sociologists sometimes conduct controlled experiments and longitudinal intervention studies, they tend to rely more on surveys and field research. Field research is the most appropriate method for studying social behaviour that cannot be measured quantitatively, that is best understood within a natural setting and that requires in-depth analysis. In surveys, information is obtained either through a questionnaire or an interview. A questionnaire is a written set of questions that survey participants fill out themselves; in an interview, a trained interviewer asks questions and records answers. Questionnaires or interviews may be composed of structured questions, i.e. questions for which a limited, predetermined set of answers is possible. Unstructured questions ask for answers in the respondents' own words. Such questions allow interviewers to probe more deeply into respondents' attitudes, feelings, beliefs and opinions.

Scientific knowledge is superior because it is based on the principles of objectivity and verifiability. *Verifiability* means that any study can be duplicated by other scientists. According to the principle of *objectivity*, scientists are expected to prevent their personal values and preferences from influencing their scientific work. Complete objectivity is impossible because all scientists have values, beliefs, attitudes and prejudices that affect their work to some extent. Subjectivity can be minimized, however, if researchers are aware of their biases and make them public.

Concluding remarks

In the opening of this chapter the sharply divergent trends in dental caries levels between developed and developing countries were considered. The causes, character and consequences of this process are fundamentally sociological in nature. These trends can be viewed from other perspectives–the clinical, biodental or biomedical point of view, for example–but the sociological approach is just as valid, in principle, and arguably provides insights that would not otherwise be achieved.

The decline in caries in the developed countries has been steady and sustained. It has occurred in countries both with and without widespread fluoridation of public water supplies, it has affected all social groups, it has taken place among regular and irregular dental users, and it is happening in successive age groups. The obvious question that arises for somebody

trained for provision of oral health care is how important clinical dental intervention has been in achieving this decline. The answer is probably–very little. The most likely causes of the decline are related to self-care, diet, education, improving standards of living, social and political stability, and a regular, consistent and sustained period of economic growth. There are strong parallels and precedents for such an analysis in the wider health area. There is substantial evidence, for example, that the virtual withering away of the infectious diseases as a major cause of death over the past century is a phenomenon largely attributable not only to the great medical breakthroughs of immunization and the antibiotic and antimicrobial drugs, but to long-term social and economic change and public health reform. Again, clinical interventions are seen to play a less important part alongside broader changes in lifestyle and economic and social conditions.

These insights into the possible causes of the dramatic decline in caries in the developed countries of the world result from the sociologist's interest in the social context of health and illness. The analysis and conclusion may be controversial and subject to further debate, but the methodology and approach are quite standard in epidemiological research.

References

Beal, J.F. (1989). Social factors and preventive dentistry. In: *The Prevention of Dental Disease* (J.J. Murray, ed.). Oxford Medical, Oxford.

Berger, P. and Luckman, T. (1967) *The Social Construction of Reality.* Penguin Books, Harmondsworth.

Durkheim, E. (1966) *The Rules of Sociological Method.* Free Press, New York.

Giddens, A. (1982) *Sociology–A brief but Critical Introduction.* Macmillan Press, London.

Gratrix, D., Taylor, G.O. and Lennon, M. (1990). Mothers' dental attendance patterns and their children's dental attendance and dental health. *British Dental Journal* **168**: 441–443.

Laher, M.H. (1990) A comparison between dental caries, gingival health and dental service usage in Bangladeshi and white Caucasian children aged 7, 9, 11, 13 and 15 years residing in an inner city area of London, UK. *Community Dental Health*, **7**: 157–163.

Marx, K. (1967) *Capital.* International, New York.

Mattin, D. and Smith, J.M. (1991) The oral health status, dental needs and factors affecting utilization of dental services in Asians aged 55 years and over resident in Southhampton. *British Dental Journal* **170**: 369–372.

Mead, G.H. (1934) *Mind, Self and Society*. University of Chicago Press, Chicago.

O'Brien, M. (1994) *Children's Dental Health in the United Kingdom 1993*. OPCS, London.

Patrick, D.L. and Scambler, G. (eds) (1982) *Sociology as Applied to Medicine*. Baillière Tindall, London.

Petersen, P.E. (1986) Community dentistry and sociology. *Scandinavian Journal Society of Medicine* **14**: 1–2.

Petersen, P.E. (1990) Social inequalities in dental health–towards a theoretical explanation. *Community Dental and Oral Epidemiology* **18**: 153–158.

Petersen, P.E. (1992) Oral health behaviour of 6-year-old Danish children. *Acta Odontolocal Scandinavica* **50**: 57–64.

Petersen, P.E. and Escheng, Z. (1994) *Oral Health Behaviour in a Group of 6-year-old Children and Parents in Wuhan City, PR China*. University of Copenhagen, Copenhagen.

Petersen, P.E. and Holst, D. (1995) Utilization of dental health services. In: *Disease Prevention and Health Promotion: Socio-dental Sciences in Action*. (H. Gift and L. Cohen, eds). Munksgaard, Copenhagen.

Petersen, P.E. and Nörtov, B. (1989) General and dental health in relation to life-style and social network activity among 67-year-old Danes. *Scandinavian Journal of Primary Health Care* **7**: 225–230.

Petersen, P.E., Hadi, R., Al-Zaabi, F.S. *et al.* (1990) Dental knowledge, attitudes and behaviour among Kuwaiti mothers and schoolteachers. *Journal Pedodontics* **14**: 158–164.

Petersen, P.E., Poulsen, V.J., Ramahaleo, J. and Ratsifaritana, C. (1991) Dental caries and dental health behaviour situation among 6- and 12-year-old urban schoolchildren in Madagascar. *African Dental Journal* **5**: 1–7.

Petersen, P.E., Kuzmina, E. and Smirnova, T. (1993) *Oral Health Behaviour Situation in 6- and 12-year-old Children and Parents in Moscow*. Russian Federation. University of Copenhagen, Copenhagen.

Petersen, P.E., Danila, I. and Samoila, A. (1995) Oral Health Behaviour, knowledge and attitudes of mothers and schoolteachers in Romania, 1993. *Acta Odontolocal Scandinavica* **53**: 363–368.

Plamping, D., Bewley, B.R. and Gelbier, S. (1985) Dental health and ethnicity. *British Dental Journal* **154**: 261–263.

Rossow, I. (1993) *Developing Health Behaviour*. Thesis. University of Oslo, Oslo.

Todd, R. and Gelbier, S. (1991) Dental caries and dental attendance patterns in Vietnamese children aged 11–12 years resident in three inner London boroughs, UK. *Community Dental Health* **8**: 163–165.

Todd. J.E. and Lader, D. (1991) *Adult Dental Health in United Kingdom 1988*. HMSO, London.

Whitehead, M. (1992) *The Health Divide*. Penguin Books, London.

Williams, S.A., Ahmed, I.A. and Hussein, P. (1991) Ethnicity, health and dental care–perspectives among British Asians: 2. *Dental Update* **18**: 205–207.

4

Health needs assessment

Aubrey Sheiham and John Spencer

Introduction

The concept of need is at the core of health planning. Planning health services is, in turn, rooted in the ethical imperative to use resources appropriately. A common assumption in the organization and provision of health services, including dental health services, which is being challenged, is that the need for health care can be objectively determined by professionals. Now it is known that health care needs may be defined in other ways, because the definition of any given state of ill health has become open to much wider interpretation than in the past. Health care needs now extend beyond a narrow clinical interpretation to issues like: the impact of ill health on individuals and on society; the degree of disability and dysfunction that ill health brings; the perceptions and attitudes of patients themselves towards ill health; and the social origins of many common illnesses. All these factors are believed to influence the utilization of health services, the development of health care techniques and, ultimately, the effectiveness of treatment.

Definitions of need

To Donabedian (1973) need describes states of the client that create a requirement for care and therefore represent a *potential* for service. Need does not always lead to use of services and use of services does not always result from need, but the existence of disease and normatively defined need does create a potential for the use of services

(Spencer, 1984). Cooper (1975) had a related definition: 'a state of health assessed as in need of treatment by a medical practitioner'. Matthew (1971) extends this service-related definition to effectiveness of treatment as 'a need for medical care exists when an individual has an illness or disability for which there is an effective and acceptable treatment or cure'. With the growing demand for 'evidence-based medicine' Matthew's definition has become widely accepted. Nevertheless, the definition which has been generally used is the taxonomy suggested by Bradshaw (1972). Namely, *'normative need'* is that which the expert or professional, administrator or social scientist defines as need in any given situation. *'Felt'* need is equated with *'want'*, expressed as the individual's own assessment of his or her requirement for health care. *'Expressed'* need or demand is felt need converted into action by seeking assistance. *'Comparative need'* is assessed by comparing the health care received by different people with similar characteristics. Additionally, *'unmet'* need is the difference, if any, between those services judged necessary to deal appropriately with defined health problems and those services actually being received (Carr and Wolfe, 1979). Need is relative to time, place and assessor (Magi and Allander, 1981).

The most commonly used type of need assessment in dental health planning is normative need because it seems to be relevant to the disease-oriented or biomedical model, which is believed to identify diseases without depending on the subjective perception of the patient.

Estimates of dental needs are expressed in terms of numbers of people, numbers of procedures, hours of work, division of labour or costs. The shortcoming of this approach has been increasingly recognized. First, professional judgements in normative need are neither value-free, nor objective. Indeed, the concept of objectivity is much less clear-cut than is often supposed (Teeling-Smith, 1973). Its methods often depend upon a consensus agreement from a number of subjective approaches. Even within those agreements, there is intraexaminer and interexaminer variability among different judgements. Second, the standard norm of measures of disease accepted by dentists, which are translated into treatment need, is not always the norm in terms of functional or social requirements of people examined. This problem occurs particularly in conditions which lack easy definition, such as occlusal disharmonies (Sheiham *et al.*, 1982). Oral health problems usually have much more to do with an individual's quality of life and personal comfort. Further, a person's dental satisfaction bears little relation to clinical assessment of his or her oral condition (Giddon *et al.*, 1976; Barenthin, 1977; Davis, 1980). Third, need which is justified by purely professional assessment is questioned in terms of human or consumer rights. Discrimination between people with the same needs cannot be morally justified. Although access and uptake of oral health services differ markedly between individuals living in the same society, as has been discussed in Chapter 3, decisions of priority in health care must be discussed publicly and should not be the sole prerogative of any single professional group or agency of government. In addition, recent developments in consumerism and marketing have highlighted the importance of patient attitudes in health care decisions. Lastly, normative need is criticized for its paradoxical approach. Although it recommends treatment, in the belief that all the sick should be helped, treatment is not obtained in many situations because of limited health care resources. 'If some of the needy receive complete care, nothing may be left for others. We cannot be endlessly generous and continue to be fair' (Acheson, 1978). This is why Fuchs (1974), an economist, described normative need as romantic rather than humanitarian. The key elements of suggested improvement in estimating needs are as follows:

- Consideration of people's need should include the utility of the procedures available to meet it and the resources that permit those procedures to be used. There has to be the probability that the use of the proposed service will lead to an acceptable outcome and resources are available to provide it. Therefore, both effectiveness and cost of health care have to be included in consideration of need.
- Measuring need should include the outcomes which underlie the need. These outcomes comprise risk of morbidity and impairment, pain and discomfort, disability and dysfunction, handicap and mortality. Attempts to meet each kind of need should lead to an acceptable overall outcome.

Expanded definitions of need attempt to include some of the values contained in the World Health Organization definition of health. This widely used definition of 'health as a state of complete physical, mental and social well-being and not merely the absence of disease or infirmity' emphasizes the non-clinical elements of health and assessment of need (World Health Organization, 1947).

Oral health needs assessment

Determining the service needs of an individual patient illustrates many of the possible approaches and issues in the assessment of oral health needs in the community. Schonfeld (1981) has described the process beginning with the individual patient's desire for dental care and decision to make a visit to a dentist where dental care would be planned. The patient's oral health would be observed and dental problems would be identified. A treatment plan would be proposed to address those problems collectively. The individual items of treatment proposed might vary among dentists. The patient's previous experiences and current expectations may also influence the planned or actual treatment delivered. Thus, two patients in similar oral health and with similar dental problems will very likely receive different dental treatment.

Where oral health needs are assessed on the basis of the nature and distribution of the oral health of a sample of the population translated into estimates of dental treatment, Schonfeld describes this as the condition-to-need approach.

Aside from the variation in assessment of oral health, considerable uncertainty surrounds guidelines for the translation process. Where the oral health needs are assessed on the basis of the nature and distribution of the treatment needs of a sample of the population, this is described as the direct treatment plan approach. Again, variation in assessment is to be expected. However, the key issue with the direct treatment plan approach is the scope for negotiation between dentist and patient to change the types and timing of dental services to be received. Making explicit the perspective of both dentist and patient and what is negotiated between them are the fundamental issues in new ways of assessing oral health needs. While condition-to-need approaches have been used to assess oral health needs, most assessment has been based on the direct treatment plan approach. Beck (1968) used the Dental Services Index with an extensive coding system based upon well-defined criteria for the direct recording of restorative needs. Davies *et al.* (1969) used a similar, but simplified method which was tested by Davies *et al.* (1973), and subsequently accepted by the World Health Organization (1977) for assessing restorative needs. Recognizing the acknowledged shortcoming of the caries experience of teeth or the decayed, missing and filled (DMF) index as a measure of need for restorative treatment (as described in Chapter 6), the method involved the direct treatment planning of an individual's need for restorative treatment as part of survey examinations. A similar pattern of development has occurred in the area of periodontal needs (Bellini, 1974; Gjermo, 1976; World Health Organization, 1978). Simplified methods of surveying for treatment needs developed by the World Health Organization (1977, 1987) are widely used by oral epidemiologists and dental public health planners.

In the direct treatment planning approach, normative need is interpreted as the quantity of dental health care which expert opinion judges ought to be consumed over a relevant period, in order for people to remain or become as dentally healthy as is permitted by existing knowledge. Normative need may be expressed in terms of items of dental service, or resource supply equivalents such as work value units or cost (Spencer, 1980). Resource supply equivalents are usually specific to various levels of dental technology, use of auxiliaries, practice organization and administration. As such they may hold little validity from one area to another (Spencer, 1984). Normative need for dental care may also be subdivided into diagnostic needs, preventive needs and disease-, disability- or dysfunction-oriented needs (Burt, 1978). The first course of treatment to eliminate the detectable dental disease meets initial needs, whilst treatment to meet dental needs after the initial course of treatment is maintenance care (Young and Striffler, 1969).

The direct treatment plan approach, in which treatment need is based on direct examination of the individual, was introduced to solve problems in the *post hoc* translation of condition-to-need estimates. In the widely used World Health Organization (1987) oral health survey manual, restorative and periodontal treatment needs are measured by using the number of surfaces needing a filling, i.e. one, two, three, four or more surfaces, crowns or extraction, and the Community Periodontal Index of Treatment Needs (CPITN; Cutress *et al.*, 1987) indices, respectively. The CPITN includes three clinical disease indicators–bleeding, calculus and probing depth. The CPITN and its precursor, the Periodontal Treatment Need System (PTNS; Bellini, 1974) were developed when the natural history of periodontal disease was believed to follow an inexorable progression from marginal gingival inflammation to periodontitis to tooth loss. Treatment need estimates were based on preventing progression by controlling the gingivitis and removal of calculus. These concepts have been challenged and may be incorrect. Another cause for concern in using the CPITN is its misuse in workforce and resource projections, as illustrated in the World Health Organization Federation Dentaire Internationale (FDI) manual *Health through Oral Health* (World Health Organization, 1989). The indicators in the CPITN are inadequately sensitive and specific as predictors and the index does not comply with the fundamental principle that the treatments recommended must be shown to be effective in positively altering the life history of the disease. The limitations of the normative approach illustrated in relation to periodontal needs extend to other dental conditions.

Limitations of oral health needs assessments
Although clinical criteria, based on professional judgement, still largely dominate the assessment of oral health status and the estimation of need,

it is increasingly recognized that there are areas where normative need is deficient. That does not mean that normative need assessment is not useful. Very few would argue that reliably diagnosed cavitation requires filling. But such consensus cannot be reached in the case of need to replace missing teeth or extract third molars. The inadequacy of normative need is also evident in the case of malocclusion, where traditional indicators require supplementation by more subjective lay assessments of need. Malocclusion is not a disease and it would be incorrect to consider any deviation from an average as an abnormality. The demarcation between acceptable and unacceptable occlusions is influenced by psychological and social factors, and methods of measuring subjective or perceived need. As discussed in Chapter 6, normative need and a service-oriented definition of need have major shortcomings. The short-comings were cogently expressed by Locker (1989, p. 76) 'from the point of view of contemporary definitions of health DMF, CPITN have serious limitations; they tell us nothing about the functioning of either the oral cavity or the person as a whole and nothing about subjectively perceived symptoms such as pain and discomfort'.

Attempts have been made to find an oral health status or condition indicator that is better than the DMF. Sheiham *et al.* (1987) proposed two alternative indices. The first was a functional measure of the number of filled and sound functioning teeth (FS-T) which gives equal weight to filled and sound teeth and no weight to decayed teeth. The second was the T-Health (tissue health), which gives arbitrary proportional weights to decayed (1), filled (2) and sound teeth (4). The weights were intended to represent the relative amounts of sound tissue in these three categories. The weightings were changed to 1, 1, 4 in a later study (Marcenes and Sheiham, 1993). Sheiham *et al.* (1987) found that the new indicators were more sensitive in identifying social and behavioural risk factors than the standard DMF, which implicitly gives equal weights of 1 to D, M and F.

It should be recognized that estimates of treatment needs obtained by using the condition-to-need or the direct treatment plan approach do not consider either the outcomes of oral diseases or the consequence of limited resources for health care. It is also possible that most of these needs would not be perceived by people themselves who, therefore, would not seek the treatments proposed. The latter observation was confirmed by the gap between the professional and patient's definitions of need (Barenthin, 1977; Reisine and Bailit, 1980; Smith and Sheiham, 1979).

Impairment, disability and handicap

The concepts of impairment, disability and handicap have become pivotal to the development of sociodental indicators. The assessment of need for orthodontic treatment will serve to illustrate how traditional indicators have been supplemented by more subjective lay assessments of need. The majority of measures of orthodontic treatment need are based on clinical examinations alone. Few have attempted to measure or even record the perceptions of the child and parent in relation to disability or handicap. Yet these subjective elements are the most important determinants of the demand for orthodontic treatment. The definition of dysfunction and disturbances of usual performance 'are matters for personal, community or national concern' (Cohen and Jago, 1979). An unacceptable occlusion can therefore be regarded as one which is disturbing to individuals, thereby impacting upon them. It is an impairment which is disabling or handicapping. What then is an impairment, what is a disability and what is a handicap?

The following definitions of impairment, disability, and handicap are based on the work of Nagi (1976), the World Health Organization (1980), Locker (1988) and Pope and Tarlov (1991). *Impairment* is a loss or abnormality of mental, physical or biochemical function either present at birth or arising out of disease or injury, such as edentulousness, periodontium loss or malocclusion. All pathology is associated with impairment, but not all impairments lead to functional limitations. Inevitably, in defining an impairment the problem of normality and deviance arises. Functional limitation is restriction in function customarily expected of the body or its component organ or system, such as limitation of jaw mobility. Discomfort extends biomedical measures, for instance, pain associated with underlying pathological processes, extra to the subjective appraisals of well-being. Discomfort involves non-observable feeling states which can be experienced even in the absence of an underlying clinical condition. *Disability* is any limitation in or lack of ability to carry out socially defined tasks and roles that individuals generally are expected to be able to do (Pope and Tarlov, 1991). Roles are organized according to how people participate in a social system, for example as teachers, parents, civil servants. Tasks are specific physical and mental actions through which an individual interacts and performs her or his roles (Pope and Tarlov, 1991). *Handicap* is concerned with the broader social effects and is defined as the disadvantage experienced by impaired and disabled people because they do not or cannot conform to the expectations of society or the social groups to which they belong. It is the disadvantage or restriction experienced by individuals in their personal and social life consequent upon disability or impairment. In this sense, a handicap results from interactions between physical impairment, the adjustment to it and the physical and social environment (Wood, 1975; Bury, 1978; World health Organization, 1980).

The relationship between impairment, disability and handicap is a continuum. A malposed or missing tooth (impairment), for example, can lead to a restriction in eating or to avoidance of hard foods (physical disability), which in turn can make people feel embarrassed (psychological disability) and avoid eating in front of others (social disability). This may be a disadvantage to the individual, leading to problems with employment and relationships.

Although this approach presents operational difficulties (it is not possible, for example, to predict that a given degree of impairment will produce a similar degree of disability or handicap), it none the less focuses attention on the importance of the sociopsychological aspects of health needs assessment. It also helps us to understand why patients with similar oral impairments will present at differing points in time from onset, and why some may never present at all.

Development of sociodental indicators

Cohen and Jago (1976) argued that clinical indicators of oral health would be greatly improved by adding a dimension of social impact. Then the indicators would encompass the broader implications of oral conditions that are more relevant to policy-makers. Clinical indices are essential for measuring oral disease; the problem arises when these indices are used as measures of health and treatment need (Sheiham *et al.*, 1982). More realistic assessments of treatment need should include the functional and the social dimensions of dental disease and an assessment of the social motivational factors which predispose people towards dental ill health and influence the effectiveness of treatment and health promotion.

The shortcomings of professionally defined need for health care have led to the development of the broader measurements of health need. A variety of sociomedical indicators have been developed and used (Andrews, 1976; Scrivens *et al.*, 1985; Hunt *et al.*, 1986; Mootz, 1986). They are multidisciplinary with major contributions from psychology, sociology, economics, operational research and biostatistics. While a great deal of effort has been devoted to the construction of valid and reliable indices of oral disease, behavioural or subjective measures of oral health have been used less frequently. There has generally been less development of alternative definitions of need in dental than there has been in general health care. Though dental ill health affects populations in epidemic proportions and they are the most prevalent group of chronic disorders, neither the definition of dental health nor current treatment need assessments correspond to or reflect the origins of dental disease.

A measure for dental need should incorporate not only clinical assessment, but also psychological and social dimensions because the presence of a clinical impairment alone is neither a necessary nor sufficient basis for need. The loss of molars, for example, is an impairment. But this does not necessarily mean that there is a need for dental treatment. A further question should be asked: is this impairment disabling? Furthermore, does it lead to handicap? If yes, then the molars need replacing. If no, then need for treatment is debatable. Apart from the clinical, psychological and social dimensions, other dimensions that should be incorporated in any measure of dental needs are social motivational factors.

A measure of dental needs should include the following:

- a clinical dimension based upon sound concepts of the life history of the diseases;
- a measure of impairment which incorporates

functional measures to assess the impacts of the impairment;

- measures of social dysfunction;
- the wants of the individual. Wants are the individuals' perceptions of their own dental needs and depend on the individual oral health, their perceptions of what is normal and what the possible benefits of treatment are, as well as on factors such as social class and education (Cooper, 1975);
- assessment of the propensity of the individual to take preventive action and the perceived barriers to prevention. Included in this is general health maintenance orientation and knowledge and attitudes about health matters;
- a prescription of effective and acceptable treatments or cures (Matthew, 1971) and the skills required to carry out the care (division of labour).

Sociodental indicators

From the concept of assessing the impact of oral conditions on daily life, Nikias *et al.* (1978) proposed sociodental indicators, which they defined as 'a measure of the extent to which oral conditions disrupt normal role functioning'. The definition was expanded by Locker (1989, p. 77) to 'measures of the extent to which dental and oral disorders disrupt normal social role functioning and bring about major changes in behaviour such as an inability to work or attend school, or undertake parental or household duties'.

Dental ill health is largely social and behavioural in origin and almost entirely preventable by social and behavioural means (Cushing *et al.*, 1986). The measurement of consequences of oral diseases is essential for a full scientific understanding of the scope of oral health problems, rational decision-making with regard to the allocation of health care resources and the evaluation of dental health services (Nikias, 1985).

From the viewpoint of utility of sociomedical information, Bice (1976) suggested that health indicators should measure variables specified by a social system model and should be scaled according to units that are relevant to decision-making criteria. Moreover, an appropriate sociodental indicator for estimating need of a population also requires high efficiency, namely, minimum time and workforce spent on administration. The identification of new

concerns tends to increase the need for further development of health indicators to monitor progress towards new goals, and so the cycle begins again. Rising expectations have led to a shift away from viewing health in terms of survival, through a phase of defining it in terms of freedom from disease, thence to an emphasis on the individual's ability to perform daily activities, and now to the current emphasis on positive themes of happiness, social and emotional well-being, and quality of life. Disruption in normal social functioning could be used as a basis for measuring the impact of dental ill health (Reisine, 1981).

In simple terms optimum oral health will include the ability to chew and eat the full range of foods native to the diet, to speak clearly, to have a socially acceptable smile and dentofacial profile, to be comfortable and free from pain, and to have fresh breath. The relative importance of these factors and their scope will vary with age, sex and the culture that determines the social norm. The sociodental indicators have examined some or all of these factors. These are described in detail.

Cushing *et al.* (1986) developed sociodental indicators by assessing the impact of dental status on perceptions of people. The impacts were categorized as function (difficulty in eating), social interaction (difficulty in communication), comfort and well-being (pain and discomfort) and self-image (dissatisfaction with aesthetics). A questionnaire based on the four categories was developed to measure the social and psychological impact of dental disease. A score for each individual was constructed from responses to questions related to these categories.

Leao (1993) selected and adapted questionnaires from Cushing *et al.* (1986) and some other indices to developed weighted sociodental indicators. Leao's approach includes questions which cover five main categories relating to the mouth and teeth; comfort; appearance; pain (symptoms); performance and eating restriction. Extra questions were added for those who wore a prosthesis. A weighting scale, based on the Nottingham Health Profile (Hunt *et al.*, 1986), was developed to find a proportional relationship between the five dimensions.

Strauss (1988) developed a 25-item Dental Impact Profile (DIP) to measure dental effects on life quality and social function. The DIP consists of four subscales: eating; health/well-being; social relations; and romance. Rosenberg *et al.* (1988) developed the Dental Functional Status. The Dental Functional Status covers lack of oral pain and discomfort and a person's ability to chew, speak and interact with people without being self-conscious about appearance. It involves four scales: psychosocial; mechanical; role limitation; and self-care, each consisting of 25 items. Rosenberg *et al.* (1988) did not attempt to assess the importance respondents attributed to the different items and dimensions in their study.

The Dental Health Index (Gooch *et al.*, 1989) is a limited measure covering three problems: pain and distress; worry or concern; and reduced social interactions. The Geriatric Oral Health Index of Assessment (GOHAI) was designed to assess oral health problems of older adults (Atchison and Dolan, 1990). It consists of 12 items grouped in one single construct and does not contain subscales. Chen (1991) related biological measures of oral status to quality-of-life indicators. The quality-of-life measure consisted of three scales: symptoms; perceived well-being; and level of functioning. An extra dimension was included for those who wore dentures. Leake (1990) developed an index of chewing ability. The five-item index is derived from questions about the ability to chew or bite five types of food. The index showed high predictive value and acceptable reproducibility.

Locker (1992) using his expanded World Health Organization (1980) model, collected data on impairment, functional limitation, pain and other symptoms and complaints, disability and handicap using different scales for each category. Locker used conventional clinical measures to assess impairment. These were accompanied by Leake's (1990) index of chewing capacity as a measure of functional limitations and a modified version of Locker and Grushka's (1987) pain inventory. Disability and handicap were assessed by a seven-item scale of social and psychological impact of oral disorders, a single item on worry caused by oral health problems and a three-item index of satisfaction with oral health. Locker regarded these as preliminary measures and called for the development of further measures of social and psychological impact.

The development of indicators based on the concepts of impairment, disability and handicap has been extended by Slade and Spencer (1994) with the Oral Health Impact Profile (OHIP). The OHIP is the first sociodental indicator to use a scaled index of the social impact of oral disorders.

This measurement is based on the theoretical model proposed by Locker (1988) and consists of 49 items grouped in seven subscales. The seven subscales include: functional limitation (for example, reduced masticatory performance); physical pain (for example, toothache); psychological discomfort (for example, self-consciousness); physical disability (for example, avoidance of foods); psychological disability (for example, reduced concentration); social disability (for example, avoiding social interaction); and handicap (for example, inability to work). The relative importance of statements within each subscale was assessed among an adult sample ranging in age from 18 to 75 and over years old.

Functional limitation was the most frequently expressed limitation among a group of edentulous older adults in South Australia surveyed by Slade and Spencer (1994). Physical pain was most prevalent among the dentate. Social disability and handicap were less frequent. Most people reported multiple forms of impact, with a mean of nearly 6 out of a maximum possible of 49 impact items. Slade *et al.* (1995) have examined trends and fluctuations in the impact of oral conditions among older adults during a 1 year period. The findings demonstrated that the majority of persons experience periods of overall stability in social impacts. However, a minority of persons experience either short-term impacts or trends of increasing or decreasing impacts over time. It would, of course, be desirable that trends of decreasing social impacts were as a result of health needs being met.

Relationship of sociodental indicators with oral health

Some sociodental indicators, mentioned above, have been compared with clinical oral status. Cushing *et al.* (1986) compared the social impact of dental disease with clinical indices of caries, periodontal and prosthetic status and treatment needs. Half of the dentate people had discomfort, one-quarter had toothache, one-fifth of males had eating restrictions and one-seventh had communication restriction and dissatisfaction with appearance of teeth. Cushing (1986) suggested that although relationships between clinical and social variables were weak, those which were significant could be used as a stepping stone to start building a picture of characteristics, both clinical and social, of people who experience dental problems. Those who reported having eating problems had a higher DMFT and fewer functioning teeth (sound plus filled teeth; Sheiham *et al.*, 1987) than those with no problems. Dental pain and discomfort were associated with higher mean decay scores. Dissatisfaction with dental appearance was associated with one or more decayed teeth and two or more missing teeth and three fewer functioning teeth. Communication restriction was associated with decay status and functioning teeth.

Rosenberg *et al.* (1988) compared the Dental Functional Status with DMFT status in a random sample of dental clinic patients. Forty-four per cent of the variance in the Dental Functional Status was explained by periodontal status, age and amount of exercise undertaken. The clinical measures for DMFT were not significant factors in defining a patient's Dental Functional Status. On the other hand, Gooch *et al.* (1989) found that there was a significant correlation between DMFT index, individuals' components of DMFT index, Russell's Periodontal Index and subjective measures of social impact. Atchison and Dolan (1990) compared the GOHIA with clinical variables in people aged 65 years and over. Those with 21–32 teeth and no removable denture felt they did not need dental treatment and presented more positive impacts. Objective clinical measures of oral health were significantly correlated.

Chen (1991) went one step further. She related separate components of the DMF to quality-of-life indicators. Of the oral health status measures, number of decayed teeth was significant for all dimensions including symptoms, perceived well being and level of functioning. The number of missing teeth was significant for well-being and function and number of filled teeth was significant for well-being. Locker (1992) analysed similar clinical measures, but added number of natural functional units and the number of decayed coronal and root surfaces. Clinical variables were weakly, but significantly, correlated with subjective measures except for pain symptoms. The number of missing teeth and mean periodontal attachment loss were significant predictors of impact scale scores.

Slade and Spencer (1995) have examined the associations between clinical oral conditions and social impact using OHIP. Edentulous persons reported significantly more social impact in four subscales: functional limitation, physical disability, social disability and handicap. Among

dentate persons, tooth loss was associated with all seven subscales of social impact. Anterior tooth loss was associated with more impact, whether or not there was replacement of the missing teeth by prosthetic units, while posterior tooth loss was associated with social impact only when there were unreplaced spaces. Decayed root surfaces were consistently associated with higher levels of social impact, while components of periodontal attachment loss had varied effects. Slade and Spencer (1995) concluded that when it was important to quantify subtle differences in outcome, the different subscales of OHIP appear most useful. Similar findings were reported using the Dental Impacts on Daily Living (DIDL) index (Leao and Sheiham, 1995). Leao (1993) demonstrated that DIDL discriminates between different subjective impacts for different groups. Respondents classified by different DMFT levels showed a significant difference in the distribution of scores for all the five dimensions in the DIDL questionnaire (appearance, comfort, performance, eating restriction and pain). The worse the oral status, the worse the subjective impact. Results of correlations between clinical oral status and subjective impact scores were consistent with the results found when the oral status of respondents was investigated for level of satisfaction. The oral status of dissatisfied subjects showed significant associations with subjective measures.

Overall, all the studies show a significant but weak association between oral status and sociopsychological measures. They present negative or positive impacts according to the different oral status and the clinical variables associated with subjective impacts are indeed relevant. Different levels of oral status have different impacts on people's daily living. In some instances, weak associations between clinical and subjective oral health indicators are to be expected given the nature of the measures employed (Locker, 1992). For example, comfort in Leao's DIDL, which includes questions about bleeding, food packing, halitosis and satisfaction with gums (all of which may be associated with filled teeth), showed a weak but significant correlation with filled teeth. This is not unexpected, given that those problems could not only be caused by filled teeth, but could be related to decayed teeth as well.

Locker (1992) maintained that the weak association of clinical variables with indicators of social and psychological impact exist because these indicators are mediated by functional and experiential variables and by sociodemographic variables. In addition, Locker maintained that when scores of subjective impacts are added together the relationships of specific impacts with clinical variables are diluted by the other impacts being added. Therefore clinical status and multiple social and psychological dimensions should be assessed simultaneously when assessing people's dental needs.

Desirable characteristics of sociodental indicators

Ware *et al.* (1981) identified five broad categories of use of the major health status measurements: measuring the efficiency or effectiveness of health interventions; assessing the quality of life; estimating the health needs of a population; improving clinical decisions; and understanding the causes and consequences of differences in health. The application of sociodental indicators for each specific purpose may vary considerably. Thus, it is essential in selecting sociodental indicators to assess needs, to see which matches the purpose and qualities of currently established indicators. There are five major factors that must be considered in choosing an instrument for measuring health status: practicality, reliability, validity and objectivity/subjectivity and whether global measures are preferable to more specific ones (Ware *et al.*, 1981). At least three major qualifications should be considered for the population need assessment for health planning:

- the index should be brief and easy to use in large populations within a reasonable time (Brazier and Lobjolt, 1991);
- scaling according to units should be relevant to decision-making criteria;
- the index should measure variables specified by a system model to provide cause-and-effect relationship information for policy-makers (Bice, 1976).

Therefore, a brief and easy-to-use indicator with an appropriate scoring system, supported by a relevant theoretical model, is what is required.

Existing subjective measures of oral health do not conform well to these criteria. Many have concentrated on understanding the causes and consequences of health differences (Rosenberg *et al.*, 1988; Locker, 1992). Some indicators focus

on a specific outcome, for example, prevalence of dental and facial pain and impacts measures (Locker and Grushka, 1987) or the index of chewing capacity (Leake, 1990). The GOHAI is designed specifically for oral health problems of elderly people (Rosenberg *et al.*, 1988). The OHIP (Slade and Spencer, 1994) and the DIDL (Leao, 1993) are the closest to the requirements. However, the OHIP, which permits the relevant statistical analysis and has a good theoretical basis, has the disadvantage of length. A simplified version of the OHIP, referred to as OHIP-S, which consists of only 14 items, has been developed, but requires further evaluation.

Items for the social impact measures described, with the exception of the OHIP (Slade and Spencer, 1994), have been grouped without being assigned weights. This is equivalent to implicitly attributing equal weighting to each of the items involved. A fundamental problem which arises from this is that some items may be more important to the construct underlying the scale than others and should therefore contribute more to the total score (Bowling, 1991). On the other hand, Streiner and Norman (1989) concluded that when the scale has more than 40 items or when items are fairly homogeneous, differential weighting contributes little, except maybe complexity to the scoring. Further tests should therefore be conducted on those measures to verify if weighting is important or not.

The use of the same panel weighting for the OHIP in different groups of populations may fail to reflect social and cultural differences. The potential existence of such cultural differences was one factor which led Slade *et al.* (1995a) to use the unweighted OHIP or simple count of impacts, in the comparison of social impact in the elderly across three countries: Australia, Canada and the USA. The findings supported other published data (similar to that reported in Chapter 3) that there are social and cultural factors influencing oral health and its impact. Among dentate people, US blacks reported the highest levels of impact for 39 of the 49 OHIP items. Blacks reported four times as many impact items as whites, while people from South Australia and Ontario had intermediate levels of social impact. For dentate people, there was a larger amount of variation between race-groups than among the three countries. This suggests the likelihood of different weightings being derived from different population groups in judging the importance of individual impacts.

While the DIDL (Leao, 1993) provides a more flexible weighting system and a total score for policy use, its empirical approach has weaker theoretical support than the OHIP and its 36 questions are still time-consuming.

Sociodental indicators and treatment

While most sociodental indicators are focused on impacts from oral disorders, Ettinger (1987) proposed that rational decision-making in dental treatment, particularly in the elderly, should include an assessment of the functional and social benefits associated with alternative treatment plans. Slade and Spencer (1994) highlighted the benefit of sociodental indicators to assess improvements in the quality of life from dental treatment. There is a need to develop outcome measures sensitive to treatment effects (Reisine and Locker, 1995) and need for dental care. Maizels *et al.* (1993) used a sociodental approach and propensity to adopt dental self-care measures to identify different dental treatment need groups. However, a new scheme for estimating dental health needs with relevant qualities has been proposed by Adulyanon *et al.* (1995). An assumption is made that more appropriate dental treatment need should be considered not only from professional judgement, but also the related sociodental impact and behavioural factors such as people's perception and propensity. The system conforms to the definition of a sociodental indicator of oral health status and treatment need, namely, indicators that assess the impacts of oral disorders, clinical status and the perceived and effective need, as well as the ability to benefit from treatment.

The theoretical framework on which the system is based is modified from the World health Organization's International Classification of Impairments, Disabilities and Handicaps (Wood, 1975; Patrick, 1976), which was modified for dental health by Locker (1988) and the Nagi system (Nagi, 1976). The main modification is that different levels of the variables are established. The system should have:

- the oral status including oral impairments which most clinical indices attempt to measure;
- the possible early negative impacts caused by oral health status–pain, discomfort, functional limitation or dissatisfaction with appearance. Any of these dimensions may lead to impacts on performance ability;
- the translation of the dimensions into impacts on the ability to perform daily activities. These are grouped into physical, psychological and social performance dimensions. This level is equivalent to disability and handicap dimensions in the World Health Organization model and disability in the Nagi system.

The system focuses on measuring the translation of the impact dimensions into impacts on the ability to perform daily activities. It is a way to screen the significant impacts, by eliminating very small negative perceptions from oral conditions which do not lead to an impact on daily performances. The screened outcomes should be more useful in the context of policy planning based on more appropriate measures of need. Lastly, it is less difficult to measure the behavioural impacts in term of performance than the feeling-state dimension. The reliability and validity of behaviourally based measures are easier to establish.

An important criterion of need is whether there is an effective treatment for the condition. Matthew (1971) considers that a need for treatment exists only if there is an effective and acceptable treatment. Apart from the issue of effectiveness, the potential for prevention by the individual should also be assessed, as this may lead to a modification of the treatment need. The use of sociodental treatment need assessments has many implications for the planning and provision of dental services. First, it encourages a shift in emphasis away from the purely mechanical to the behavioural aspects of treatment. Second, it supports the development of a health-oriented model of care in preference to the treatment model that dominates current dental services. Third, it promotes the adoption of preventive behaviour by populations. Fourth, it guarantees the higher effectiveness of treatment and a greater degree of long-term success. Some other advantages include a better division of labour in providing dental care and an improvement in the use of scarce resources (Sheiham *et al.*, 1982). In summary, measures of need should include the impact of ill health upon individuals, the degrees of dysfunction and the perceptions and attitudes of patients.

The need for care is widespread, while cure is rare (Cochrane, 1972). The point on the distribution at which therapy begins to do more good than harm should be established. Therefore, in addition to measurement of oral health status and their perceived impacts, behavioural factors affecting health gain from dental therapies should be included in needs estimations. These behavioural factors are the appropriate use of service and delays in seeking treatment (Locker, 1989), propensity to carry out preventive behaviours and self-care (Maizels *et al.*, 1993) and compliance with treatment instructions. These additional dimensions to health and illness behaviour (defined in Chapter 3), could provide a behavioural and environmental consideration within health needs assessment.

Most definitions of need have emphasized the need for treatment. Little attention has been given to the needs for the promotion of health and the primary prevention of disease. Since health/sickness and function/dysfunction can each be conceived as being on a single continuum parallel to one another (Bergner *et al.*, 1979), attention should be given to the needs of people at all points along the continuum and not just to those at the sickness and dysfunction ends. The advantage of this approach is that it makes possible a much more comprehensive treatment of the important issue of needs as well as indicating how they may be incorporated into planning for the attainment of health and well-being.

A number of factors need to be taken into consideration when assessing the relative importance of different types of normative need. They are:

- The life-threatening conditions. In life-threatening oral conditions, treatment or further investigation is essential even without the impact being assessed. Among oral health conditions, only oral cancer or precancerous lesions, fractures of jaw, and severe infections are life-threatening and come under this category;
- Chronic progressive conditions. Some professional clinical judgements are based on the intention to prevent progression of irreversible impairments. Here, impact related to such impairments is not of prime importance in assessing need;
- The perceived impact without normative need. Treatment planning in clinical dentistry is an art rather than a science. Few criteria or systems have been developed for evaluation of

the appropriateness of the overall treatment strategy.

There is a gap between professional and lay perception of treatment need. Oral disorders, like many other chronic degenerative disorders, do not have a single causal factor. Professional treatment has a limited role in such cases. The counselling or negotiating role between dental professional and client becomes more important in the process of treating ill health. Therefore, it is prudent to assess propensity and psychological and social factors as well as health and illness behaviours. The social structure and the individual's social status direct how symptoms are expressed and acted upon. A biopsychosocial model of health proposes that diseases are influenced not only by the underlying pathology, but also by the individual's perceptions, personality and stress (Engel, 1980).

Patterns of behaviours play important roles in personal treatment planning and, therefore, in treatment need estimation of the population. Health behaviour of the patient is important in various dental treatments consideration. This indicates that the mere presence of disease or symptoms, irrespective of their severity, is not always sufficient to stimulate the seeking of professional care (Andersen and Newman, 1973; Hannay, 1980; Locker, 1988). Social, psychological and organizational factors are involved in the process which ends with a consultation. Models describing health behaviour are discussed in detail in Chapter 12.

The effectiveness of treatment

Sackett and Snow (1979) caution that the strategies applied to change compliance behaviour must meet at least three preconditions: the diagnosis must be correct; the therapy must do more good than harm; and the patient must be an informed, willing partner in the execution of all interventions. Clinical judgement includes the balancing of probabilities for benefit and harm.

The treatment which is professionally judged to be that needed for a specific impairment, should be evaluated for its effectiveness. The need for health technology assessment arises from the concern that health technology may neither be used wisely, nor produce the expected health benefit (White and Antzcak-Bouckoms, 1995). Many studies using the randomized controlled trial have given ample warnings of how dangerous it is to assume that well-established medical therapies which have not been tested are always effective (Cochrane, 1972). Few dental therapies have been subjected to rigorous randomized controlled trials, and there are limited quantitative assessments of effectiveness. Where analyses have been done, using systematic reviews, most commonly done treatments, such as removal of supragingival calculus and orthodontics, were found to be relatively ineffective without unrealistic compliance regimens (Shaw *et al.*, 1991; Antczak-Bouckoms *et al.*, 1989; Addy and Koltai, 1994). Considerations of dental treatment effectiveness should be based on investigation of available therapy appraisal data, as well as the possible resources and qualified personnel to perform such treatment effectively in each planning setting.

Use of health needs assessment to plan oral health care

Health needs assessments have long been considered useful in planning oral health care. While the foregoing discussion has emphasized the limitations of a single normative perspective of health needs, the increasing range of indices that are combining clinical assessment with social and psychological factors within sociodental indicators will aid the appropriate application of health needs assessments to planning.

Use of health needs assessments in planning oral health services could include:

- investigating the natural history and consequences of disease;
- assessing the burden of illness and health care needs of communities and populations
- determining health goals, objectives and priorities;
- allocating and managing health care resources;
- assessing intervention strategies and evaluating the impact of services (White and Henderson, 1976).

As dentistry responds to changing concepts of health and broadens the previously unidimensional biological model of health and disease toward a multi-dimensional model of health and needs (Locker and Miller, 1994), the opportunity for useful application of health needs assessment broadens.

The iterative measurement loop

A number of theoretical frameworks are available to provide linkage between the applications of health needs assessments. One that will be presented is the Iterative Measurement Loop (Tugwell *et al.*, 1984). The iterative measurement loop is a framework to assist organizing information about to whom health services should be provided in order effectively and efficiently to reduce the burden of illness, disability and handicap (Fig. 4.1).

An underlying assumption is that the identification and critical appraisal of evidence about the effectiveness of health care are necessary as part of reducing the burden of illness. Its approach was influenced by Cochrane's (1972) emphasis on effectiveness and efficiency and Sackett's (1980) methodological considerations for health care evaluation. While the iterative measurement loop preceded the new emphasis on effectiveness-based health care, it shares a similar origin and perspective. The iterative measurement loop is comprised of seven steps organized in a loop that build to a targeted logical progression from hypothesis generation, through prevention or treatment, to assessment of the impact of treatment of individual patients and provision of services to a community.

Summary

Needs are assessed in order effectively and efficiently to reduce the burden of illness, disability and handicap. Assessments of needs should include clinical, social and psychological dimensions except for life-threatening oral conditions, such as malignancies and chronic progressive conditions such as cavitated carious lesions. Measures of impact are redundant in such cases as some treatment should be done, in consultation with the patient. For all other clinical conditions, measures of physical, social and psychological impacts should be incorporated into the measure of need. The wants of individuals are included routinely. There are a range of sociodental indicators available from which to choose to assess impacts of oral conditions on daily living. They have been validated on a range of populations.

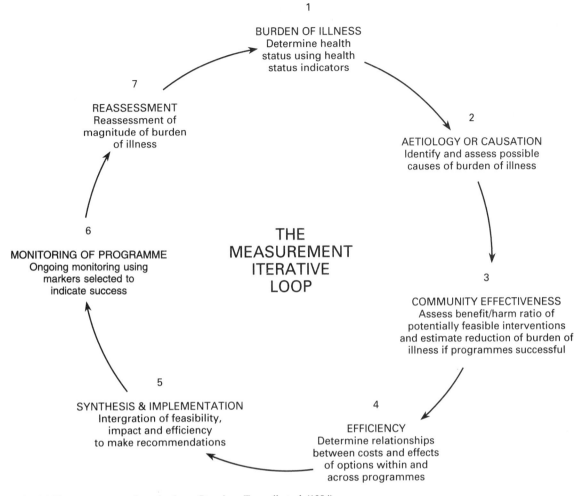

Fig. 4.1 The measurement iterative loop. Based on Tugwell *et al.* (1984).

The optimal benefit from any needs assessment, and oral health care plan on which it is based, depends on a high level of diagnostic accuracy, dental health provider compliance with guidelines for managing oral and dental diseases and patient concerns, as well as patient compliance with diet control, oral hygiene and use of fluorides. Unless evidence-based dental care is provided, needs may be incorrectly redefined leading to a recurring spiral of more and more complex treatments. Efficiency can be achieved if the appropriate interventions are provided to those who would benefit from them with the optimal use of resources. Tasks should be matched with the skills of operators. Population-wide health promotion will reduce inequities and increase the numbers of people who would benefit by making healthier choices easier.

References

Acheson, R.M. (1978) The definition and identification of need for health care. *Journal of Epidemiology and Community Health* **32**: 10–15.

Addy, M. and Koltai, R. (1994) Control of supragingival calculus. *Journal of Clinical Periodontology* **21**: 342–346.

Adulyanon, S., Tsakos, G. and Sheiham, A. (1995) *Integrating Socio-behavioural Factors into Dental Treatment Needs Estimations*. Unpublished report. London: Department of Epidemiology and Public Health, University College London.

Andersen, R.F. and Newman, J.F. (1973) Societal and individual determinants of medical care utilization in the

United States. *Milbank Memorial Fund Quarterly Health Society* **51**: 95–124.

Andrews, F.M. (1976) *Social Indicators of Well being.* Plenum Press, New York.

Antczak-Bouckoms, A., Tulloch, J., White, B. and Capilouto, E. (1989) Methodological considerations in the analysis of cost effectiveness in dentistry. *Journal of Public Health Dentistry* **49**: 215–222.

Atchison, K. A. and Dolan, T. A. (1990) Development of the geriatric oral health assessment index. *Journal of Dental Education* **54**: 680–687.

Barenthin, I. (1977) Dental health status and dental satisfaction. *International Journal of Epidemiology* **6**: 73–79.

Beck, D.J. (1968) *Dental Health Status of the New Zealand Population in Late Adolescence and Young Adulthood; A Survey Conducted by the Dental Health Division of the Department of Health.* Department of Health, Special Report Series No. 29. Government Printer, Wellington, New Zealand.

Bellini, H.T. (1974). The time factor in periodontal therapy; a pilot study correlating time and plaque, calculus, pocket depth and number of teeth. *Journal Periodontal Research* **9**: 56–61.

Bergner, M. Bobbitt, R.A., Kressel, S. *et al.* (1979) The sickness impact profile: conceptual formation and methodology for the development of a health status measure. In: *Socio-medical Health Indicators* (Elinson, J. and Siegman, A.E., eds), pp. 9–31. Baywood, Farmingdale, New York.

Bice, T.W. (1976) Comments on health indicators: methodological perspectives. *International Journal of Health Services* **6**: 509–519.

Bowling, A. (1991) *Measuring Health: A Review of Quality of Life Measurements Scales.* Open University Press, Milton Keynes.

Bradshaw, J.S. (1972) A taxonomy of social need. In: *Problems and Progress in Medical Care.* Seventh Series. (McLachlan, G., ed.). pp. 69–82. Oxford University Press.

Brazier, M. and Lobjoit, M. (eds) (1991) *Protecting the Vulnerable: Autonomy and Consent in Health Care.* Routledge, London.

Burt, B.A. (1978) *A Method for Comparing the Expenditures on two Alternative National Dental Programs for Persons aged 6–21.* University of Michigan, School of Public Health, Ann Arbor, MI.

Bury, M.R. (1978) *Perspectives in Disablement.* Paper presented at Medical Commission on Rehabilitation, Southampton (mimeo).

Carr, W. and Wolfe, S. (1979) Unmet needs as sociomedical indicators. In: *Sociomedical Health Indicators* (Ellinson, J. and Siegman, A.E., eds). Baywood, Farmingdale, pp. 33–46.

Chen, M.I. (1991) *Oral Health and Quality of Life: A Social Perspective.* Paper presented at the 30th World Congress of the International Institute of Sociology, Kobe, Japan, 1991 (mimeo).

Cochrane, A.L. (1972) *Effectiveness and Efficiency: Random Reflections on Health Services.* The Nuffield Provincial Hospitals Trust, London.

Cohen, K. and Jago, J.D. (1976) Toward the formulation of socio-dental indicators. *International Journal of Health Services* **6**: 681–687.

Cohen, L.K. and Jago, J.D. (1979) Toward the formulation of socio-dental indicators. In: *Sociomedical Health Indicators* (Ellinson, J. and Siegman, A.E., eds), Baywood, Farmingdale, pp. 165–182.

Cooper, M.H. (1975) *Rationing Health Care.* Croom Helm, London.

Cushing, A. (1986) *The Development of Socio-dental Indicators of Oral Health Status and Needs.* PhD thesis. University of London, London.

Cushing, A.M., Sheiham, A. and Maizels, J. (1986) Developing socio-dental indicators–the social impact of dental disease. *Community Dental Health* **3**: 3–17.

Cutress, T.W., Ainamo, J. and Sardo-Infirri, J. (1987) The community periodontal index of treatment needs (CPITN) procedure for population groups and individuals. *International Dental Journal* **37**: 222–233.

Davies, G.N., Horowitz, H.S. and Wada, W. (1973) The assessment of dental caries for public health purposes. *Community Dental Oral Epidemiology* **1**: 68–73.

Davies, G.N., Kruger, B.J. and Homan, B.T. (1969) Dental survey of children in country districts of Queensland. *Australian Dental Journal* **141**: 153–161.

Davis, P. (1980) *The Social Context of Dentistry.* Croom Helm, London.

Donabedian, A. (1973) *Aspects of Medical Care Administration: Specifying Requirements for Health Care.* Harvard University Press, Cambridge, MA.

Engel, G.L. (1989) The clinical application of the biopsychological model. *American Journal of Psychiatry* **137**: 535–544.

Ettinger, R. (1987) Oral disease and its effect on the quality of life. *Gerodontics* **3**: 103–106.

Fuchs, V.R. (1974) *Who shall live? Health, Economics and Social Choice.* Basic Books, New York.

Giddon, D.B., Moser, M., Colton, T. and Bulman, J. (1976) Quantitative relationships between perceived and objective need for health care–dentistry as a model. *Public Health Reports* **91**: 508–513.

Gjermo, P. (1976) The assessment of needs for periodontal treatment. *International Dental Journal* **26**: 41–45.

Gooch, B.F., Dolan, T.A. and Bourque, L.B. (1989) Correlates of self-reported dental health status upon enrollment in the Rand health insurance experiment. *Journal of Dental Education* **53**: 629–637.

Hannay, D. (1980) The iceberg of illness and trivial consultations. *Journal of the College of General Practitioners* **30**: 551–554.

Hill, A.B. (1971) *Principles of Medical Statistics,* 9th ed. Lancet, London.

Hunt, S.M., McEwen, J. and McKenna, S.P. (1986) *Measuring Health Status.* Croom Helm, London.

Leake, J.L. (1990) An index of chewing ability. *Journal of Public Health and Dentistry* **4**: 262–267.

Leao, A. (1993) *The Development of Measures of Dental Impacts on Daily Living.* PhD. thesis. University of London, London.

Leao, A. and Sheiham, A.L. (1995) Relation between clinical dental status and subjective impacts on daily living. *Journal of Dental Research* **74**: 1408–1413.

Locker, D. (1988) Measuring oral health: a conceptual framework. *Community Dental Health* **5**: 3–18.

Locker, D. (1989). *An Introduction to Behavioural Science and Dentistry.* pp. 73–89. Routledge, London.

Locker, D. (1992) The burden of oral disorders in a population of older adults. *Community Dental Health* **9**: 109–124.

Locker, D. and Grushka, M. (1987) The impact of dental and facial pain. *Journal of Dental Research* **66**: 1414–1417.

Locker, D. and Miller, Y. (1994) Evaluation of subjective oral health status indicators. *Journal of Public Health Dentistry* **54**: 167–176.

Magi, M. and Allander, E. (1981) Towards a theory of perceived and medically defined need. *Sociology of Health and Illness* **3**: 49–71.

Maizels, J., Maizels, A. and Sheiham, A. (1993) Sociodental approach to the identification of dental treatment-need groups. *Community Dental and Oral Epidemiology* **21**: 340–346.

Marcenes, W.S. and Sheiham, A. (1993) Composite indicators of oral health: functioning teeth and the number of sound-equivalent teeth (T-Health). *Community Dental and Oral Epidemiology* **21**: 374–378.

Matthew, G.K. (1971) Measuring need and evaluating services. In: *Portfolio for Health* McLachlan, G., ed). Oxford University Press, Oxford.

Mootz, M. (1986) Health indicators. *Social Science and Medicine* **22**: 255–263.

Nagi, S.Z. (1976) An epidemiology of disability among adults in the United States. *Milbank Memorial Fund Quarterly* **54**: 439–467.

Nikias, M.K. (1985) Oral disease and the quality of life. *American Journal of Public Health* **75**: 11–12.

Nikias, M., Sollecito, M. and Fink, R. (1978) An empirical approach to developing multi dimensional oral status profiles. *Journal of Public Health Dentistry* **38**: 148–158.

Patrick, D.L. (1976) Constructing social metrics for health status indexes. *Internationa Journal of Health Services* **6**: 443–453.

Pope, A.M. and Tarlov, A.R. (1991) *Disability in America. Toward a National Agenda for Prevention.* National Academy Press, Washington DC.

Reisine, S.T. (1981) Theoretical considerations in formulating sociodental indicators. *Social Science and medicine* **15A**: 745–750.

Reisine, S.T. and Bailit, H.L. (1980) Clinical oral health status and adult perceptions of oral health. *Social Science and Medicine* **14**: 597–605.

Reisine, S. and Locker, D. (1995) Social, psychological and economic impacts of dental conditions and treatments. In: *Disease Prevention and Oral Health Promotion: Sociodental Sciences in Action* (Cohen, L.K. and Gift, H.C., eds). pp. 33–71. Munksgaard, Copenhagen.

Rosenberg, D., Kaplan, S., Senie, R. and Badner, V. (1988) Relationship among dental functional status, clinical dental measures, and general health measures. *Journal of Dental Education* **52**: 653–657.

Sackett, D.L. (1980) On the evaluation of health services. In: *Preventive Medicine and Public Health,* 11th edn. (Last, J., ed). Appleton Century Crofts, New York.

Sackett, D.L. and Snow, J.C. (1979) The magnitude of compliance and non-compliance. In: *Compliance in Health Care* (Haynes, R.B., Taylor, D.W. and Sackett, D.L., eds). pp. 11–22. Johns Hopkins University Press, Baltimore.

Schonfeld, W.H. (1981) Estimating dental treatment needs from epidemiological data. *Journal of Public Health Dentistry* **41**: 25–32.

Scrivens, E., Cunningham, D., Chailton, J. and Holland, W. (1985) Measuring the impact of health interventions: a review of available instruments. *Effective Health Care* **2**: 47–59.

Shaw, W C., Richmond, S., O'Brien, K.D. and Brook, P. (1991) Quality control in orthodontics: indices of treatment need and treatment standards. *British Dental Journal* **170**: 107–112.

Sheiham, A., Maizels, J.E. and Cushing, A.M. (1982) The concept of need in dental care. *International Dental Journal* **32**: 265–270.

Sheiham, A., Maizels, J. and Maizels, A. (1987). New composite indicators of dental health. *Community Dental Health* **4**: 407–414.

Slade, G.D. and Spencer, A.J. (1994) Development and evaluation of the Oral Health Impact Profile. *Community Dental Health* **11**: 3–11.

Slade, G.D. and Spencer, A.J. (1995) *Clinical Conditions Associated with Social Impact among older South Australians.* Unpublished report. Chapel Hill, NC: Department of Dental Ecology, University of North Carolina, 14pp.

Slade, G.D., Spencer, A.J., Locker, D. et al. (1996) Variations in the social impact of oral conditions among older adults in South Australia, Ontario and North Carolina. *Journal of Dental Research* (accepted for publication 1/2/96).

Slade, G.D., Hoskin, G.W. and Spencer, A.J. (1995b) Trends and fluctuations in the impact of oral conditions among older adults during a one year period. *Community Dental and Oral Epidemiology* (accepted 8/1/96).

Smith, J. and Sheiham, A. (1979) How dental conditions handicap the elderly. *Community Dental and Oral Epidemiology* **7**: 305–310.

Spencer A.J. (1980) The estimation of need for dental care. *Journal of Public health Dentistry* **40**: 311–327.

Spencer, A.J. (1984) *Evaluation of Changing Normative Needs for Dental Care in Planning for the Delivery of Dental Care to the Australian Adolescent Population.* PhD. thesis. University of Melbourne. Melbourne

Strauss, R.P. (1988) The patient with cancer: social and clinical perspectives for the dentist. *Spec-Care-Dentist* **8**(3): 129–134.

Strauss, R.P. and Hunt, R.J. (1993) Understanding the value of teeth to older adults: influences on the quality of life. *Journal of American Dental Association* **124**: 105–110.

Streiner, D.L. and Norman, G.R. (1989). *Health Measurement Scales: A Practical Guide to their Development and Use.* Oxford University Press, New York.

Teeling-Smith, G. (1973) *Health Economics and Cost–benefit Analysis in Health Planning and Organization of Medical Care.* pp. 34–45. World Health Organization, Copenhagen

Tugwell, P., Bennett, K.J., Sackett, D. and Haynes, B. (1984) Relative risks, benefits and costs of intervention. In: *Tropical and Geographic Medicine.* (Warren, K.S., and Mahmoud, A.A.F., eds), McGraw Hill, New York. pp. 1097–1113.

Ware, J.E., Brook, R.H., Davies, A.R. and Lohr, K.N. (1981) Choosing measures of health status for individuals in general populations. *American Journal of Public Health* **71**: 620–625.

White, K.L. and Henderson, M.M. (eds) (1976) *Epidemiology as a Fundamental Science; Its Uses in Health Services Planning, Administration, and Evaluation.* p. 215. Oxford University Press, New York.

White, B.A. and Antzcak-Bouckoms, A. (1995) Improving oral health through systematic reviews and meta-analysis. In: *Disease Prevention and Oral Health Promotion: Socio-dental Sciences in Action* (Cohn, L.K. and Gift, H.C., eds), pp.455–479. Munksgaard, Copenhagen.

Wood, P.H.N. (1975) *Classification of Impairments and Handicaps.* WHO/ICD9/REVCONF/7515. World Health Organization, Geneva. (mimeo).

World Health Organization (1947) *The Constitution of the World Health Organization.* WHO Chronicle 1.29, Geneva: World Health Organization.

World Health Organization (1977) *Oral Health Surveys. Basic Methods.* 2nd ed. World Health Organization, Geneva.

World Health Organization (1978) *Epidemiology, Etiology and Prevention of Periodontal Diseases.* Technical Report. series 621. World Health Organization, Geneva.

World Health Organization (1980) *International Classification of Impairments, Disabilities and Handicaps.* World Health Organisation, Geneva.

World Health Organization (1987) *Oral Health Surveys. Basic Methods.* 3rd ed. World Health Organization, Geneva.

World Health Organization (1989) *Health Through Oral Health: Guidelines for Planning and Monitoring Oral Health Care.* Quintessence, London.

Young, W.O. and Striffler, D.F. (1969) *The Dentist, his Practice and his Community,* 2nd edn, p. 185. Saunders, Philadelphia.

5

Basic principles and methods of oral epidemiology

Flemming Scheutz

Introduction

Epidemiology is a central medical science that studies the distribution and determinants of health-related states or events in specified populations, and the application of this study to control health problems. The study of the distribution of diseases or health-related events is essential for the planning and evaluation of health services and as a first and basic part of an epidemiological study. The essence of epidemiology is, however, to study *outcomes* in relation to *exposure* status. The expression *exposure* means any of an individual's characteristics or any agent with which the individual comes in contact that may be important for the individual's health. Thus, we study the association between exposure and disease by studying the determinants of health-related conditions or events which may be of genetic, environmental, biological, social or psychological nature. To identify the determinants and events, groups of people are analysed, aiming to learn why some individuals develop disease and others do not. Analytical epidemiology is essential for preventive medicine, where the objective is to intervene to the benefit of the community and the individual, and for the evaluation of health services by setting priorities and allocating scarce health care resources efficiently.

The concept of causation is an essential part of epidemiology. Some of the criteria that have been suggested and may be used to establish a causal relationship are given in Table 5.1.

A *temporal relationship* is critical since a cause must precede an outcome in time. However, a temporal relationship may be difficult or impossible to ascertain when measurements of the potential cause and the outcome are made at the same point of time, as in case-control and cross-sectional studies. Factors suspected to be causes may turn out to be caused by the disease. The argument for *strength of association* is that strong associations should be more likely to be causal than weak associations but the strength of an association may be a characteristic dependent on the relative prevalence of other risk factors. A *dose–response relationship* may or may not be present, and if present, it may be caused by confounding. We talk about *consistency* when we observe an association in different studies under different circumstances. A causal association may, however, be present without consistency because some effects are seen only under unusual circumstances.

Biologically trained individuals tend to focus on the *biological plausibility*, i.e. the proposed causal association should be consistent with our current knowledge about biology and the disease

Table 5.1 Selected criteria for a causal relationship

Temporal sequence
Strength of association
Dose–response relationship
Consistency
Biological plausibility
Specificity
Analogy
Experimental evidence

process. By *specificity* we mean that a cause has a single effect. However, most causes have multiple potential effects. A simple *analogy* is that if, for example, one drug causes cleft palate, another drug could also. *Experimental evidence* is a strong argument for a causal relationship. Unfortunately, such evidence is seldom available in epidemiology where we observe human populations.

The concept of cause

The concept of cause has been a source of much controversy. A cause of a disease can be defined as an event, characteristic or circumstance, or combinations of these that play a significant role in the occurrence of the disease. A *sufficient* cause inevitably produces or initiates a disease whereas a cause is termed *necessary* if disease cannot develop in its absence. It may be difficult to establish causation for diseases which occur years after first exposure. A sufficient cause in our field is very seldom a single factor, but comprises several components. For example, sugar could be considered a cause of dental caries, but not a sufficient one since the type of sugar and the manner and frequency of sugar intake must be specified (see Chapter 13). Sugar intake may not lead to dental caries in everyone; who are the susceptible individuals or those at risk? To determine that, we may need to consider amount and type of plaque, enamel characteristics, type and composition of the microbiological flora, genetic characteristics or fluoride intake. Although it is improbable that all causal components of a disease are known, there is a tendency to ascribe the same risk to individuals who have a similar set of known component causes. Hidden or unknown causal components of a disease force us to assign an average risk value to individuals exposed to a set of risk factors. Such a concept of causes in medicine could be called *deterministic*.

A schematic illustration of constellations of component causes is shown in Figure 5.1. Each set of component causes is sufficient to produce disease, but component causes may play a role in one, two or all three causal mechanisms. Let us assume that the factors A, B and C are common among all people and D is rare. Despite the fact that all factors are causes, the factor D could emerge as an important determinant, because those individuals with D would be assigned a greater risk than those without. An example of this situation would be if D were a genetic determinant, for example, a genetic tendency for high cholesterol levels is, proportionately, a minor explanation of the incidence of myocardial infarction. The strength of a cause is thus determined by the relative occurrence of component causes. A *deterministic* concept of causation leads to multifactorial disease models and points towards research aiming to study several component causes and a close collaboration between epidemiological, biological, psychological and sociological research. For example, in oral health there is a complex set of social and psychological factors that in our field may produce associations between variables such as diet, oral cleanliness, cigarette smoking, drinking habits, occupational exposure, social status, educational status, age, sex and so on. If we adopt such a concept in oral epidemiology futile discussions about a disease and its cause that have been common would occur less frequently.

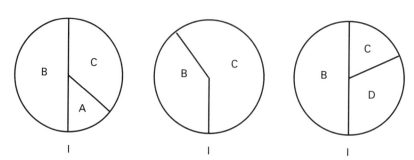

Fig. 5.1 Conceptual schematization of deterministic causal models in epidemiology. See text for details.

Diagnostic testing

If we had perfect diagnostic tools our ability to classify individuals as either diseased (or at risk) or as healthy (or not at risk) would increase from zero toward certainty as we collected new meaningful pieces of information during the diagnostic process. Unfortunately, this is not the case. In fact, it is much more common that our decisions are rather uncertain and based upon probability, because the information to which we have access is incomplete or inaccurate. Nevertheless, our diagnostic procedures aim at confirming or rejecting the hypothesis that disease is present.

Ideally, a positive diagnostic test indicates that the disease or condition is present and a negative test result indicates that the disease or condition is absent. However, tests are not perfect. Let us consider a test result that is either positive or negative. After the test is performed, one of four scenarios can occur, as shown in Figure 5.2.

Whether disease is present or absent–the *true* disease status–is determined by the best available diagnostic method, referred to as the gold standard. In cell *a* of Figure 5.2, the disease or condition of interest is present and the test result is positive, or true positive. In cell *d*, the disease is absent, and the test is negative, or true negative. In other words, there is no misclassification, since the test results agree with disease status. Cell *b* represents persons without disease who have a positive test result. These persons are misclassified and considered to be false positive. The persons in cell *c* have the disease, but since tests incorrectly suggest that disease is absent, they are designated as false negative. Any diagnostic test can be evaluated in this manner. The first step in the evaluation of a test is thus to select the gold standard, i.e., determine the true disease status or condition of interest. In a hypothetical example, Figure 5.3, we could compare the test results obtained in a high risk group to the results obtained if the patients' true disease status was determined subsequently.

The *sensitivity* and *specificity* of the test describe the performance of the test relative to true disease status or the gold standard. The sensitivity is defined as the fraction or percentage of persons with the disease who have a positive test result, or the probability of a positive test given that disease is present. Sensitivity is calculated as follows:

$$\text{Sensitivity} = \frac{\text{True positives}}{\text{True positives} + \text{False negative}}$$

$$= \frac{a}{a+c}$$

Using the data from Figure 5.3, the sensitivity and its 95% confidence interval (CI) of the test is:

$$\text{Sensitivity} = \frac{49}{49+12} = 0.80 \ (95\% \ \text{CI} = 0.68\text{--}0.89)$$

The higher the sensitivity, the more likely the test is to detect persons with the disease or condition of interest. In the hypothetical

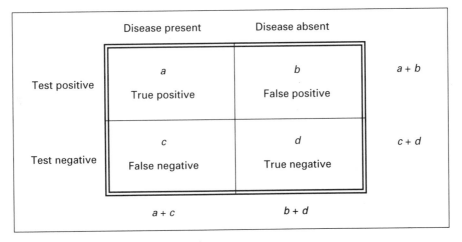

Fig. 5.2 Results of a diagnostic test and disease status.

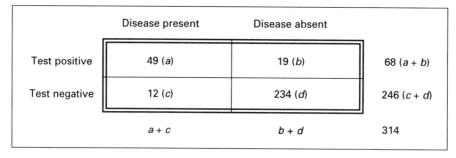

Fig. 5.3 Hypothetical example of a diagnostic test and disease status.

example, 0.80 or 80% of all diseased patients had a positive test result.

Specificity is defined as the percentage of persons without the disease or condition of interest who have negative test results, or the probability of a negative test result given no disease. Specificity is calculated as follows:

$$Specificity = \frac{True\ negatives}{True\ negatives + False\ positives}$$

$$= \frac{d}{d+b}$$

Using the data from Figure 5.3, the specificity of the test is:

$$Specificity = \frac{234}{234+19} = 0.92\ (95\%\ CI = 0.88–0.95)$$

The higher the specificity, the more likely it is that persons without the disease or condition of interest will be excluded by the test. Together, sensitivity and specificity express the validity of a test–its ability to measure what is wanted.

Positive and negative predictive values

Sensitivity and specificity describe the accuracy of a test whereas the *positive predictive value* (PV+) and the *negative predictive value* (PV−) estimate the probability of disease or condition of interest among people given a certain test result. The PV+ and the PV− are more useful parameters to understand given that a screening procedure is in place. The PV+ estimates how likely it is that a disease or condition of interest is present if the test is positive.

Referring again to Figure 5.2, PV+ is calculated as follows:

$$PV+ = \frac{True\ positives}{True\ positives + False\ positives} = \frac{a}{a+b}$$

The PV+ is the percentage of persons who have both the disease and a positive test result among all the persons with positive test results. The calculation of the PV+ in the example in Figure 5.3 is:

$$PV+ = \frac{49}{49+19} = 0.72\ (95\% = 0.60–0.82)$$

The average probability of disease or the prevalence in this sample prior to the test was 61 out of 314 individuals, or 0.19. After the test, the probability of disease for individuals with positive test results increased to 0.72.

The negative predictive value (PV−) is the probability of no disease if the test is negative. The general formula for the calculation of PV− is:

$$PV− = \frac{True\ negatives}{True\ negatives + False\ negatives} = \frac{d}{d+c}$$

For the hypothetical data in Figure 5.3, PV− is:

$$PV− = \frac{234}{12+234} = 0.95\ (95\%\ CI = 0.91–0.97)$$

Before the test, the likelihood of no disease in this sample was 253 unaffected individuals out of 314 persons, or 80.6%, whereas after a negative test result the probability of no disease increased to 95%.

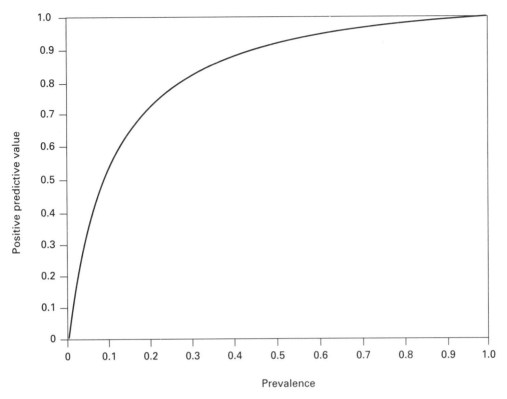

Fig. 5.4 Illustration of the influence of disease prevalence on the positive predictive value.

In addition to recognizing that tests are not perfect, it is important to note that the usefulness of a test changes as the clinical situation changes. The pretest probability of disease in an individual, or the prevalence of disease in the population, greatly influences the predictive value. Given the same sensitivity and specificity of a test, the PV+ increases with prevalence, as illustrated in Figure 5.4. Therefore, relatively fewer persons will be misclassified as diseased in populations with a high disease prevalence.

The importance of the disease prevalence on the PV + 1 for a given test can also be seen from the following formula:

$$PV+ = \frac{\text{Sensitivity} \times \text{prevalence}}{\text{Sensitivity} \times \text{prevalence} +}$$
$$(1 - \text{prevalence}) \times (1 - \text{specificity})$$

If the sensitivity and the specificity of a test and the fraction of test-positive individuals are known, the following formula can be used to calculate the true prevalence:

Prevalence =

$$\frac{\text{Fraction of test positives} + (\text{specificity} - 1)}{\text{Sensitivity} + (\text{specificity} - 1)}$$

Using the data from Figure 5.3:

$$\text{Prevalence} = \frac{0.2166 + (0.9249 - 1)}{0.8033 + (0.9249 - 1)} = 0.19$$

Dichotomization of clinical findings is common. However, test results often occur along a continuum and do not have just positive or negative outcomes. Therefore, we have to choose a *cut-off point*, dichotomizing between normal and abnormal. Different cut-off points change a test's sensitivity, specificity and positive and negative predictive values. A plot of the true-positive and false-positive fractions resulting from varying the diagnostic threshold value, called a receiver operating characteristic (ROC) curve, can be useful since it gives an understanding of the compromises that have to be made in deciding on an appropriate cut-off point.

Screening

When the posterior probability of disease has been calculated for either a positive or negative test result, the usefulness of the test for screening purposes can be further considered. The aim of screening a population is to detect the disease or predictors of disease at an early stage. Two important aspects should be noted. First, the aim is to detect diseased persons before symptoms occur. Second, if treatment is initiated at the time of detection by screening, as opposed to the time of routine diagnosis, there should be an improved chance of survival. Let us, for example, look at oral cancer. It is known that the length of survival from time of diagnosis is related to the size of the tumour and the amount of spread of the cancer. By screening asymptomatic individuals some cases of oral cancer will be detected earlier, and these individuals should survive longer.

However, this alluring logic has two important biases–*lead-time bias* and *length-biased sampling*. The time from early diagnosis by screening to routine diagnosis is defined as the lead time. Length-biased sampling occurs when disease detected by a screening programme is less aggressive than disease detected without screening. On average, oral cancers detected by screening may be less aggressive than those detected when symptoms appear. This occurs because less aggressive cancers typically grow more slowly than more aggressive cancers. The length of time during which the cancer is detectable by screening is therefore greater for slow-growing cancers. To overcome lead-time bias and length-biased sampling, the true benefit of a screening programme must be evaluated by estimating disease-specific rates among individuals who are either randomly assigned to a screening programme or who receive no screening. Some essential requirements for a screening programme are given in Table 5.2.

Measures of disease frequency

Prevalence and incidence

Prevalence is the number of *existing* cases in a population. Prevalence estimates are calculated by dividing the number of affected individuals, or cases, by the total number of persons in the population. The expressions *point prevalence* and *period prevalence* are used to distinguish between two subtypes of prevalence.

Point prevalence =

$$\frac{\text{Number of cases at a particular time}}{\text{Total population at that time}}$$

Period prevalence =

$$\frac{\text{Number of cases during a specified period}}{\text{Total population during that period}}$$

(usually at the mid-point of the period)

Prevalence estimates are obtained from cross-sectional studies or derived from registers. *Incidence* is the number of new cases or events during a specified period of time. Prevalence depends on duration and previous incidence, because old as well as recent cases are included in the calculation of prevalence. When the incidence and duration of a disease are reasonably constant, the following relationship exists:

Prevalence = Incidence × duration

Therefore, prevalence may change over time if there are changes in incidence, duration or the number of susceptible persons. Prevalence, like risk, ranges between 0 and 1 and has no units. A typical example from oral epidemiology is to calculate the prevalence of individuals with

Table 5.2 Requirements before launching a screening programme

The morbidity or mortality must have public health importance

Early intervention must be known to improve prognosis

The screening test or procedure must be highly sensitive and specific

The disease prevalence in the target population must be sufficiently high

The test procedures must be acceptable for the population

Adverse effects, including psychological and ethical aspects, caused by the test should be minimal

The natural history of the condition should be adequately understood in order to determine the best time to apply the screening test

There should be an agreed policy on whom to treat as patients

An appropriate treatment for those detected must be available

The cost–benefit and cost-effectiveness must be favourable

caries in a particular age group in a community. For example, if there were 221 12-year-olds in a particular geographic area in August 1994 and 41 children were diagnosed as having dental caries, the point prevalence estimate of dental caries in August 1994 was:

$$\text{Prevalence} = \frac{41}{221} = 0.186 \text{ or } 18.6\%$$

Prevalence estimates are useful for descriptive purposes, community diagnosis, administrative purposes and health planning. They have the potential to arouse suspicion about the determinants of disease, and serve as a basis for the formulation of hypotheses. The principal drawback of prevalence estimates is that information about the outcome and exposure is collected at the same time. This severely limits the possibilities for an evaluation of a causal relationship between an exposure and an outcome.

The *incidence rate* (IR), sometimes called incidence density, reflects the occurrence of *new* cases of disease during a given period of time. To estimate the IR, a population is observed in a time period, and the number of new cases is counted together with the total person-time. The total person-time is the total time the individual

in the population is at risk of developing disease during the study. The formula for calculating IR is:

$$IR = \frac{\text{New cases}}{\text{Person-time}}$$

To illustrate calculation of person-time and IR, consider the small hypothetical group of 8 people in Figure 5.5. Person 1 develops disease 7 years after entry into the study. Since subjects contribute person-time only while at risk, the person-time for patient 1 was 7 years, at which time disease developed. Person 2 contributed with 5 years until the study ended. The total person-time is simply obtained by addition of the time contributed by each subject. The total number of person-time was $7+5+7+6+1+5+2+5=38$. As the number of new cases was 3, the incidence rate is:

$$IR = \frac{3}{38} \text{ cases per person-time}$$

$$= 0.079 \text{ cases per person-time}$$

If the time unit was years, the rate could alternatively be expressed as 79 cases per 1000 person-years by multiplying the numerator and denominator by 1000.

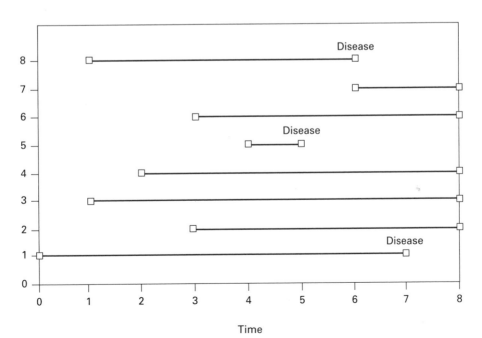

Fig. 5.5 Hypothetical study of a group of 8 individuals in a given time period.

Cumulative incidence proportion (CIP) is a measure of new cases accumulated during a specific period of time in a population at risk. It could also be considered as the probability or the average *risk* an individual has of developing disease in the specified time interval. The risk is estimated by observing a particular population for a defined period of time, the risk period. The estimated risk is a proportion where the numerator is the number of new cases of disease and the denominator is the unaffected population or population at risk:

$$CIP = \frac{\text{New cases of disease during time interval}}{\text{Persons at risk at beginning of time interval}}$$

By definition all members of the population under observation are free of disease, at risk, at the beginning of the observation period. CIP has no unit, and ranges from 0 (no new cases occur) to 1 (when all members of the population become affected).

In order to illustrate the calculation of risk, consider a hypothetical study of 123 subjects' risk of developing oral candidiasis after being diagnosed as seropositive for antibody to human immunodeficiency virus (HIV-1). Each individual was examined for oral candidiasis and found free of disease at the time of enrolment. The study started at the beginning of 1987 and all subjects were followed for 3 years, during which 21 patients were diagnosed with oral candidiasis at least once. The cumulative incidence proportion for a 3-year period was:

$$CIP = \frac{21}{123} = 0.17 \text{ or } 17\%$$

In order to calculate the CPI as straightforwardly as in this example, no members of the population at risk must be lost during follow-up. If that is the case the risk will have to be calculated in another way.

Rates, proportions, odds, risks, ratios and differences

In a *rate* there is a distinct relationship between the numerator and the denominator; usually time is a part of the denominator. A rate such as 79 cases per 1000 years does, of course, not require that we actually have an observation period of 1000 years. The estimate could, for example, be derived by observing 79 cases among 500 people over a 2-year period. An appropriate time unit is selected for the denominator. It should be noted that an assumption is that the number of new cases is the same in different time bands. A *proportion* ranges from 0 to 1 (or as a percentage from 0 to 100). A proportion (P) can also be expressed as *odds*. In general the relationship between probability and the corresponding odds is:

$$Odds = P/(1 - P)$$

$$P = odds/(1 + odds)$$

Odds, which may vary from zero to infinite, is an important expression in epidemiology, in particular in case-control studies. Odds expresses the ratio of the probability of an event occurring to the probability of the event not occurring. In epidemiology *risk* expresses the probability of a certain event in a specified time period. These measures have different applications. Risk is most useful if interest focuses on the probability that an individual will become ill over a specified period of time. IRs are preferred if interest focuses on the rapidity with which new cases arise. Rates and risks are not identical, but they are associated: the larger an IR, the higher the risk (CIP) in the specified time period.

A *ratio* is obtained by dividing one quantity with another such as the IRs in two populations. We obtain an estimate of the disease frequency in a population compared to the disease frequency in another population. Typically one of the populations is exposed to a risk factor while the other is not. In this way we get an estimate of the importance of the exposure or risk factor for disease outcome. If the IR of new decayed surfaces is 1.5 per year in group A and 0.4 per year in group B, the *incidence rate ratio* is 3.8. Thus the IR is nearly 4 times larger in group A than in group B. If CIPs are compared, the ratio is named a *relative risk* (RR). IRs can also be compared by the absolute difference of disease outcome between the two groups– *incidence rate difference* (IRD). In the example the IR difference is $1.5 - 0.4 = 1.1$ per year, or the individuals in group A had an average of 1.1 more new decayed surfaces per year than those in group B.

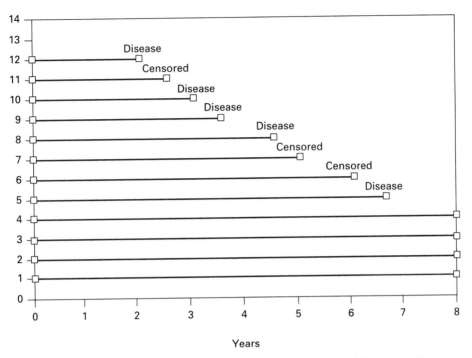

Fig. 5.6 Hypothetical study of a group of 12 individuals in a given time period with censoring of 3 individuals.

Calculation of risk time

In Figure 5.5 it was easy to calculate the total person time, because we were able to follow all 8 individuals. However, in follow-up studies, also called cohort studies, it is common that some individuals leave the study for a variety of reasons, such as death, moving away, deciding to discontinue participation or the study simply ends. Such observations are called censored. In the small hypothetical study in Figure 5.6, where 5 persons became diseased and 3 were censored, we wanted to describe the prognosis up to 8 years after treatment. However, we do not have complete information for all individuals. Therefore we cannot calculate CIP as 3/12, but we can calculate the IR using all the information we collected. The censored individuals contribute with their risk time until censoring, and those who became diseased until disease is observed. The total risk time is 65 years, and the incidence rate 3/65 = 0.0462 per year or 5 per 100 years. In this hypothetical study calculation of the time interval was years, and we had a fixed population. Using computers it is possible to calculate the risk time accurately even in dynamic populations, when people migrate to and from the population.

Survival in epidemiology

Survival rate is the proportion of survivors or the probability of remaining alive (or healthy) for a specific length of time. For a chronic disease such as oral cancer, 1-year survival and 5-year survival are often used as indicators of the severity of disease and the prognosis. If the 5-year survival for oral cancer is 0.32, it indicates that 32% of the patients survive at least 5 years after diagnosis. Survival analysis is used in epidemiology to describe the prognosis, and to compare treatments and outcome in different populations. The observation time is complete for the participants (or study units) in which the event occurs during the study. For the remaining participants the observations are censored, i.e. the observation time ends either at the end of the study or they are lost in the follow-up.

Survival analysis can be carried out using the *Kaplan-Meier* method or the *actuarial* method. The first method aims at giving an exact description of the sequence of survival in a cohort. The second method is an approximate description of the survival because the observation period is divided into time intervals, for example 1 year. If an observation is censored, the number of persons at risk in that interval are reduced by subtracting half of the censored observations. It is thus assumed that the censored observations contribute half of the risk in the time interval.

Variability and bias

Obviously we wish to be as *precise* as possible in our measurements in epidemiological studies. If we adhere to a deterministic view on causality, as described in the beginning of this chapter, complete knowledge about all relevant component causal factors would make it possible for us to predict all outcomes perfectly. However, ignorance and inadequate information leave us with a great amount of unpredictability of the outcome. Such unpredictability cannot be distinguished from random error, and we therefore treat this *variability* as being due to chance. We can improve the precision of a study by increasing the size of the study. However, when planning study size we have to balance the value of increased precision against the greater cost of a larger study. It is therefore of pre-eminent interest to assess the size of a planned study. Detailed examples are given in Chapter 9.

Validity concerns the degree to which we measure what we intend to measure or our study reaches a correct conclusion. It is common to distinguish between two types of validity–*internal validity* and *external validity* or *generalizability*. Internal validity reflects the validity concerning the actual individuals in the study, whereas external validity pertains to individuals outside the study population. A study is internally valid if it provides a true estimate of effect in the population studied. If the results are not valid in the study population, then there is little reason to expect that they will apply to other populations. Internal validity is often improved by restricting the type of individuals to be included in a study and the circumstances in which it is performed. In this way the impact of factors extraneous to the research questions is reduced. Many types of bias can destroy the internal validity of a study, but it is common to

put them into one of three categories: *selection bias*, *information bias* and *confounding*.

In a descriptive investigation the reported occurrence of a disease, for example dental caries, can be biased for several reasons. The sample we study may not be representative of the population we wish to describe. If that is the case, our estimate of the amount of dental caries in the population will not be correct, and we talk about *selection bias*. In most studies we do not get information from all members of our sample. For various reasons some people do not wish to participate and a response rate as low as 80% is not uncommon. Since the non-responders and the responders usually differ with regard to the factors we wish to study there may be bias in our study. This bias cannot be reduced by increasing the sample size. It may happen that we have information about some characteristics of the non-responders that may allow us to speculate about the direction of the bias. However, it remains speculative. In a cohort study, the major potential selection bias is loss to follow-up, and certain types of people are more likely than others to drop out. Selection bias is of particular importance in case-control studies where we select the cases and non-cases in a setting in which the exposure has already occurred. For example, we may decide to use existing (prevalent) cases at the onset of the study regardless of duration of their disease or decide to use newly diagnosed (incident) cases. If the risk factor of interest is a prognostic factor too, use of prevalent cases can lead to a biased conclusion.

Information bias (or misclassification) can occur when there are errors in obtaining the required information. The misclassification may be differential or non-differential. When the error in classification of exposure or disease status is independent of the level of the other variable, the misclassification is called non-differential. Non-differential misclassification may occur in a case-control study if the participants' recollection of exposure is not related to whether the participants have the disease or condition of interest or not. The participants may answer a question about the exposure with a socially acceptable but inaccurate response. Consider a case-control study of periodontal disease in which the exposure of interest is poor oral hygiene. Regardless of disease status, respondents may overreport the measures they take to increase their oral cleanliness because

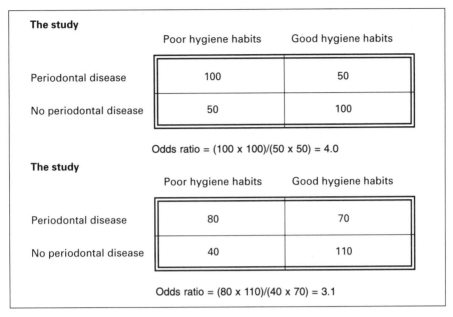

The study

	Poor hygiene habits	Good hygiene habits
Periodontal disease	100	50
No periodontal disease	50	100

Odds ratio = (100 x 100)/(50 x 50) = 4.0

The study

	Poor hygiene habits	Good hygiene habits
Periodontal disease	80	70
No periodontal disease	40	110

Odds ratio = (80 x 110)/(40 x 70) = 3.1

Fig. 5.7 Illustration of non-differential misclassification in a hypothetical case-control study of the association between poor oral preventive behaviour and periodontal disease.

they know that good oral hygiene is much more socially acceptable. What happens when this kind of non-differential misclassification occurs is that the differences between the study groups are blurred as illustrated in Figure 5.7.

In this case, the association we observe between the exposure, poor oral hygiene and periodontal disease will be less than an unbiased estimate. In general, non-differential misclassification tends to introduce bias towards the null hypothesis. We will underestimate the association between exposure and disease or maybe find no association at all.

Differential misclassification occurs when the misclassification of one variable depends upon the status of the other. In a case-control study, this type of misclassification can occur if the information on exposure status depends on whether or not the individual had the disease. If a case with rampant dental caries is more likely to overestimate the level of a particular harmful diet than a non-case subject, then a biased result might be found. The study would tend to overestimate the association between that particular diet and rampant caries (Fig. 5.8).

Two common types of differential information bias are often referred to as *recall bias* and *interviewer bias*. Recall bias results from the participants' ability to recall previous events and exposure. Mothers of children with a cleft palate may well recall previous exposures better than other mothers. Recall bias is a possibility in case-control studies where people have to remember something in the past. Interviewer bias may occur when an interviewer knows the research objectives. The interviewer may explore the responses from the cases more thoroughly than those from non-cases and may even unknowingly send subtle signals by body language or voice. Therefore, it is desirable to blind the interviewers to the research hypothesis, although this may be impossible in a case-control study. The terminology of bias in relation to the type of study and misclassification of exposure and outcome can be summarized as in Figure 5.9.

External validity

External validity is the extent to which the results of a study are generalizable. Conclusions reached in a narrow environment may or may not be applicable to more general situations. Generalization of study results obtained in restricted surroundings and highly selected study groups will be incorrect when estimating the efficiency of interventions. Experimental clinical trials evaluating biological efficacy of new

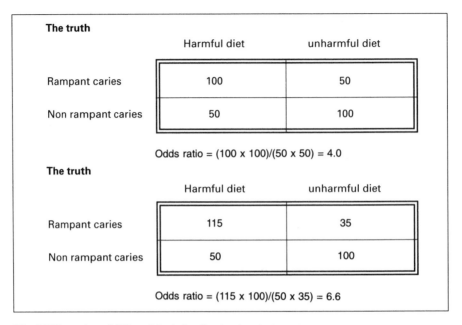

Fig. 5.8 Illustration of differential misclassification in a hypothetical case-control study of the association between diet and rampant caries.

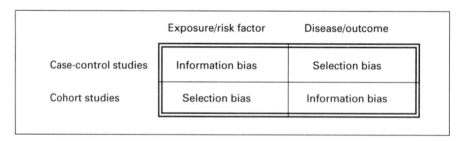

Fig. 5.9 Schematic illustration of bias in relation to type of study.

agents or procedures in preventing or treating disease should be followed up with pragmatic clinical trials evaluating community efficiency conducted under real-life conditions. However, this ideal scenario is not always followed and distinctions are blurred such that we are often faced with the question as to whom do the study results apply apart from the specific groups followed? Many tend to believe that generalization from an epidemiological study is dependent on the study population being a representative sample of a target or parent population, in the statistical sense of a sample. However, that is not the case, although this concept has had a heavy influence on many epidemiological studies. Scientific reasoning

should not just be a matter of mechanical aspects of sampling. Instead, we should rather determine the valdity of a generalization by informed interpretation and judgement of the information we have at hand. In fact, if we were to demand representativeness of the study populations in epidemiological studies, few studies would pass such a test.

Confounding

In its simplest form, analytical epidemiology compares the disease outcome in groups of individuals with different exposure. If a study is to be considered valid the amount of disease should be the same if the exposure is of no

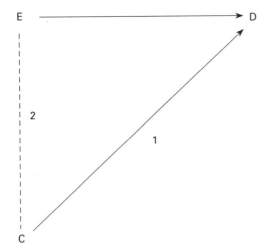

Fig. 5.10 Schematic presentation of confounding where C is confounder(s), E is exposure and D is disease or outcome.

importance. That is the case when all other risk factors of importance for the outcome are distributed equally between the two groups. An unbalanced distribution of risk factors among exposure categories, exposed and unexposed, is called a *confounder*. Confounding refers to the mixing of the effect of an extraneous variable with the effects of the exposure and disease or condition of interest. Confounding can be illustrated as in Figure 5.10. D is the effect or outcome, E is the exposure and C a potential confounder. A confounder must be an independent risk of disease and it must be associated with both the exposure and the disease under study, but it must not be a link in the causal chain between the exposure and the disease.

We know that plaque is a risk factor for the development of periodontal disease. However, smoking seems to be a risk factor too, and we know that smoking is associated with a poorer oral hygiene. An unadjusted estimation between the presence of plaque and periodontal disease will therefore reflect the population's smoking habits too, because there will be more individuals with poor hygiene among the smokers than among the non-smokers. Smoking will be a confounder. Variables such as age, gender and social status are often treated as potential confounders in epidemiological studies, because many diseases occur with diverging frequency in men and women, in different age groups and in the various

socioeconomic segments of society. Such variables are rather risk indicators, not causes. They are proxy variables for hidden and unknown causes. We may, however, be able to adjust for these causes by adjusting for such proxy variables.

The goal of any epidemiological study is to provide a valid conclusion. In order to accomplish this objective, complete attention must be given to all aspects of the study, from the inception through design and data collection to analysis and final reporting of results. Bias can be introduced at any of these stages leading to erroneous results. It is useful to look for potential sources of bias and to consider their possible impact. To keep abreast of scientific developments in dentistry, clinicians should, as part of their training, develop critical skills to assess the literature accurately. Clinicians must be able to judge whether results can be generalized to their particular practice. Understanding the potential problems with measurements and bias in medical research improves our ability to decide on appropriate preventive and therapeutic strategies as scientists, administrators and clinicians.

Types of epidemiological studies

Having described the terminology in oral epidemiology, it is now possible to apply that understanding to categorize types of studies. Although the distinctions are not always clear-cut, epidemiological research can be categorized according to whether the primary focus is on describing the distributions of disease or on analysing its determinants (Table 5.3).

All study designs involve some descriptive or

Table 5.3 Overview of epidemiological design strategies

Descriptive studies
Observational studies
    Case reports
    Case series
    Populations (correlational studies)
    Cross-sectional surveys
Analytical studies
Observational studies
    Case-control studies (unmatched and matched)
    Cohort studies (prospective and historical)
Experimental studies
    Intervention studies
    Clinical trials

analytic type of comparison of exposure and disease status. In analytic studies, however, the comparison is explicit, since groups of individuals are sampled principally to determine whether or not the risk of disease is different for individuals exposed compared to individuals not exposed to a particular factor. By matching we make a study group and a comparison group comparable with respect to extraneous factors. The goal is not to make the groups similar in all respects. A matching scheme strives to improve statistical efficiency and eliminate bias from the effect of interest.

The two basic types of analytic epidemiological studies are the *cohort* and the *case-control* study. Each design offers certain advantages and disadvantages. It is often possible to investigate a particular hypothesis using either a case-control or cohort study design. The choice of which type of design to use to study a particular exposure–disease relationship depends on the nature of the disease under investigation, the type of exposure and the available resources. For example, the case-control design is particularly efficient for investigation of a relatively rare disease since it selects a group of individuals who have already developed the outcome. Prospective cohort studies observe the subsequent development of disease over time; therefore this design is best suited to investigations of outcomes that will appear in sufficiently large numbers over a reasonably short period during follow-up. Experimental studies can be intervention studies or clinical trials and may be viewed as a particular type of prospective cohort studies, because participants are identified on the basis of their exposure status and followed to determine whether they develop disease or not. Well designed and conducted experimental studies can provide the most direct epidemiological evidence on whether an exposure causes a disease.

Cross-sectional studies

In *cross-sectional* studies we can look at distributions of variables within the sample. Cross-sectional designs are suitable to describe variables and their distribution patterns. Cross-sectional studies can also be used to look for potential associations, but to decide which variables are risk factors and which are outcomes depends on the hypotheses of the investigator, rather than on the study design.

Concerning constitutional factors such as age, sex and race, the decision is easy because they cannot be altered and therefore are generally predictors. For most variables, however, the decision is more difficult.

Cross-sectional studies are relatively fast and inexpensive to carry out and may be included as the first step in a cohort study or intervention study at little or no added cost. A weakness of cross-sectional studies is the difficulty of establishing causal relationships from data collected in this time frame. A series of cross-sectional studies of a single population observed at several points in time, called *serial surveys*, is sometimes used to draw inferences about changing disease patterns over time. A good example is the use of oral health data to look at changes from one decade to the next. This design is not a cohort design because it does not follow a single group of people over time.

Cohort studies

Cohort studies, also called *follow-up studies* or *longitudinal studies*, are observational studies where measurements are made more than once on the members of the cohort. In a cohort study we choose or define a sample of study subjects who do not have the outcome of interest at the beginning of the follow-up; or they have the potential to develop new disease, e.g. in caries studies, subjects have or will be erupting surfaces at risk. The objective of a cohort study is to compare the incidence of disease among those *exposed* to a factor with the IR among those *not exposed* to this factor in order to assess whether this exposure influences the outcome. As we collect information about the total person-time, i.e. the amount of time contributed by the participants, during the follow-up and about the outcome, we can calculate the incidence of the disease or condition of interest.

The design of a cohort study can either be *prospective* or *historical*, as illustrated in Figure 5.11. Historical studies are sometimes called *retrospective*, but the terminology historical is preferable to avoid any confusion. In a historical cohort study, information about exposure status was recorded some time in the past and the outcome, usually disease experience, is studied up to the present time. In a prospective cohort study, the exposure status of individuals is determined at the present time and the outcome is studied from now into the future. In cohort

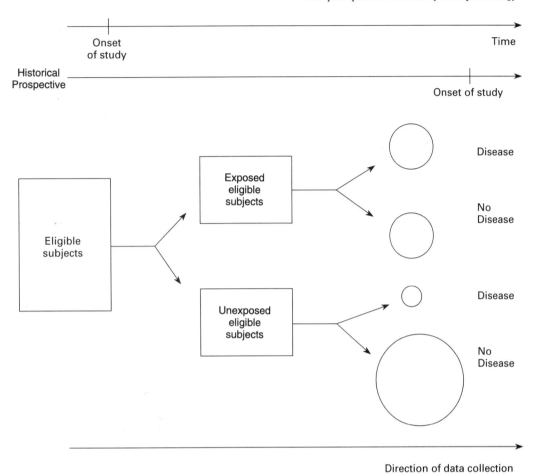

Fig. 5.11 Schematic presentation of the design of a prospective and a historical cohort study.

studies, as in other analytical studies, we formulate the hypothesis to be investigated, e.g. that poor social status is a risk indicator for poor oral health. The group of individuals to be studied must be identified, e.g. children with poor and favourable social status, respectively. The exposure, the outcome and potential confounders should be defined together with their measurement. Finally, the results must be analysed and the findings interpreted. As for any other study design, it is essential that clear hypotheses are formulated. Cohort studies are often carried out after similar hypotheses have been explored in cross-sectional or case-control studies since cohort studies tend be both expensive and time-consuming because they involve follow-up of a large number of persons for a long period of time. The study hypothesis

will specify which exposure and outcomes will be studied.

Individuals are classified according to whether they are (or have been) *exposed* or *unexposed* to the factor of interest, which is thought to be associated with the outcome. *Exposure*, also called a risk factor, is used in a very general sense. In dentistry some exposures could be: sugar; plaque; hepatitis B virus; fluorides; tobacco; working in a particular industry; being a member of a poor socioeconomic group; living in a particular region; particular microorganisms. Often we can classify those in the exposed group according to the degree of exposure. For example, the exposed can be classified by amount or frequency of sugar per day, amount of plaque, prevalence of hepatitis B infection in the patient population.

In cohort studies the incidence rate of disease in exposed and unexposed groups is compared. If these incidence rates are different it may indicate that the exposure either causes or prevents the disease. To make valid inferences it is necessary to assume that factors other than the exposure under study, which may be associated with the risk of disease, are equally distributed in the two groups. In principle, the only way to ensure a similar distribution of other potential risk factors in the groups is to carry out a randomized controlled trial. In randomized controlled trials the study participants are randomized to either the *exposed* group or to the *unexposed* group. Provided the size of the study is sufficiently large, the only difference between the groups will then be the exposure, and any differences in outcome can therefore be attributed either to chance or to the exposure. In an *observational* study, like a *cohort* study, study participants are, however, not randomized to the groups. Thus, differences in disease incidence may be due to factors unrelated to the exposure of interest. Therefore, efforts should be made to select study groups that are as comparable with respect to risk factors for the outcome under study, other than the exposure itself. A problem which may arise in cohort studies is whether the controls are truly unexposed. The classification of exposure depends on the available information and there may be inaccuracies, giving us poor quantitative estimates of exposure. The major advantage of historical cohort studies is that much of the information is already available, so reducing study length, even if the interval between exposure and outcome is long, as, for example, oral cancer. However, it is important to consider possible misclassification of exposure against the saving in time and changes of exposures over time.

In a *prospective cohort study* we collect data on exposure as part of the study. This allows us to use appropriate measurement methods and to minimize bias in exposure classification. Changes in exposure during follow-up and the interdependence of repeated measurements on the same individual may be handled by statistical packages. If the outcome of interest has a short latency, time lag until effects of exposure appear may be of little importance. An additional advantage of prospective cohort studies is that several risk factors and confounding variables can be accurately measured.

The outcome of interest must be identical for those exposed and those not exposed and should not be influenced by knowledge of the exposure status in any way. Attempts should be made to *blind* investigators with respect to information about whether individuals belong to the exposed or the unexposed group. If this is not done, measurement bias can occur. A particularly vital aspect in cohort studies is that as many as possible of the members in the cohort are followed up. Some members will inevitably be lost, but serious efforts must be made to trace all participants because incomplete follow-up may introduce selection bias, since people who leave a study are usually different from those who stay.

Collecting information from each person on many confounding variables can be a major task and may hinder the conduct of a cohort study. In historical cohort studies information on confounding variables is frequently not available. In prospective cohort studies the collection of data on potential confounders can be built into the design of the study. For example, if we want to study whether dentists have an increased risk of contracting a particular disease according to subspeciality, it is for example necessary to assess whether the exposed and unexposed groups have a similar risk of contracting the disease in their leisure time. If they do not, then statistical adjustment for differences must be made.

Analysis and interpretation

In cohort studies we calculate the IR or the CIP of the outcome in the exposed and unexposed cohorts and compare these disease measures. This makes it possible to calculate measures of RR, either as a rate ratio or a risk ratio, as shown in Table 5.4.

If there are more than two levels of exposure the trend of disease incidence at various levels of exposure can be studied.

In case of confounding, adjustment of the RR and the rate ratio must be made. As in other observational studies, we must assess possible bias (including misclassification of exposure and/or disease status), possible residual confounding and the potential influence that these may have on the observed results. A single study cannot be expected to provide sufficient evidence for a causal association between exposure and outcome. Additional proof is consistency of findings by other researchers and evidence from other types of study, e.g.

Table 5.4 Analysis of cohort studies by risks (cumulative incidence proportion; CIP) and by rates (incidence rate; IR)

Risks				Rates		
	Exposed	*Unexposed*			*Exposed*	*Unexposed*
Cases	a	b		Cases	a	b
Non-cases	c	d		par	par_1	par_0

Risk in exposed $(CIP_1) = a/(a+c)$
Risk in unexposed $(CIP_0) = b/(b+d)$
Risk ratio $= CIP_1/CIP_0$
Risk difference $= CIP_1 - CIP_0$

Rate in exposed $(IR_1) = a/par_1$
Rate in unexposed $(IR_0) = b/par_0$
Rate ratio $= IR_1/IR_0$
Rate difference $= IR_1 - IR_0$

par = Person-time at risk.

descriptive studies and *case-control studies*. The best proof is provided by a *randomized intervention study* reporting a reduction in disease by removal of the exposure, but such randomized interventions are often impossible to carry out for various reasons. The main one is that it is unethical to expose people experimentally to factors which may increase their risk of acquiring a disease. It occurs, however, that inference can be based on so-called *natural experiments* such as the large population studies. The large-scale studies of the effects of fluoride on dental health are one example. They contributed to our knowledge about dental decay, showing that there was an association between fluoride levels in water and dental health. Subsequent intervention studies confirmed the hypothesis.

Case-control studies

Case-control studies are, like cohort studies, designed to assess the association between an outcome, usually disease, and an exposure. Case-control studies are also called *case-referent* studies to stress that the controls do not serve as control in the same sense as the unexposed group in cohort studies. The major characteristic that distinguishes a case-control study from a cohort study is that the selection of study participants is based upon their disease status and not exposure status. Cases are selected from among those persons who have the disease of interest and non-cases from those who have not. The general principle involved is that the likelihood of a case being included in the study must not depend on whether that case was exposed to the risk factor of interest. Non-cases are chosen independent of exposure, and the cases and non-cases are examined to assess association between exposure and disease. In an optimally designed case-control study, cases are selected from a clearly defined population, sometimes called the *study base* or *source population* and the non-cases from the same population. The basic design of a case-control study is shown in Figure 5.12.

The criteria for the source population of those who have the disease (the cases) and who do not have the disease (the non-cases) should be specified. For example, cases might be sampled at random from all patients within a geographic region, who are diagnosed with oral cancer. The source population comprises those living in that region and cases may be found in population-based disease registers or identified at hospitals. In practice the selection of cases is often straightforward, whereas the difficult part in the design of a case-control study relates to the selection of the non-cases. The goal is to identify people at risk who represent the same population as the cases.

In case-control studies we can select *incident cases* (newly diagnosed) or *prevalent cases* (previously existing cases). In retrospective case-control studies we are restricted to use prevalent cases. The odds for being a case or not being a case based on existing cases may be different from that of becoming a case or not becoming a case based on prospective incidence data. In prevalent cases exposure may affect the prognosis or the duration of illness. If it does, then the exposure status of existing, prevalent cases, will tend to differ from that of all cases. Let us hypothesize that the use of a particular medicine prolongs the duration of oral candidiasis. Prevalent cases with oral candidiasis would then tend to have a higher reported use

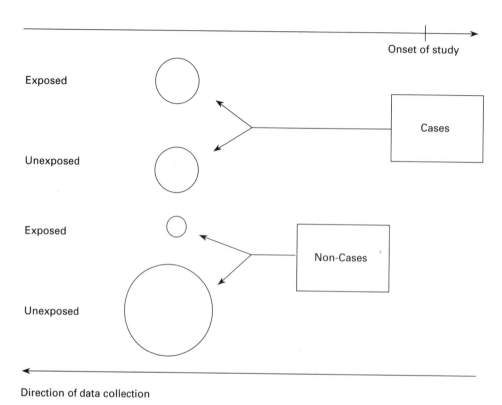

Onset of study

Exposed

Cases

Unexposed

Exposed

Non-Cases

Unexposed

Direction of data collection

Fig. 5.12 Schematic presentation of the design of a case-control study.

of this type of medicine than would all cases with this disease. A case-control comparison of medicine use would then be distorted by an inflated estimate for the cases.

A particular case-control study design is a case-control study within a cohort study, called *a nested case-control study*. In a traditional cohort study, all study individuals are subject to the same procedures, but we could also follow the cohort until a sufficient number of cases develop and then collect more detailed information, but only for the cases and for a sample of the non-cases, not for all members of the cohort. This approach is particularly useful when dealing with expensive procedures that would otherwise have to be made on many individuals. In an unmatched case-control study data can be arranged as in Figure 5.13, when only two levels of exposure are analysed. Each subject can be classified into one of four groups defined by disease and exposure status.

Although data arrangement resembles that of a cohort study, when incident cases are sampled during follow-up, the underlying approach to

sampling differs, and the analysis must account for these differences. Case-control studies cannot give estimates of the IR or prevalence, because the fraction of the subjects with disease has been determined by how many cases and how many non-cases the researchers choose to sample. An outcome that occurs infrequently can be oversampled and thus constitute a large proportion of the study sample. This possibility of oversampling cases is in fact why case-control studies are efficient for the study of rare diseases. One trade-off is that the risk of the outcome cannot be estimated.

Odds ratio

With the notation introduced in Figure 5.13, the probability that a case was exposed previously is estimated by:

$$\text{Case exposure probability} = \frac{\text{Exposed cases}}{\text{All cases}}$$

$$= \frac{a}{a+b}$$

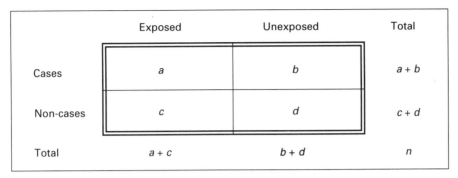

	Exposed	Unexposed	Total
Cases	a	b	a + b
Non-cases	c	d	c + d
Total	a + c	b + d	n

Fig. 5.13 Summary of data collected in an unmatched case-control study.

The odds of exposure for cases represents the probability that a case was exposed by the probability that a case was not exposed. The odds are estimated by:

Odds of case exposure =

$$\frac{\text{Exposure cases}}{\text{All cases}} \bigg/ \frac{\text{Unexposed cases}}{\text{All cases}} = \frac{a}{a+b}$$

Similarly, the odds of exposure among non-cases are estimated by:

$$\text{Odds of non-case exposure} = \frac{c}{d}$$

The odds of exposure for cases divided by the odds of exposure for non-cases are expressed as the odds ratio. Substituting from the preceding equations, the odds ratio is estimated by:

$$\frac{\text{Odds of case exposure}}{\text{Odds of non-case exposure}} = \frac{a}{b} \bigg/ \frac{c}{d} = \frac{a \times d}{b \times c}$$

Odds ratio is sometimes termed the exposure odds ratio or the cross-product, because it results from dividing the product of entries on one diagonal of this table by the product of entries on the cross-diagonal. What case-control studies do provide is an estimate of the strength of the association between exposure and disease outcome. Odds ratios are discussed in more detail in Chapter 9.

Intervention studies

The model for an intervention study is the randomized controlled trial. A key characteristic of an intervention study is that it includes at least one comparison group, against which the effect of the intervention under study is compared. The aim of the intervention study is to obtain two groups which are similar in all respects other than the preventive or therapeutic measure under study. Unless this is done, the underlying differences between the study groups may be responsible for any differences in outcome. Information from intervention studies provides the best assessment of the effect of an intervention because confounding can be avoided. The collection of baseline data on the study participants is essential and should include all the variables that are known or thought to affect the outcome of interest. The participants are then allocated to the two treatments. The best way to avoid selection biases is entirely to remove the element of human choice from the allocation process using random allocation of the participants to the groups, with the allocation not being known in advance to either the participants or the person doing the enrolment. Often we must use a modified method of randomization called stratified random allocation, in which the participants are separated into different subgroups or strata based on key risk factors or indicators. Study participants are then randomly selected for each group from within each of these strata.

In so-called *before/after studies*, the outcome is compared before an intervention has been introduced with the outcome after its introduction. This design involves the use of historical controls. However, with this design it is not possible to rule out that changes might have occurred irrespective of the intervention. The *before/after studies* are often used in evaluations of health services. Their potential can be maximized by careful monitoring of changes other than the intervention. It might also be useful to monitor changes in the outcome of interest in the general population and compare them with the changes in the intervention population.

Confounder control

Confounding can to some extent be evaluated in the analysis of the results. Therefore it differs from selection bias and information bias. Presence of confounding is demonstrated by a change in the estimated strength of association between exposure and the disease or condition of interest when the effects of extraneous variables are taken into account. There are two accepted methods for dealing with potential confounders. The first is to consider them in the design of the study; the second is to evaluate and adjust for confounders during the analysis. In the study design we can match for potential confounders, or we can restrict the sample to limited levels of the potential confounders. For various reasons caution is warranted concerning a matched design. Matching ensures only that there is no statistical association between exposure and the factors for which we have matched, but there may still be confounding from the factors we have matched for. If we choose to restrict our sample we cannot later evaluate the importance of those factors on which the restricting was based. Our second option to control confounding is to assess for confounding in the analysis phase and adjust if necessary by *stratification* or by using *multivariable analysis* such as multiple logistic regression.

A detailed presentation of statistical methods used in studies of community oral health is provided in Chapter 9 where many of the issues raised in this chapter are expanded and further examples given. A clear understanding of the methodological and statistical basis on which we make decisions in planning for oral health should be complemented by an appreciation of societal structure (given in Chapter 3); health economic realities (given in Chapter 10) and the principles of how we organize and deliver oral health care (given in Chapter 16).

Further reading

Armstrong, B.K., White, E. and Saracci, R. (1994) *Principles of exposure measurement in epidemiology.* Oxford University Press, Oxford.

Bader, J.D. (ed). (1990) *Risk assessment in dentistry.* University of North Carolina, Chapel Hill, NC.

Beaglehole, R., Bonita, R. and Kjellström, T. (1993) *Basic Epidemiology.* World Health Organization, Geneva.

Clayton, D. and Hills M. (1993) *Statistical Models in Epidemiology.* Oxford University Press, Oxford.

Greenberg, R.S., Daniels, S.R., Eley, J.W. *et al.* (1993) *Medical epidemiology.* Prentice Hall, New Jersey.

Greenland, S. (1990) Randomization, statistics, and causal inference. *Epidemiology* 1:421–429.

Henneken, C.H. and Buring, J.E. (1987) *Epidemiology in Medicine.* Little, Brown, Boston, MA.

Hosmer, D.W. and Lemeshow, S. (1989) *Applied Logistic Regression.* John Wiley, New York.

Hulley, S.B. and Cummings, S.R. (1988) *Designing Clinical Research.* Williams & Wilkins, Baltimore, MD.

Kahn, H.A. and Sempos, C.T. (1989) *Statistical Methods in Epidemiology.* Oxford University Press, Oxford.

Kleinbaum, D.G. (1994) *Logistic Regression. A Self-learning Text.* Springer Verlag, New York.

Kleinbaum, D.G., Kupper, L.L. and Morgenstern, H. (1982) *Epidemiologic Research. Principles and Quantitative Methods.* Lifetime Learning Publications, London.

Kleinbaum, D.G., Kupper, L.L. and Muller, K.E. (1988) *Applied Regression Analysis and Other Multivariable Methods.* Duxbury Press, Belmont, CA.

Last, J.M. (1988) *A Dictionary of Epidemiology.* Oxford University Press, Oxford.

Lwanga, S.K. and Lemeshow, S. (1991) *Sample Size Determination in Health Studies.* World Health Organization, Geneva.

Olsen, J. and Trichopoulos, D. (eds) (1992) *Teaching Epidemiology. What you should know and what you could do.* Oxford University Press, Oxford.

Olsen, J., Overvad, K. and Juul, S. (1994) *Analytisk epidemiology.* Munksgaard, Copenhagen.

Rothman, K.J. (1986) *Modern Epidemiology.* Little, Brown, Boston, MA.

Schlesselman, J.J. (1982) *Case-control Studies.* Oxford University Press, New York.

Schwartz, D. and Lellouch, J. (1967) Explanatory and pragmatic attitudes in therapeutic trials. *Journal of Chronic Disease* 20:229–236.

Stamm, J.W., Stewart, P.W., Bohannan, H.M. *et al.* (1991) Risk assessment for oral diseases. *Advances in Dental Research* 5:4–17.

Wilson, J.M.G. and Jungner, G. (1968) *Principles and Practice of Screening for Disease.* World Health Organization, Geneva.

World Health Organization (1992) *Health Research Methodology. A Guide for Training in Research Methods.* World Health Organization, Regional Office for the Western Pacific, Manila.

6

Public health aspects of oral diseases and disorders

Dental caries

Helen Whelton and Denis M. O'Mullane

Introduction

The Latin word *caries* means rottenness. Dental caries is a localized destruction of the tooth tissue by microorganisms. It has been recorded in *Homo sapiens* since palaeolithic times and apparently increased during the neolithic period. In ancient humans caries was located mainly at the cementoenamel junction or in the cementum, in contrast to more modern times where dental caries is primarily located in pits, fissures and in the smooth surfaces of the teeth. Over the centuries various theories have been proposed for the aetiology of dental caries. These included worms, humours and the vital chemical and septic theories. Later the chemoparasitic proteolytic and the proteolysis-chelation theories were proposed. It is now established that dental caries is a multifactorial disease and results from a combination of four principal factors (Fig. 6.1), host and teeth factors, microorganisms in dental plaque, principally *Streptococcus mutans* and substrate, principally sucrose. The fourth factor, time, is relevant because, even in the presence of the other three factors, the development of dental caries is a relatively slow process and clinically visible destruction of the enamel (cavitation) takes up to 4 years to develop (Newbrun, 1983; Pitts 1983).

The measurement of dental caries

The DMF index, which is a record of the number of decayed, missing and filled teeth (DMFT) or surfaces (DMFS) in permanent teeth was first described by Klein and Palmer (1937) and has now gained global acceptance. For deciduous teeth, because of the difficulty in distinguishing between teeth extracted for caries and natural exfoliation, especially in children aged over 5 years, variations such as the def (decayed, indicated for extraction, filled) and df (decayed filled) have been used (Burt and Eklund, 1992).

The major advantage of the DMF index is that, because of its widespread use worldwide over the past 60 years, it provides a reasonably accurate historical account of changes in the

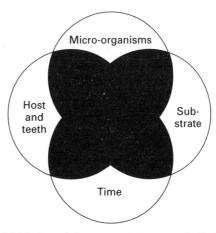

Fig. 6.1 The four circles represent diagrammatically the parameters involved in the carious process. All four factors must be acting concurrently (overlapping of the circles) for caries to occur. From Newbrun (1983), with permission.

prevalence of dental caries. The limitations of the DMF index have been widely recognized. For example, difference still exists between US and European researchers on the method of scoring the decayed (D) component of the index, the former using a sharp probe, the latter a blunt one. Another disadvantage is that the DMF index does not take account of the number of teeth or surfaces at risk in different subjects. The missing (M) component also presents problems amongst adults, for whom the reason for missing teeth is not easy to establish. Perhaps the major difficulty with the DMF index nowadays is the fact that in many studies the F component dominates the scores; fillings have been inserted by dental professionals who vary enormously in their decisions on when to intervene in the carious process and place a filling. Despite these and other limitations, however, the traditional DMF index is recommended for continued use in epidemiological studies of dental caries. Changes in the pattern of dental caries however and also advances in methods of diagnosing caries need to be taken into account when recording and reporting caries studies in the future but without affecting the ability to make historical and international comparisons. The decline in the prevalence of dental caries had made the mean DMFT for a group less informative and frequency distributions with standard deviations are essential in reports of prevalence and incidence caries studies. Perhaps also with the change in the pattern of dental caries, more use should be made of the vast amount of information collected in dental caries studies. For example, in many studies caries is recorded at the very early stage–the white spot? stained fissure to a small cavity to gross cavitation filling or extraction. However, when analysing and reporting the data the grades from cavitation upwards are aggregated when calculating the mean scores per person in the group. This practice would seem an inefficient method of analysing and reporting data, which requires much training and time and resources to collect. As pointed out by Backer Dirks (1966), the power to discriminate between preventive strategies and products in longitudinal cohort studies is likely to be enhanced if the movement of lesions from one grade to the next (including reversals) is taken into account in the analysis and fully reported. The advancing technology in methods of recording precavitation carious lesions is likely to emphasize further the need for

this change in analysis and reporting methods. There has been a welcome recent trend to record levels of healthy teeth and surfaces rather than disease. In adults, for example, the mean number of natural teeth present, the percentage of subjects with more than 20 natural teeth present, the percentage of subjects with 18 or more sound, untraumatized, untreated teeth have been reported (Todd and Lader, 1991; O'Mullane and Whelton, 1992).

For a number of reasons, including the increased retention of natural teeth into old age, interest in root surface caries has increased. Despite this increased interest however, there is no consensus on the methods to be used when recording root surface caries in epidemiological studies. The dilemma was perhaps best highlighted in a report by De Paola *et al.* (1989). They showed how prevalence figures varied depending on which methods are used; the percentage of subjects affected varied between 23 and 85% depending on which method of recording root surface caries was used. At a symposium on this issue (Welton, 1990) at the 1989 International Association for Dental Research (IADR) international meeting the problems associated with recording, analysing and reporting root surface caries data were highlighted. It was recommended that an attempt be made to establish a worldwide consensus on these issues. Also it was suggested that when reporting on root surface caries data, information on the number of teeth present, the number with gingival recession (i.e. with exposed roots), the number of exposed roots with root surface caries (Katz, 1980) and also the percentage edentulous in the group being studied should be routinely presented (Aherne *et al.*, 1990).

The prevalence of dental caries

Levels of dental caries remained low until the 17th century (Hardwick, 1969). Skeletal data collected in England show that the prevalence of dental caries increased dramatically towards the end of the 17th century (Moore and Corbett, 1971, 1973, 1975) and, as in other developed countries, continued to increase until the early 1970s. The only break in this increase came about during the mid 40s and early 50s and coincided with the reduced availability of sucrose as a result of food rationing imposed during and following World War II. Since the mid 1970s reports from developed countries worldwide have shown that the prevalence of dental caries in children and adolescents has declined (Marthaler, 1990, 1995; Glass, 1991; Naylor, 1994). One of the most comprehensive caries data sets is that collected in the UK where national surveys of children's dental health were conducted in 1973, 1983 and 1993 (Downer, 1994) as well as local surveys coordinated by the British Association of Community Dental Health (Pitts and Palmer, 1994). In 1973 the mean DMFT of 12-year-olds in England and Wales was 4.8 whilst in 1992 the corresponding figure was 1.2. The oral health programme of the World Health Organization (WHO) has collated results of epidemiological studies conducted in different countries over the last 20 years through its Global Data Bank. Whilst these latter data confirm a decline in the prevalence of dental caries in children and adolescents resident in developed communities, there is evidence of an increase in dental caries in some developing countries. The most recent data published by the WHO Global Data Bank (1995) show that of the 178 countries for which data were available, 25% were categorized as having very low levels of dental caries (a mean DMFT of 0.0–1.1), 42% as low (DMFT 1.2–2.6), 30% as moderate (DMFT 2.7–4.4), 13% as high (DMFT 4.5–6.5) and 2.1% as very high (DMFT > 6.6). Further details describing trends in dental caries prevalence in both children and adults are given in Chapter 8.

There is now increasing evidence that whilst caries levels have declined in developed countries in the past 20 years there continues to be a large at-risk group for whom caries remains a major problem (Johnson, 1991). Recent reports confirm that in many communities 80% of dental caries is occurring in 20% of the population and has given rise to the risk strategy for the prevention of dental caries as compared with the whole population approach. This is described further in Chapter 1. Perhaps the most widely reported at-risk group are those in the lower socioeconomic groups amongst whom higher caries levels are consistently reported. Recent data from the UK add further to the mounting evidence that dental caries is now largely a disease affecting deprived sections of society (Gratrix and Holloway, 1994; Ellwood and O'Mullane, 1995). For example, high-caris-risk communities tend to bottle-feed their babies, wean them earlier, use infant feeding bottles longer and give babies fruit juices more regularly. Parents in these high-risk caries communities tend to have considerably more social and financial problems and their children have poorer school attendance records and greater consumption of confectionery after school. All of these indicators of dental caries are linked with deprivation and poverty, two conditions which seem unlikely to change for many residents of developed communities in the near future. Strategies such as water fluoridation and increased availability of low-cost fluoride toothpastes (Davies *et al.*, 1995) are more likely to benefit these deprived children than dental health messages to their parents entreating them to alter their lifestyles (Gratrix and Holloway, 1994).

Prevention of dental caries

There have been major advances in understanding how fluoride works to prevent caries and this new knowledge has led to a more rational approach to the use of fluorides (O'Mullane, 1994). When the relationship between fluoride intake and decreased caries prevalence was first recognized it was assumed that the method of action was due to the incorporation of fluoride into the enamel during enamel formation: that, in chemical terms, it involved substitution of the hydroxyl ion with the fluoride ion in hydroxyapatite, leading to the formation of fluorapatite (McClure and Likins, 1951). Fluorapatite was deemed to be less soluble in acid and this reduction in acid solubility of enamel was attributed to larger apatite crystals, better crystallinity and the buffering action of fluoride released from enamel crystals during the early stages of acid attack. It was believed that in order for fluorapatite to be formed it was necessary for the fluoride ion to be present during amelogenesis and hence systemic fluoride was essential. However, later work using sophisticated enamel biopsy and fluoride analysis techniques revealed no simple relationship between enamel fluoride levels and caries experience. Further epidemiological evidence supported this view, in that caries reductions were found in teeth already erupted at the start of fluoridation programmes (Ast *et al.*, 1950; Collins and O'Mullane, 1970). It would seem, therefore, that reduced enamel solubility is not the sole factor involved in the cariostatic action of fluoride (Browne *et al.*, 1977) and furthermore, several studies have failed to demonstrate any relationship between fluoride levels of surface enamel and decreased caries levels (Kidd *et al.*, 1980).

Also during the 1970s understanding of how a carious lesion develops began to change. Initially it was believed that the carious lesion developed as a slow, persistent ongoing process; that it started as a microscopic change leading to a whitespot lesion, which inevitably progressed to a cavity. It is now known that this is not the case and that whitespot lesions and other early carious lesions can remineralize. A whitespot lesion therefore can behave in three different ways; it can progress to a cavity, remain static or reverse (remineralize). The carious process is a delicate balance between demineralization and remineralization and in the mouth there is a constant see-saw between these two phenomena depending on the cariogenic challenge present. The presence of fluoride has been to slow demineralization and also to promote the process of remineralization; indeed the healed lesion has been found to be more resistant to caries attack than a similar unchallenged site (Koulourides *et al.*, 1980). There is also evidence to show that low levels of fluoride in plaque affect plaque metabolism (including glycolysis) in such a way that acid production is reduced. These advances in knowledge, therefore, have changed our thinking on how fluoride works in caries prevention and clearly have a bearing on the rational use of fluoride and have important public health implications. It is now known that its effect is largely therapeutic and its action mainly topical, although some pre-eruptive effect, especially in pits and fissures, has also been demonstrated (Groeneveld *et al.*, 1990).

It would appear, therefore, that fluoride has its most effective use in caries prevention when a low level of fluoride is constantly maintained in the oral cavity. An important reservoir of this fluoride is in plaque, though some is also found in saliva, on the surfaces of the oral soft tissue, and in loosely bound form on the enamel surfaces. Fluoride strategies aimed at regular, low-level exposure to fluoride in order to maintain the ambient level of fluoride in the oral cavity are superior for caries prevention in public health terms to professional applications with high-concentration fluoride products. The latter are most appropriate for selective use on caries-susceptible individuals. In public health, they are less cost-effective, logistically more difficult to target to the needy members of the community and need to be applied at regular intervals to be more effective.

A number of studies have reported that in industrialized countries many parents begin brushing their children's teeth from a very young age, in many societies before the age of 1 year. Reports show that early use of fluoride toothpaste is associated with increased levels of questionable to very mild fluorosis (Osujii *et al.*, 1988; Milson and Mitropoulos, 1990; Riordan, 1993). Further details on enamel opacities are given later in this chapter. Despite the fact that these enamel changes are not an aesthetic problem and are not of public health significance, there have been suggestions that the level of fluoride in toothpastes for young children should be lowered to less than 500 p.p.m. (Rock, 1994). However, there are two important points worth noting in this regard. First there is evidence that caries levels in the deciduous teeth of young children in some countries are increasing (O'Brien, 1994). Second there is no evidence that toothpastes containing less than 500 p.p.m. fluoride will be effective in preventing dental caries (World Health Organization, 1994). It would indeed be ironic that in finding a solution to a problem which is not of public health significance, caries levels in children could increase as a result.

The choice between population strategies such as water fluoridation which are aimed at reducing dental caries in the population as a whole and risk strategies designed to target preventive programmes, such as fissure sealing at high-risk caries groups, has received considerable attention during the past decade. Many caries risk assessment studies have been undertaken with a view to identifying at an early age those subjects who will develop high caries levels in the future (Beck *et al.*, 1992). Many predictors have been employed to predict future caries levels in permanent teeth, such as caries levels in deciduous teeth and salivary factors such as flow rate buffering capacity and residual volume, calcium and phosphate levels and also *Streptococcus mutans* and lactobacillus counts. To date, success has been limited and the application of a risk strategy in the prevention of dental caries is still questionable. The number of subjects predicted by the test as being likely to develop caries and who do not (false positives) and those predicted by the test as being very unlikely to develop caries and who do (false negatives) continues to be excessively high for the successful implementation of a risk strategy for the prevention of dental caries. Despite these uncertainties however, many preventive programmes currently in place contain a combination of population and high-risk strategies.

The evidence linking dietary sugars and dental caries is unequivocal (Rugg-Gunn, 1993), hence numerous dental health education programmes have included advice to reduce the frequency of intake of foods and drinks sweetened with sugars. These factors are thoroughly reviewed in Chapter 13. Dental health education is part of oral health promotion and dental health education programmes have been conducted on a regular basis in many developed countries in the recent past. There are three main messages currently used in dental health education (Health Education Authority, 1989):

- Reduce the frequency of intake of foods and drinks sweetened with sugar.
- brush teeth regularly with a fluoride toothpaste.
- Visit a dental professional regularly.

These three desirable behaviours are regarded as crucial to good oral health. It would seem that some success can be claimed in the case of the latter two measures; however, in the case of altering behaviour relating to sugar consumption, as stated earlier, success to date has been modest.

The improvement in knowledge of the aetiology of dental caries together with study of the recent decline in caries levels and the reasons for this decline form the basis of a rational approach to the prevention of dental caries. The main approaches are described in further detail as follows: fluorides, in Chapters 7 and 14; fissure sealing and plaque control in Chapter 7; dietary choice in Chapter 13; dental health education in Chapter 12; dental health promotion in Chapters 11 and 15.

The management of dental caries

Dentistry is a relatively new profession. Its growth can be traced directly to the developing technology for the management of dental caries which affected over 90% of the population at the end of the 19th century and up to the 1970s. The passing of the Dentists Acts in 1878 in the UK occurred at about the same time as the establishment of the first dental school in Maryland, USA. Over the past 120 years new dental schools have been constructed throughout the world and a close look at their curriculum will show that a very large part of the training provided for dentists has been concerned with the mechanical repair of the destruction caused to the hard tissues by dental caries. In many countries the percentage of the gross national product spent on health services is of the order of 6–8%, though in the USA it is 11% (Burt and Eklund, 1992). The percentage of the total health budget spent on dental services varies generally between 0.5 and 2.0% (Downer *et al.*, 1994). Hence in financial terms the cost of treating dental disease is substantial.

The approach to the treatment of dental caries has changed considerably. Extension for prevention and other principles of cavity preparation, proposed at the early part of the 20th century and followed assiduously by generations of dentists, is now giving way to the minimal tissue removal approach (Elderton, 1990). Developments in the prevention of dental caries and also new knowledge of how the caries lesion develops and progresses have meant that in many educational establishments the minimum intervention approach is being promoted. The role of fluoride in halting the progress of the early caries lesions and its role in the remineralization of these lesions has also been important in this change of philosophy. Development of new methods for the diagnosis of caries, particularly the carious lesion in its early stages, is also likely to affect the management of the carious lesion in the future. The use of bitewing radiographs and their sensible interpretation, fibreoptic transillumination, the electric caries monitor and other diagnostic aids are increasingly making an impact on the practice of dentistry. As pointed out by Elderton (1994), however, these new scientific developments and approaches are not necessarily affecting the management of dental caries amongst the practising profession as a whole. It would appear that the gap between new scientific and philosophical approaches and their implementation in everyday life is large. The science transfer programmes being established by the IADR are one example of the dental research community's efforts to bridge the time lag between new scientific developments and their use in the everyday practice of dentistry.

During the past 10 years questions have been raised about possible health risks associated with use of dental amalgam, the traditional method of restorations of carious cavities in posterior teeth. The issue has occasionally received negative media attention, resulting in considerable public anxiety about the possible toxic effects of slow leakage of small amounts of mercury from amalgam fillings. In fact there is no evidence to show an association between the presence of amalgam fillings in the mouth and any disease or condition (Jones, 1994). It is estimated that over 200 million US citizens have amalgam fillings in their mouths. In England and Wales it is estimated that approximately 50% of the population receive at least one amalgam filling each year and in the former West Germany it has been estimated that 38 million persons received an amalgam filling annually. Clearly, if amalgam presented a health hazard then many of the millions worldwide who have amalgam fillings would have shown signs of various illnesses associated with mercury poisoning. There is in fact no evidence of such happenings. There are aesthetic reasons of course in continuing the search for tooth-coloured materials such as posterior composite resins to replace dental amalgam. However, there is no justification for replacing satisfactory amalgam restorations on the basis that they represent a health hazard.

The widely reported decline in the prevalence of dental caries in children and adolescents over the past 20 years can have a negative impact on future public financing of research aimed at further reductions due to a misplaced wave of optimism amongst decision-makers and funding agencies who believe that the caries problem is as good as solved. It is true that nowadays in many industrialized countries about 50% of children aged 5–12 years have never experienced dental caries. This of course means that 50% have had dental caries, some to a level experienced by the corresponding age groups 20 or 30 years ago. As pointed out by Bowen and Tabak (1993): 'it is difficult to imagine any other circumstances where 50 per cent of a population suffering a disease would evoke such an aura of success'. Dental caries continues to be a major public health problem, is the source of considerable pain and suffering for many, especially amongst the poor and the deprived,

and its management represents a large proportion of the health budgets worldwide. Efforts to prevent dental caries must continue.

References

Aherne, C.A., O'Mullane, D.M. and Barrett, B.E. (1990) Indices of root surface caries. *Journal of Dental Research* **69**:1222–1226.

Ast, D.B., Finn S.B. and McCafferty I. (1950) The Newburgh-Kingston caries fluorine study. I, Dental findings after three years of water fluoridation. *American Journal of Public Health* **40**:116–124.

Backer Dirks, O. (1966) Posteruptive changes in dental enamel. *Journal of Dental Research* **45** (suppl.):503–511.

Beck, J.D., Weintraub, J.A., Dicnes, J.A. *et al.* (1992) University of North Carolina, caries risk study: Comparisons of high risk prediction and risk prediction and high etiology models. *Community Dental and Oral Epidemiology* **20**:313–321.

Bowen, W.H. and Tabak, L.A. (1993) *Cariology for the Nineties*. University of Rochester Press, Rochester, New York.

Brown, W.E., Gregory, T.M. and Chow, L.C. 1977. Effects of fluoride on enamel solubility and cariostasis. *Caries Research* **11** (suppl. 1):118.

Burt, B.A. and Eklund, S.A. (1992) *Dentistry, Dental Practice and the Community*. W. B. Saunders, Philadelphia.

Collins, C. and O'Mullane D. (1970) Dental caries experience in Cork city school children age 4–11 years after 4½ years of fluoridation. *Journal of the Irish Dental Association* **16**:130–134.

Davies, R.M. Holloway,, P.J. and Ellwood R.P. (1995) The role of fluoride dentifrices in a national strategy for the oral health of children. *British Dental Journal* **179**: 84–87.

De Paola, P.F., Soparkar, P.M. and Kent, R.L. Jr (1989) Methodological issues relative to the quantitation of root surface caries. *Gerodontology*, **8**:3–8.

Downer, M.C. (1994) Caries prevalence in the United Kingdom. *International Dental Journal* **44**:367–370.

Downer, M.C., Belbier, S. and Gibbons (1994) *Introduction to Dental Public Health*. F.D.I. World Press, London.

Elderton, R.J. (1990) *Evolution in Dental Care*. Clinical Press, Bristol.

Elderton, R.J. (1994) The effect of changes in caries prevalence on dental education. *International Dental Journal* **44**:445–450.

Ellwood, R.E. and O'Mullane D.M. (1995) The association between oral deprivation and dental caries in groups with and without fluoride in their drinking water. *Community Dental Health* **12**:18–22.

Glass, R.L. (1982) The first international conference on the declining prevalence of dental caries. The evidence and the impact on dental education, dental research and dental practice. *Journal of Dental Research* **61** (suppl.):1301–1383.

Gratrix, D. and Holloway, P.J. (1994) Factors of deprivation associated with dental caries in young children. *Community Dental Health* **11**:66–70.

Groeneveld, A., Van Eck A. and Backer Dirks O. (1990) Fluoride in caries prevention: is the effect pre or post operative? *Dental Research* **69**, 751.

Hardwick, J.L. (1969) The incidence and distribution of caries throughout the ages in relation to the Englishman's diet. *British Dental Journal* **108**: 9–17.

Health Education Authority (1989) *The Scientific Bases of Dental Health Education*, 3rd edn. Health Education Authority, London.

Johnson M.W. (ed. (1991) *Risk Makers for Oral Diseases, volume 1, Dental Caries*. Cambridge University Press, Cambridge.

Jones, D.W. (1994) The enigma of amalgam in dentistry. *British Dental Journal* **177**:159–170.

Katz, R.V. (1980) Assessing root caries in populations: The evaluation of the root caries index. *Journal of Public Health Dent* **40**: 7–15.

Katz, R.V., Hazen, S.P., Chilton, N.W. and Mumma, R.D. Jr. (1982) Prevalence and intra-oral distribution of root caries in an adult population. *Caries Research* **16**:265–171.

Kidd E., Thylstrup, A., Fejerskov, O. *et al.* (1980) Influence of fluoride in surface enamel and degree of dental fluorosis on caries development *in vitro*. *Caries Research* **14**:196.

Klein, H. and Palmer, C.E. (1937) *Dental Caries in American Indian children*. Public Health bulletin no. 239. US Government Printing Office.

Koulourides, T., Keller, S., Manson-Hing L. *et al.* (1980) Enhancement of fluoride effectiveness by experimental cariogenic priming of human enamel. *Caries Research* **14**:32.

McClure, F.J. and Likins, R.C. (1951) Fluorine in human teeth studied in relation to fluorine in the drinking water. *Journal of Dental Research* **30**:172–176.

Marthaler, T.M. (1990) Caries status in Europe and future trends. *Caries Research* **24**: 381–396.

Marthaler, T.M. (1995) The prevalence of dental caries in Europe, update 1990–1995. *Caries Research* **30**: 237–255.

Milson, K. and Mitropoulos, C. (1990) Enamel defects in 8-year-old children in fluoridated and non-fluoridated parts of Cheshire. *Caries Research* **24**:285–289.

Moore, W.J. and Corbett, M.E. (1971) The distribution of caries in ancient British populations 1. Anglo Saxon period. *Caries Research* **5**:150–158.

Moore, W.J. and Corbett, M.E. (1973) The distribution of caries in ancient British populations 2. Iron age, Romano, British and medieval periods. *Caries Research* **7**:139–153.

Moore, W.J. and Corbett, M.E. (1975) The distribution of dental caries in ancient British populations. 3. The 17th century. *Caries Research* **9**:163–172.

Naylor, N.M. (1994) Second international conference on declining caries. *International Dental Journal* **44** (suppl.):363–458.

Newbrun, E. (1983) *Cariology*. Williams & Wilkins, Baltimore.

O'Brien, M. (1994) *Children's Dental Health in the United Kingdom 1993*. HMSO, London.

O'Mullane, D.M. (1993) Are we using epidemiology effectively? In: *Cariology for the Nineties* (Bowen, W.H. and Tabak, L.A., eds) pp. 51–60. University of Rochester Press, New York.

O'Mullane, D.M. (1994) Introduction and rationale for the use of fluorides for caries prevention. *International Dental Journal* **44**:257–261.

O'Mullane, D.M. and Whelton H. (1992) *Oral Health of Irish Adults 1989–90*. Stationery Office, Dublin.

Osujii, O., Leake, M., Chipman G., Mikoforuh., G., Loener, D. and Levine, M. (1988) Risk factors for dental fluorosis in a fluoridated community. *Journal of Dental Research* **67**:1488–1492.

Pitts, N.B. (1983) Monitoring of caries progression in permanent and primary posterior approximal enamel by bitewing radiography. *Community Dental and Oral Epidemiology* **11**:228–235.

Pitts, N.B. and Palmer J.D. (1994) The dental caries experience of 5–12 and 14-year-old children in Great Britain. Surveys coordinated by the British Association for the Study of Community Dentistry in 1991/92, 1992/93 and 1990/91. *Community Dental Health* **11**:45–52.

Riordan, P.J. (1993) Dental fluorosis, dental caries and fluoride exposure among 7-year-olds. *Caries Research* **27**:71–77.

Rock, W.P. (1994)–Young children and fluoride toothpaste. *British Dental Journal* **117**:17–20.

Rugg-Gunn, A.J. (1991) *Sugarless – The Way Forward*. Elsevier Applied Science, London.

Rugg-Gunn, A.J. (1993) *Motivation and Dental Health*. Oxford Medical Publications, Oxford.

Todd, J.E. and Lader, D. (1991) *Adult Dental Health 1988*. HMSO, London.

Welton, H. (1990) *Proceedings: Symposium 'Root Surfaces Caries' Preface. Journal of Dental Research* **69**(5): 1194.

World Health Organization (1994) *Fluorides and Oral Health*. Technical report series 846. WHO, Geneva.

World Health Organization (1995) *Oral Health Programme*. 12 Yr. Book/95.3. WHO, Geneva.

Periodontal diseases

Taco Pilot

Periodontal diseases: what is the problem?

Changing concepts on the progression of periodontal diseases

During the 1980s, a major conceptual advance was made related to the progression of destructive periodontal diseases. The more traditional concept was replaced by the new concept of risk for periodontal destruction. The traditional concept was of *continuous progression* of chronic inflammation: when plaque control was not perfect, gingivitis would develop; the process would proceed into the deeper layers of the periodontium, slowly but continuously progressing. It advanced for all persons and all teeth, with loss of attachment to the terminal stages of the disease when extraction was inevitable. In the traditional concept, periodontal disease was believed to be the main cause of tooth loss after the age of 40 and, therefore, the main contributor to edentulousness in middle age. The current *concept of risk* for periodontal destruction acknowledges the cause-and-effect relationship between the microbial plaque and the inflammatory reaction in the gingiva. However, the disease is considered to progress in relatively short episodes of rapid tissue destruction, sometimes followed by some repair, and mostly by prolonged periods of quiescence.

There is still much scientific debate as to which model of progression is the best one. However, there is consensus that loss of attachment is neither evenly distributed within the dentition, nor in the population. Throughout the scientific debate, dental plaque is still considered to be the cause of most, if not all types of periodontal diseases. *Dental plaque* is the important factor in the whole chain of events which leads from the healthy periodontium to tooth loss because of periodontal diseases. But the attack from bacterial plaque and the resistance of the host accounts for a variety of disease patterns. Periodontal diseases result from an imbalance between potentially pathogenic microbes and the nature and efficacy of the local and systemic host responses. Pathogens are necessary but not sufficient for disease to occur. The pathogens must be actively producing virulence factors and the host must be susceptible to a sufficient number of them–beyond a threshold which will vary with subject, sites and time–for periodontal breakdown to occur.

Risk for periodontal destruction, risk factors and risk groups

There must be varying degrees of risk involved, as the definition of risk is the probability of an event occurring within a given period of time. Some people are more exposed to risk factors than others or have less resistance to risk factors. It is likely that the variation with regard to risk for periodontal destruction within and between populations is best represented and described on a continuous scale (Fig. 6.2). It may even be in a normal distribution which–like so many biomedical distributions–is slightly skewed towards one end (Rose, 1985). Most diseases can be depicted in this way, certainly those that have multifactorial causes or influences. Examples are cardiovascular and respiratory diseases, but also the ailments caused through traffic accidents and resulting from occupational hazards or injuries. The question remains then: what are the factors determining the frequency distribution of risk for periodontal breakdown? Are the people in the tail of the distribution curve there because of normal chance variation or are identifiable factors causing people to end up in this tail?

A *risk factor* is causally related and increases the probability of occurrence of disease. In the present case, the issue is not the reversible gingivitis, but the destructive periodontitis. Risk factors can be modified, e.g. smoking. *Disease determinants* however cannot be modified, e.g. race and gender. In recent reviews and consensus conferences it has been confirmed that race and gender *per se* do not make substantial contributions to the variations in prevalence and severity of periodontal diseases around the world. There exists some genetic predisposition associated with severe periodontitis in some

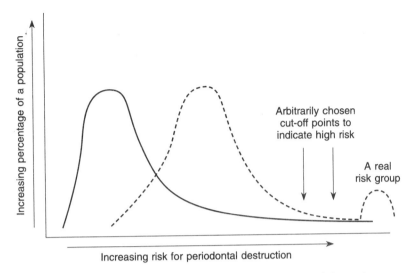

Fig. 6.2 Potential distribution curves of persons at risk of periodontal destruction.

relatively rare diseases. A range of acquired systemic diseases increases susceptibility for destructive periodontal diseases. The most frequently cited examples are diabetes and acquired immune deficiency syndrome (AIDS; human immunodeficiency virus or HIV infection). Insulin-dependent diabetes mellitus may influence periodontal health, especially if the diabetes is poorly controlled. As a result of compromised defence mechanisms, an HIV-infected person is likely to become a target for several infectious diseases, including periodontal diseases. Usual as well as unusual manifestations of common periodontal diseases may occur.

Some periodontal destruction might be related to emotional stress. One could make a case for the potential influence of stressful life-events. But it is very difficult to prove a straightforward relationship. Nutrition is still an area to be investigated. However, all of the above explains at present only a very small part of the periodontal destruction in the world. When discussing oral health at the community level, one should concentrate on the prime risk factors and the most important risk groups. Then the message becomes relatively simple. All available evidence strongly supports the opinion that plaque control is essentially the only decisive factor in the prevention and treatment of the vast majority of periodontal diseases.

Smoking is an additional risk factor. There is consensus in the literature that tobacco smoking is associated with aggravated periodontal breakdown. Hence heavy smokers and long-term smokers should be considered a *risk group*. Two special risk groups need to be considered. While age *per se* seems not be a risk factor, it is easy to see that in older age cohorts more periodontal destruction will be prevalent. The life-time accumulation of the effects of periodontal diseases is apparent. The number of medically compromised persons is increased. Many elderly people frequently use medicines which might have an adverse side-effect on the periodontal tissues. Physical and mental handicaps are frequent. And with many of the elderly belonging to groups of the frail, the functionally dependent or the institutionalized, there will be problems in oral hygiene, whether it is self-care or performed by the nursing staff.

There is another risk group. It is most likely that the negative effects of the (potential) risk factors culminate at the tail end of the population distribution; people represented here are more exposed to risk factors and/or have less resistance to them. Health inequalities are obviously related to social and environmental inequalities. This also applies to periodontal destruction as there might be a concentration of the mentally, physically and genetically handicapped persons at the tail end of the scale for risk; those who are socially and educationally deprived, the lower socioeconomic strata of every population where many ailments, diseases and handicaps seem to accumulate. Economic and social deprivation is not only an issue in connection with deprived areas in the big cities of the industrialized countries. Basically the same applies to large sections of the populations in many developing countries.

Diagnostic tests and predictors of progression

Diagnostic tests are a much-debated issue in periodontology. It is necessary to distinguish between *indicators* of current destructive disease activity, for diagnosis of current disease or monitoring the effect of therapy and *predictors* of future periodontal breakdown, for prognosis of disease activity in a future period of life.

Progress in research on indicators of disease activity could assist in providing better, more effective and more efficient periodontal care. There is progress in the areas of tests for disease activity and of tests for specific infection, which are certainly not the same. Quite a number of 'test kits' for disease activity are commercially available, but the debate on their practical usefulness is ongoing. They might assist in monitoring the success of treatment and identifying those who need a detailed examination. Such developments will certainly benefit a small group of patients in the population, but it is questionable whether they will bring progress on a population base, let alone on a world scale. The really important area is the one of predictors of future breakdown. One would like to have clinical or laboratory measurements that are able to predict future periodontal breakdown in subjects with an intact periodontium or at least be able to identify subjects at a very early stage of one of the destructive periodontal diseases. The consensus is that, although some progress has been made, at present no biotechnology for prognostic indicators is available that can be recommended for general use in a practice or as a screening tool for populations.

However, some progress has been made and it seems that the clinician and the public health planner have two predictors which could be applied with reasonable confidence. Healthy gingiva–not bleeding on gentle probing–seems to be a good predictor of the maintenance of periodontal *health* (Lang *et al.*, 1990; Joss *et al.*, 1994). Papapanou *et al.* (1989) reported on the progression of periodontal disease in a Swedish population assessed radiographically over a 10-year period. Subjects most affected by bone loss at entry were the ones most prone to develop further disease progression. This observation

was confirmed in a Japanese population by Lindhe *et al.* (1989) and Haffejee *et al.* (1991). Past experience seems to be a predictor for future breakdown. This phenomenon is what some researchers call 'attachment loss for age'. The amount of loss of periodontal attachment, or alveolar bone, is compared to the age of the patient (the time the tooth has been present in the mouth). Severe destruction early in life is an indicator of more destruction later in life. It is a other diseases and ailments, for example, eye diseases, back pains, diseases of the respiratory tract. It is not surprising that periodontal diseases follow suit.

Periodontal diseases: public health problem?

Periodontal epidemiology

The main concern in periodontology seems to be the slowly progressing, chronic inflammatory adult periodontitis. But are periodontal diseases a public health problem? Or more specifically, is periodontal breakdown a public health problem–a problem of major proportions, worldwide? The first step is to obtain an overview of present periodontal conditions around the world. For most industrialized countries, a two-level approach can be followed. Elaborate descriptions of periodontal health and disease conditions (some with a longitudinal component, some on a national representative basis) have been published in the 1980s and 1990s for a number of countries: in northern Europe, e.g. Denmark, Germany, Ireland, the Netherlands, Norway, Sweden, Switzerland, the UK (e.g. Pilot and Miyazaki, 1991). Large surveys have been published for the USA. New Zealand provides an example of frequent national surveys on periodontal health. Results of detailed periodontal surveys are available for only a few developing countries, e.g. China, Kenya, Sri Lanka, Tanzania.

Most of these surveys provide considerable detail and depth. The results could be applied in the process of planning for periodontal care, perhaps also in neighbouring countries where such detailed surveys have not been carried out. However, international comparison is difficult to perform because of the different, often elaborate methods applied. Some of these studies provide indepth details, which are of great value for the researcher, but superfluous to the public health decision-maker: more details do not always assist in making decisions!

A less complex and internationally established method of estimating levels of periodontal conditions in populations, which is widely used, is the WHO Community Periodontal Index of Treatment Needs or CPITN (Cutress *et al.*, 1987). In less than a decade, the CPITN has become an established index and has generated considerable data to identify, in populations, periodontal conditions for which specific interventions might be considered. By 1995, there were an estimated 500 publications in scientific journals and reports contributing to the accumulated results of CPITN data; most of the results are incorporated into a WHO data bank. At the Global Oral Data Bank (GODB) at WHO headquarters in Geneva, the results of CPITN surveys from many countries are received, analysed and stored. Together they provide a frame of reference for the evaluation of periodontal conditions in populations and population subgroups. The WHO publication *Periodontal Profiles* (World Health Organization, 1994) first appeared in 1990 and is regularly updated. Profiles are published for three so-called key age groups: adolescents (15–19 years), adults (35–44 years) and an older age cohort (65–74 years).

The periodontal problem on a world scale

The detailed information available for some countries and the CPITN periodontal profiles have provided an insight into the magnitude of the periodontal disease problem on a world scale, its prevalence and severity, at least up to an age of around 60 years. In adolescents (15–19 years) bleeding on probing and calculus are the most frequently observed conditions. It is evident that the levels of calculus are on average much higher in most developing countries than in the industrialized countries. Pocketing of 4 or 5 mm deep is present in most of the populations surveyed. But with a few exceptions, e.g. surveys from some Caribbean islands, specific Indian populations in the USA and some African populations, it affects only a small minority of the sample and then only in one or two sextants. From surveys in adults (around age 40), it appears that completely healthy subjects are virtually absent in most surveys. Calculus and pocketing of 4 or 5 mm deep are the most

frequently observed conditions. With a few exceptions, the percentages of persons and the mean number of sextants per person affected by pockets of 6 mm or deeper are small. In most surveys the percentage of people affected is 15% or less; quite a number of surveys indicate 5% or less. Even more important, in persons with pockets of 6 mm or deeper, it is mostly in two sextants only. A pocket 6 mm deep means a loss of periodontal attachment of some 4 mm, which by some researchers is considered the threshold of tooth survival, especially in the furcation area of the molar teeth.

It is interesting to note the absence of clear differences for the more severe stages of periodontal diseases in this age category between industrialized and developing countries. The view that periodontal diseases are much more a problem of developing countries seems to be true only in terms of poorer oral hygiene and considerably greater calculus retention. There are a number of exceptions, but the relative similarity in deep pocketing around the world is far more striking. Thus, generalized periodontal destruction is very rare in adolescents and unusual among adults around age 40. For certain, not all gingivitis progresses into periodontitis; there is less periodontal destruction in adults than it was the tendency to believe some 20 years ago.

Therefore, periodontal diseases are not the major cause of tooth loss before age 50 and not the major reason for edentulousness before age 60. For the majority of people, the progress of periodontal destruction seems to be compatible with the retention of a natural functioning dentition into older age. However, the periodontal problem is still of considerable magnitude and importance as bleeding on probing is widely encountered in the younger age groups. Furthermore, 5–15% of populations affected by a serious, irreversible condition (4 mm attachment loss, pockets of 6 mm or deeper, threatening tooth life) is high, compared with most other diseases that afflict humanity. In addition, it should be stressed that reliable epidemiological data on the periodontal health of older age groups are scarce, also for CPITN. But even more, these are difficult to interpret. In some industrialized countries, there is still considerable tooth loss and high levels for edentulousness are encountered because of the lifelong accumulated effects of dental caries, and of the treatment techniques and philosophies of the past. The critical age of tooth longevity (Hellden *et al.*, 1989) in relation to progressing periodontal destruction seems to have shifted from 35–40 years (which was believed some decades ago) to 50, and may be now around 60 years. It may be that the young adults of today (with far less caries than earlier generations) will also become 'happy survivors', with regard to periodontal diseases. However, as yet, there are insufficient epidemiological data to support such a statement. Nor is there scientific evidence for a worldwide decline in the prevalence and severity of periodontal diseases. Epidemiologists might have obtained a better perspective of the problem which permits a more optimistic outlook. And it is well-documented that periodontal health in adolescents and adults has improved in some industrialized countries, notably in north-west Europe. But an increasing number of elderly persons will retain more teeth, for longer, at risk to periodontal destruction, which increases the periodontal problem (see for review, e.g. Pilot and Miyazaki, 1991).

Treatment needs and goals for periodontal health

To what extent is periodontal destruction a public health problem? This question also relates to the definition of health and to what can be considered a reasonable and attainable goal. Wennström *et al.* (1990) have proposed that the goal of periodontal care in society should be defined as the control of the development of destructive periodontal disease in order to prevent loss of function of the tooth/dentition throughout life, rather than the prevention and/or elimination of *all* clinical signs of periodontal inflammation. Thus, some plaque, calculus, gingivitis and even attachment loss can be accepted, as long as this does not threaten the proper function and the survival of the dentition. This proposal has been translated into a tentative model for decision-making regarding periodontal treatment needs, based on the amount of remaining periodontal bone support in relation to age. The goal for this decision-making model is considered to be a maintained alveolar bone height at the age of 75 years corresponding to at least one-third of the root length (other goals or levels could be substituted). In Figure 6.3 the model has been depicted in a simplified form. By assuming that the alveolar bone level at 25 years is 'normal', one can draw a line which is the critical limit of the level of alveolar bone between age 25 and 75 years. As long as the alveolar bone is coronal of the critical limit, the tooth (person) is considered safe. As soon as the resorption of the alveolar bone goes so fast that the level comes apical of the critical limit, the tooth (person) might be considered at risk and intervention should be considered. Periodontal treatment need would then be considered as the amount of treatment necessary to obtain or maintain the above-described health goal.

The strategy towards community periodontal health

The main emphasis should clearly be on a strategy towards the population. The major goal should be prevention, or at least reduction of

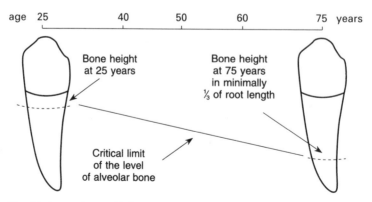

Fig. 6.3 A tentative model for decision-making in periodontal care. Based on Wennström *et al.* (1990).

the rate of attachment loss. Prevention in populations means shifting of distributions on the scale of risk towards reduced exposure to risk and reducing rates of progression. If the population could be moved towards more awareness of periodontal health and disease and towards more effective oral hygiene, it might be able to shift the vast majority away from gingivitis, which always has the potential danger of developing into destructive periodontitis. The costs of an awareness campaign for improved oral hygiene are relatively low and harmful side-effects are few. Toothbrushing is supporting gingival health and improving appearance and it is widely accepted by the public in most parts of the world. Healthy gingivae facilitate the good quality of restorative procedures and favour the prognosis of dental treatment in general. Furthermore, healthy gingivae are pleasant to look at and prevent bad breath. Many will be grateful for the improvement in social functioning, well-being and enjoyment.

Prevention campaigns in periodontology should be concentrated on the younger age groups for two reasons. First, the prevention component of lifestyle should be induced and accepted at a young age. Second, as one cannot detect the real risk patient at a young age (attachment loss for age), one might as well consider them all for the time being as belonging to the potential risk group. Isolated campaigns specifically to improve oral hygiene will not be very (cost) effective. A general approach of health promotion based on social, educational and economic development will have a better chance of long term and lasting effects. In this respect, oral hygiene should not be a periodontal health/disease issue, but a normal part of bodily hygiene and grooming behaviour. It should relate to well-being, appearance and social acceptability. The driving force to improve periodontal health might be commercial advertising for toothpastes rather than professional (oral health) intervention.

Professional removal of calculus supports better oral hygiene through self-care in the individual. However, one should be reluctant to propose professional cleaning at regular intervals for everybody, because then everybody is made a patient for life, which is not necessary in periodontology. And for many populations it is totally unrealistic economically to propose regular scaling on a population basis. Scarce resources would be far better applied to stimulate reduction of plaque levels through self-care. In the future, improvements in toothpastes–additions of antiplaque, anticalculus, antigingivitis agents–might further assist in effective self-care. A small yearly decrease of, for example, only 3% (in volume of plaque or in calculus scores) would have a tremendous cumulative effect for the next generation of adolescents.

References

Cutress, T.W., Ainamo, J. and Sardo Infirri, J. (1987) The community periodontal index of treatment needs (CPITN) procedure for population groups and individuals. *International Dental Journal* 37:222–233.

Haffajee, A.D., Socransky, S.S., Lindhe, J. *et al.* (1991) Clinical risk indicators for periodontal attachment loss. *Journal of Clinical Periodontology* 18: 117–125.

Hellden, L., Salonen, L. and Gustafsson, I. (1989) Oral health status in an adult Swedish population. *Swedish Dental Journal* 12:45–60.

Joss, A., Adler, R. and Lang, N.P. (1994) Bleeding on probing. A parameter for monitoring periodontal conditions in clinical practice. *Journal of Clinical Periodontology* 21:402–408.

Lang, N.P., Adler, R., Joss, A. and Nyman, S. (1990) Absence of bleeding on probing–an indicator of periodontal stability. *Journal of Clinical Periodontology* 17: 714–721.

Lindhe, J., Okamoto, H., Yoneyama, T. *et al.* (1989) Periodontal loser sites in untreated adult subjects. *Journal of Clinical Periodontology* 16: 671–678.

Papapanou, P.N., Wennström, J.L. and Gröndahl, K. (1989) A 10 year retrospective study of periodontal disease progression. *Journal of Clinical Periodontology* 16: 403–411.

Pilot, T. and Miyazaki, H.M. (1991) Periodontal conditions in Europe. *Journal of Clinical Periodontology* 18: 353–357.

Rose, G. (1985) Sick individuals and sick populations. *International Journal of Epidemiology* 14:32–38.

Wennström, J.L., Papapanou, P.N. and Gröndahl, K. (1990) A model for decision making regarding periodontal treatment needs. *Journal of Clinical Periodontology* 17:217–222.

World Health Organization. (1994) *Periodontal Profiles. An Overview of CPITN Data in the WHO Global Oral Data Bank.* WHO, Geneva.

Recommended reading: proceedings of (consensus) conferences

Chilton, N.W. (ed.) (1986) Proceedings of the conference on clinical trials in periodontal diseases. *Journal of Clinical Periodontology* 13:335–549.

Guggenheim, B. (ed.) (1988) *Periodontology Today*. Karger, Basel.

Johnson, N.W. (ed.) (1991) *Periodontal Diseases. Markers of Disease Susceptibility and Activity*. Cambridge University Press, Cambridge.

Löe H and Brown L.J. (ed.) (1993) *Classification and Epidemiology of Periodontal Diseases*. Periodontology 2000, vol. 2. Munksgaard, Copenhagen.

Lang, N.P. and Karring, T. (ed.) (1994) *Proceedings of the First European Workshop on Periodontology*. Quintessence, London.

Pilot, T. and Purdell Lewis, D.J. (ed.) (1992) *Guidelines for Community Periodontal Care*. FDI World Dental Press, London.

Proceedings of the Conference on 15 years of CPITN (1994) Outcomes and issues. *International Dental Journal* **44** (suppl. 1):52–59.

Proceedings of the International Conference on periodontal research (1987) *Journal of Periodontology Research* **22**:161–254.

Proceedings of the Third North Sea Conference on Periodontology (1991) *Journal of Clinical Periodontology* **18**:352–498.

Oral cancer

Martin C. Downer

Epidemiology of oral cancer

The term oral cancer is most frequently taken to include squamous cell carcinoma of the lip (ICD 140), tongue (ICD 141), gum (ICD 143), floor of mouth (ICD 144) and unspecified parts of the mouth (ICD 145; Johnson and Warnakulasuriya, 1993). The ICD numbers refer to the World Health Organization's classification of diseases (1977). The epidemiology of cancer is usually described in terms of the yearly incidence of new cases and mortality per 100 000 of a given population. Most data are derived from cancer registries, established over the years in many countries and regions of the world. While internationally coordinated efforts are made continually to improve standards and consistency of reporting (Parkin and Muir, 1992), the completeness and accuracy of registration are known to vary substantially.

The nine most common cancers in the industrialized world in 1980 in order of rank were lung, colon/rectal, breast, stomach, prostate, bladder, lymphatic system, mouth/pharynx and uterus (Parkin *et al.*, 1988). There are approximately 2000 newly diagnosed cases of oral cancer in England and Wales each year with an incidence of 4.5 per 100 000 (Office of Population Censuses and Surveys, 1994). In the UK it represents 1–2% of total cancer incidence. On the other hand, in parts of India carcinoma of the tongue in particular is the most common form of cancer and overall, oral cancer comprises 30–50% of total cancer incidence. The tongue is the most frequently involved oral site in the England and Wales population while floor of the mouth ranks second with about half the number of cases (Johnson and Warnakulasuriya, 1993).

Oral cancer incidence increases with age. The rates for mouth cancer (ICD 143–145) among males in England and Wales, for example, rise steadily from 0.1 per 100 000 in the 25–29-year age group to 12.3 in those aged 85 years and over (Parkin *et al.*, 1992). Males in a given population almost invariably have higher age-specific incidence rates than females for all types of oral cancer, as illustrated in Table 6.1. Exposure to sunlight has been implicated as a major risk factor for lip cancer (Lindquist and Teppo, 1978), with fair-skinned, male outdoor workers being particularly affected. The other important factor is exposure to tobacco, particularly from pipe smoking.

For intraoral disease the two main risk factors are tobacco use and alcohol consumption (Macfarlane, 1993). Diets high in fat (Marshall *et al.*, 1992), a low intake of foods containing vitamin A, or its precursor β-carotene, and iron deficiency are also important predisposing factors (Johnson and Warnakulasuriya, 1993). In addition, dietary fibre and vitamin C intake have been found to have an inverse association with oral cancer risk and, importantly, some protective effect from vitamin C has been shown, among heavy smokers in particular (Macfarlane, 1993).

Table 6.1 Incidence rates of oral cancer per 100 000 population in selected locations (1983–87) by site, gender and ethnic group (where specified), age-standardized to the world population

Site, gender and ethnicity	England and Wales	France (Bas-Rhin)	USA	Bermuda	India (Ahmedabad)	Japan (Miyagi)
Lip (ICD 140)						
Male	0.5	0.4			0.6	0.2
Female	0.1	0.1			0.5	0.1
White male			2.3			
White female			0.2			
Black male			0.1	0.0		
Black female			0.1	0.0		
Tongue (ICD 141)						
Male	1.0	10.2			14.0	1.6
Female	0.5	0.8			2.2	0.6
White male			2.7			
White female			1.2			
Black male			3.6	16.3		
Black female			1.1	1.1		
Mouth (ICD 143–145)						
Male	1.4	13.4			6.1	0.9
Female	0.6	1.1			3.7	0.4
White male			3.5			
White female			1.8			
Black male			4.9	12.1		
Black female			1.5	1.4		

From Parkin *et al.* (1992), with permission.

Both smoking and alcohol consumption are important independent risk factors (Wynder *et al.*, 1957; Brugere *et al.*, 1986; Blot *et al.*, 1988) and there is evidence that their combined effect is greater than the sum of the risks from exposure to either on its own (Rothman and Keller, 1972; Brugere *et al.*, 1986; Franceschi *et al.*, 1990). A dose–response relationship between tobacco smoking and oral cancer has been demonstrated in the investigations cited as well as by others (Graham *et al.*, 1977; Franco *et al.*, 1989; Zheng *et al.*, 1990) while differential relative risks according to type of use, type of tobacco and tar content have also been shown (Merletti *et al.*, 1989; Franceschi *et al.*, 1990; La Vecchia *et al.*, 1990).

Variations in oral cancer incidence, like those in Table 6.1, between geographical regions and countries suggest differential population exposures to specific risk factors. For example, the exceptional rates for intraoral cancer in Bas-Rhin, France, also reflected to some extent elsewhere in that country, notably Calvados, have been attributed to the high consumption of crudely distilled spirit. High incidence rates in India are associated with the habit of betel-quid chewing where the addition of tobacco to the quid is the critical factor. Tobacco chewing among Indians carries a higher risk than smoking, possibly due to the enhanced topical action of nitrosamines which are present in higher concentration in exudations from betel-quid than in tobacco smoke (Johnson and Warnakulasuriya, 1993). In the USA an increased risk from the use of smokeless tobacco (snuff-dipping), after controlling for smoking habits, has been revealed in national cancer survey data. Nevertheless, snuff-dipping in the USA is far less prevalent than betel-quid chewing in India. The higher incidence rates for intraoral cancer shown among black compared with white males in the USA, and the singularly high rates among black males in Bermuda (Table 6.1), are likely to be related to social deprivation which is associated with increased alcohol and tobacco use, and poor nutrition.

Oral precancer

Although oral cancer often apparently arises *de novo*, there are also a number of clinically identifiable precursor lesions which constitute a detectable preclinical phase. The most important of these are leukoplakia, erythroplakia and lichen planus. Potentially malignant lesions such as leukoplakia and other conditions associated with a high risk may be present in up to 5% of the population over 40 years of age in industrialized countries (Bouquot and Gorlin, 1986; Axéll, 1987; Bánóczy and Rigo, 1991; Kleinman *et al.*, 1991). However, their rates of malignant transformation are generally low. The proportion of leukoplakias which have been reported as undergoing malignant change in follow-up studies varies from 0.1 to about 10% (Einhorn and Wersäll, 1967; Silverman *et al.*, 1976; Bánóczy, 1977). An overall rate of transformation of 2–4% for leukoplakia and 1% for lichen planus could be regarded as reasonable estimates for industrialized countries. It has also been established that a patient with leukoplakia has a greater chance of developing cancer than a person without a lesion, with an estimated relative risk of 7 in women and around 5 in men (Silverman *et al.*, 1976). In addition, about 3-6% of patients have lesions diagnosed clinically as leukoplakia which are found at biopsy to be carcinoma (Waldron and Shafer, 1975).

It may take 10–15 years for a leukoplakia to progress to oral cancer (Speight and Morgan, 1993), although it is not possible to predict accurately from their clinical appearance those lesions that will. The most important determinant of the relative risk of malignant change is the presence of epithelial dysplasia on histological examination; various clinical features of leukoplakia to do with colour (red speckling) and texture (roughened, nodular surface) correlate to some extent with degrees of severity of dysplastic change. The location of lesions is also significant. The lateral border of the tongue, floor of the mouth, lower buccal sulcus and alveolus, and angle of the mouth are the sites most at risk (Speight and Morgan, 1993). Because of the potentially lethal nature of precancerous lesions, which are generally without symptoms of pain or discomfort, it is important that apparently healthy people with the disease are identified and kept under continuing clinical supervision.

Public health issues

In the 1990s a number of important public health issues pertaining to oral cancer emerged. First, in several industrialized countries analyses of registration data showed that incidence and mortality were increasing. Pronounced upward trends in men in particular were observed in Scotland by Boyle *et al.* (1993) and in England and Wales by Hindle *et al.* (1994) among people aged 35–64 years, possibly associated with rising alcohol consumption since cigarette smoking had declined. Second, despite many advances in surgical techniques and rehabilitation for oral cancer patients, it was apparent that there had been no improvement in prognosis for many decades (Stell and McCormick, 1985). The incidence to mortality ratio for oral cancer in the late 1980s was 2.21 and was comparable to that of 2.07 for cancer of the cervix and 2.79 for melanoma. The annual registrations of new cases were 1982, 4496 and 3119 respectively for these diseases (Johnson and Warnakulasuriya, 1993).

However, there was also some encouragement from knowledge that small lesions and precancerous lesions can be treated conservatively whereas the treatment of advanced lesions is associated with substantial physical and psychological morbidity, and the prognosis is poor. Evidence from a large European cancer study (Platz *et al.*, 1986) indicated, for example, that for two patients aged between 50 and 70 years with lesions differing only in size, the median survival time is reduced by 4 years for the patient with a lesion greater than 4 cm in diameter. Poor survival is in part due to a failure to detect small lesions since at least 60% of patients present with lesions over 2 cm in diameter and, coincidentally, 60% of patients die from their disease within 5 years (Hindle and Nally, 1991). It would seem that the key to better quality and length of survival is more effective detection of disease at a premalignant stage or when the invasive lesion is small. This supposition, combined with our knowledge of the risk factors for oral cancer, has major public health implications.

Primary prevention

With such well-known risk factors as tobacco and alcohol (carrying an attributable risk of 75-95%) it is theoretically possible to prevent a substantial proportion of oral cancers (Cancer Research Campaign, 1993). Even for patients who already have precancerous lesions, there is encouraging evidence from a large primary intervention trial in India that the chance of these undergoing malignant change is reduced if the patients can be persuaded to curtail their dependence on tobacco (Gupta *et al.*, 1992). Findings from a study in Sri Lanka (Warnakulasuriya, 1984) cited by the Cancer Research Campaign (1993) suggest that using primary health care workers to educate adults not to indulge in the habit of betel-quid chewing may be five times more cost-effective in reducing mortality than providing high-technology treatment for those with disease. The benefits of educating children not to take up the chewing habit are likely to be considerably greater. In industrialized countries reducing smoking and alcohol consumption is a general health promotion strategy. Thus health promotion directed towards lowering the incidence of oral cancer is reinforced by general health policy through a common risk factor approach (Downer, 1994).

Secondary prevention

The value of case-finding in the control of oral cancer and precancer cannot be stressed too highly. Patients whose cancer is detected at an early stage generally have much longer survival times than those presenting with late-stage disease. Also, very importantly, their treatment will usually be less radical, with a prospect of better quality of life in after years.

In the early 1990s a UK working group considered the possibility of population screening as a preventive strategy (Speight *et al.*, 1993) since oral cancer and precancer appeared to fulfil many of the criteria of suitability for such a programme proposed by Wilson and Jungner (1968). For example, high-risk groups of the population can be identified (Speight and Morgan, 1993), the disease has a recognizable and detectable early or presymptomatic stage (i.e. precancer), and there is a simple test (thorough, systematic clinical examination of the oral mucosa) which is safe and acceptable to the population. Oral cancer screening is predicated on the supposition that early detection will increase survival and quality of life, yet there are still many unanswered questions relating to its costs, benefits, effectiveness, feasibility and appropriateness. This led the working group to conclude that there was insufficient evidence at the time to recommend a national screening programme, like those for breast and cervical cancer for example, without further research.

Challenges in oral cancer prevention

In seeking to achieve success in patient counselling, public education and uptake of screening alike, health care workers face considerable difficulties. The population groups at highest risk to oral cancer are those who are the most refractory in accepting and acting on preventive advice and also the least likely to respond to an invitation to be screened in a doctor's or dentist's surgery. This applies particularly to the elderly in lower socioeconomic groups, full denture wearers, and heavy smokers and drinkers. As a baseline, one study has shown that there is confusion and lack of knowledge among members of the public about the most important risk factors for cancer (Bhatti *et al.*, 1995). Many are misinformed and a third may be unaware that cancer can affect the mouth. People will be unlikely to understand the need for preventive measures such as avoiding smoking, reducing their consumption of alcoholic beverages and having their oral mucosa examined regularly for signs of the disease if they have little idea about its nature, prognosis and the common aetiological agents (Blinkhorn and Jones, 1993).

Screening for oral cancer and precancer has its own peculiar features. Because of the low prevalence of lesions, there is a reasonable assumption that screening will tend, inherently, to generate a high frequency of false-positive registration (Downer, 1994). Nevertheless, given the seriousness of the disease, it is obligatory to select screening criteria of high sensitivity even though this may produce a substantial number of false-positive misclassifications. The consequences of false-positives are of considerable importance: first, unwanted costs are incurred through these cases needing to be referred to secondary care services for full diagnostic follow-up. Second, distress may be caused to the misclassified patients who are left in a state of uncertainty as they await the outcome of the full diagnostic procedure which may also involve some discomfort from the removal of tissue for biopsy. Thus there are implications from false-positive misclassification for both the cost-effectiveness of the programme and the emotional well-being of the patients involved (Marteau, 1990; Brown, 1992).

However, experience with pilot oral cancer screening programmes suggests that in practice, even examiners without specific training tend to record low numbers of false-positives (Downer *et al.*, 1995; Jullien *et al.*, 1995a, 1995b). Another important consideration in screening for oral cancer and precancer is the response or uptake rate (also known as compliance) among the target population both to the offer of screening and to follow-up for those designated positive and referred (Jullien *et al.*, 1995b). Directing the programme to high-risk groups is likely to be the most cost-effective strategy in terms of yield per unit cost, but poor compliance among these groups may severely threaten the economic viability of screening. The pilot programmes conducted in the workplace (Downer *et al.*, 1995), where clients were screened conveniently on site, secured better compliance than those with postal invitations (Jullien *et al.*, 1995b). A poor response to invitational screening for oral cancer and precancer was also found in a 60-year-old population in Japan (Ikeda *et al.*, 1995). Although a number of strategies can be adopted to improve compliance in such programmes (Jullien *et al.*, 1995b), it is probable that screening people opportunistically during routine dental or health check-ups is a more appropriate approach.

Finally there is the question of factors that can bias our assessment of the value of screening for oral cancer and precancer (Chamberlain, 1993). Client self-selection bias results from the fact that participants are most likely to come from upper socioeconomic groups who are knowledgeable and concerned about health matters and unlikely to have disease. Lead-time bias is the phenomenon whereby, through early detection, screening may bring forward the diagnosis of oral cancer yet without altering the time of death. It may suggest that a screened group has a better survival rate than an unscreened control, which would be a spurious conclusion. Length bias results from the case mix of cancers available for detection in the presymptomatic phase containing a disproportionate number of slower-growing tumours. This is because many fast-growing ones will move too quickly through that phase to be picked up by a screening test repeated at, say, yearly intervals. Conversely, some screen-detected tumours may be so indolent that they would never have been diagnosed in the person's lifetime in the absence of screening. These aspects have been considered further in Chapter 5.

Future directions

As with any public health programme, screening for oral cancer and precancer and supporting health promotional initiatives, can only be evaluated fully in a prospective randomized controlled trial. However, the cost and logistical difficulties of organizing and managing such an operation and of carrying out a comprehensive economic appraisal are formidable. Very large numbers of subjects would need to be followed over a long time period in order to measure significant changes in incidence and mortality.

An alternative, though less satisfactory approach might be the setting up of some large demonstration projects which would rely on intermediate outcome measures as their method of assessment. Initially, an increased number of new registrations over and above expected local incidence rates (yield) and a substantially higher proportion of small lesions among new cases registered (improved stage distribution) would be necessary to indicate that an effect was being achieved (Chamberlain, 1993). Increased public and professional knowledge and awareness, and certain process measures such as high programme uptake or improved attendance for opportunistic examination among vulnerable sections of the population, might also constitute surrogate measures of success.

Several promising lines of health services research in the area of oral cancer detection merited inclusion among priorities put forward in the mid 1990s for research and development in primary dental care in the British National Health Service (Breckenridge, 1994). The research avenues have the potential at least to screen out and reject strategies that are unlikely to succeed and thereby save time and money. It has been stated that from a public health point of view, the diseases with the highest priority would be those which are the most dangerous and those which are the most prevalent provided the latter present a therapeutic problem (Pindborg, 1977). Diseases in the former class are typified by oral cancer. This is one of the few lethal diseases that dentists may encounter professionally and, as well as having cognizance of its clinical features, all should be aware of its epidemiology, aetiology and natural history, its impact as a public health problem, and the possibilities for its control. It is hoped that new research will help us to find solutions to counteract the upward trend in oral cancer incidence and mortality.

References

Axéll, T. (1987) Occurrence of leukoplakia and some other oral white lesions among 20 333 adult Swedish people. *Community Dental and Oral Epidemiology* **15**:46–51.

Bánóczy, J. (1977) Follow-up studies in oral leukoplakia. *Journal of Maxillofacial Surgery* **5**:69–75.

Bánóczy, J. and Rigo, O. (1991) Prevalence study of oral precancerous lesions within a complex screening system in Hungary. *Community Dental and Oral Epidemiology* **19**:265–267.

Bhatti, N.S., Downer, M.C. and Bulman, J.S. (1995) Public knowledge and attitudes on oral cancer: a pilot investigation. *Journal of the Institute of Health Education* **32**:112–117.

Blinkhorn, A.S. and Jones, J.H. (1993) Behavioural aspects of oral cancer screening. *Community Dental Health* **10** (suppl. 1):63–69.

Blot, W.J., McLaughlin, J.K., Winn, D.M. *et al.* (1988) Smoking and drinking in relation to oral and pharyngeal cancer. *Cancer Research* **48**:3282–3287.

Bouquot, J.E. and Gorlin, R.J. (1986) Leukoplakia, lichen planus, and other oral keratoses in 23 616 white Americans over the age of 35 years. *Oral Surgery* **61**:373–381.

Boyle, P., Macfarlane, G.J. and Scully C. (1993) Oral cancer: necessity for prevention strategies. *Lancet* **342**:1129.

Breckenridge, A. (1994) *Report to the Central Research and Development Committee of the Advisory Group on R & D Priorities in Relation to Primary Dental Care.* Oral Health Services Research Unit, University of Liverpool, Liverpool.

Brown, M. (1992) Sensitivity analysis in the cost-effectiveness of breast cancer screening. *Cancer* **69** (suppl.):1963–1967.

Brugere, J., Quenel, P., Leclerc, A. *et al.* (1986) Differential effects of tobacco and alcohol in cancer of the larynx, pharynx and mouth. *Cancer* **57**:391–395.

Cancer Research Campaign (1993) *Oral Cancer.* Factsheets 14.1–14.5. CRC, London.

Chamberlain, J. (1993) Evaluation of screening for cancer. *Community Dental Health* **10** (suppl. 1):5–11.

Downer, M.C. (1994) Today's proposals, tomorrow's answers? In: *Introduction to Dental Public Health* (Downer, M.C., Gelbier, S. and Gibbons, D.E. eds), pp. 106–126. FDI World Dental Press, London.

Downer, M.C., Evans, A.W., Hughes Hallett, C.M. *et al.* (1995) Evaluation of screening for oral cancer and precancer in a company headquarters. *Community Dental and Oral Epidemiology* **23**:84–88.

Einhorn, J. and Wersäll, J. (1967) Incidence of oral carcinoma in patients with leukoplakia of the oral cavity. *Cancer* **20**:2189–2193.

Franceschi, S., Talamini, R., Barra, S. *et al.* (1990) Smoking and drinking in relation to cancers of the oral cavity, pharynx, larynx and esophagus in Northern Italy. *Cancer Research* **50**:6502–6507.

Franco, E.L., Kowalski, L.P., Oliveira, B.V. *et al.* (1989) Risk factors for oral cancer in Brazil: a case-control study. *International Journal of Cancer* **43**:992–1000.

Gupta, P.C., Mehta, F.S., Pindborg, J.J. *et al.* (1992) Primary intervention trial of oral cancer in India: a 10-year follow-up study. *Journal of Oral Pathological Medicine* **21**:433–439.

Hindle, I. and Nally, F. (1991) Oral cancer: a comparative study between 1962–67 and 1980–84 in England and Wales. *British Dental Journal* **170**:15–19.

Hindle, I., Downer, M.C. and Speight, P.M. (1994) Necessity for prevention strategies in oral cancer. *Lancet* **343**:178–179.

Ikeda, N., Downer, M.C., Ozowa, Y. *et al.* (1995) Characteristics of participants and non-participants in annual mass screening for oral cancer in 60-year-old residents of Tokoname City, Japan. *Community Dental Health* **12**:83–88.

Johnson, N.W. and Warnakulasuriya, K.A.A.S. (1993) Epidemiology and aetiology of oral cancer in the United Kingdom. *Community Dental Health* **10** (suppl. 1):13–29.

Jullien, J.A., Downer, M.C., Zakrzewska, J.M. *et al.* (1995a) Evaluation of a screening test for the early detection of oral cancer and precancer. *Community Dental Health* **12**:3–7.

Jullien, J.A., Zakrzewska, J.M., Downer, M.C. *et al.* (1995b) Attendance and compliance at an oral cancer screening programme in a general medical practice. *Oral Oncology European Journal of Cancer* **31B**:202–206.

Kleinman, D.V., Swango, P.A. and Niessen, L.C. (1991) Epidemiologic studies of oral mucosal conditions– methodologic issues. *Community Dental and Oral Epidemiology* **19**:129–140.

La Vecchia, C., Bidoli, E., Barra, S. *et al.* (1990) Types of cigarettes and cancers of the upper digestive and respiratory tract. *Cancer Causes Control* **1**:69–74.

Lindquist, C. and Teppo, L. (1978) Epidemiological evaluation of sunlight as a risk factor of lip cancer. *British Journal of Cancer* **37**:983–989.

Macfarlane, G.J. (1993) *The Epidemiology of Oral Cancer.* Thesis. University of Bristol, Bristol.

Marshall, J.R., Graham, S., Haughey, B.P. *et al.* (1992) Smoking, alcohol, dentition and diet in the epidemiology of oral cancer. *Oral Oncology European Journal of Cancer* **28B**:9–15.

Marteau, T. (1990) Reducing the psychological costs. *British Medical Journal* **301**:26–28.

Merletti, F., Boffetta, P., Ciccone, G. *et al.* (1989) Role of tobacco and alcoholic beverages in the etiology of cancer of the oral cavity/oropharynx in Torino, Italy. *Cancer Research* **49**:4919–4924.

Office of Population Censuses and Surveys (1994) *Cancer Statistics Registration.* Series MB1 no. 21. Her Majesty's Stationery Office, London.

Parkin, D.M. and Muir, C.S. (1992) Comparability and quality of data. In: *Cancer Incidence in Five Continents,* vol. VI (Parkin, D.M., Muir, C.S., Whelan, S.L. *et al.*, eds.), pp. 45–55, IARC scientific publications No. 120. International Agency for Research on Cancer, Lyon.

Parkin, D.M., Laara, E. and Muir, C.S. (1988) Estimates of the worldwide frequency of sixteen major cancers in 1980. *International Journal of Cancer* 41:184–197.

Parkin, D.M., Muir, C.S., Whelan, S.L. *et al.* (1992) *Cancer Incidence in Five Continents.* vol. VI. IARC scientific publications No. 120. International Agency for Research on Cancer, Lyon.

Pindborg, J.J. (1977) Epidemiology and public health aspects of diseases of the oral mucosa. *Journal of Dental Research* 56:14–19.

Platz, H., Fries, R. and Hudec, M. (1986) *Prognoses of Oral Cavity Carcinomas. Results of a Multi-centre Retrospective Operational Study.* Hanser, Munich.

Rothman, K.J. and Keller, A.Z. (1972) The effect of joint exposure to alcohol and tobacco on the risk of cancer of the mouth and pharynx. *Journal of Chronic Disease* 25:711–716.

Silverman, S., Bhargava, K., Mani, N. *et al.* (1976) Malignant transformation and natural history of oral leukoplakia in 57 518 industrial workers in Gujarat, India. *Cancer* 38:1790–1795.

Speight, P.M. and Morgan, P.R. (1993) The natural history and pathology of oral cancer and precancer. *Community Dental Health* 10 (suppl. 1):31–41.

Speight, P.M., Downer, M.C. and Zakrzewska, J. (eds) (1993) Screening for oral cancer and precancer. Report of a UK working group. *Community Dental Health* 10 (suppl. 1):1–89.

Stell, P.M. and McCormick, M.S. (1985) Cancer of the head and neck: are we doing any better? *Lancet* II:1127.

Waldron, C. and Shafer, W. (1975) Leukoplakia revisited: a clinicopathological study of 3256 oral leukoplakias. *Cancer* 36:1386–1392.

Warnakulasuriya, K.A.A.S. (1984) Utilization of primary health care workers for the early detection of oral cancer and precancer cases in Sri Lanka. *Bulletin of the World Health Organization* 62:243–250.

Wilson, J.M.G. and Jungner, G. (1968) *Principles and Practice of Screening for Disease.* Public health papers. no. 34. World Health Organization, Geneva.

World Health Organization (1977) *Manual of the International Statistical Classification of Diseases, Injuries, and Causes of Death (Based on the Recommendations of the Ninth Revision Conference).* WHO, Geneva.

Wynder, E.L., Bross, J.J. and Feldman, R.M. (1957) A study of the etiologic factors in cancer of the mouth. *Cancer* 10:1300–1323.

Dental trauma

J.O. Andreasen and F.M. Andreasen

The prevalence of dental trauma

Unlike caries and periodontal disease, reliable data on the frequency and severity of dental trauma are lacking in most countries. In a recent compilation on the existing data on dental trauma it appears that the prevalences of traumatic dental injuries at the age 6 in four countries were found to centre around 30% (range 16–40%), whereas prevalences in 12-year-old individuals centred around 20% (range 4–33%; Andreasen and Andreasen, 1994; Tables 6.2 and 6.3). These figures can be expected to represent a minimum as most studies have been of a cross-sectioned nature whereby previous injury is to a certain extent dependent upon information from either the child or parents which can entail a significant underscoring (Andreasen and Ravn, 1972). In contrast to caries where a significant decrease in caries activity has been found over the past two decades, the opposite is found in regard to dental trauma (Todd, 1973, 1983, Fig. 6.4). In fact trauma can now in many countries be considered a greater threat than caries to the health and preservation of anterior teeth. In conclusion, the epidemiology implies that at least in some countries about every second child will become injured before the age of 12.

Table 6.2 Prevalence of traumatic dental injuries to primary teeth in 5-year-olds (From Andreasen and Andreasen, 1994)

			Sex	
Author	*Year*	*Country*	*M*	*F*
Andreasen and Ravn	1974	Denmark	31.3	24.6
Garcia-Goday *et al.*	1983	Dominican Republic	33.6	28.9
Forsberg and Tedestam	1990	Sweden	28.0	16.0
Sanchez and Garcia-Goday	1990	Mexico	40.0	

Table 6.3 Prevalence of traumatic dental injuries to permanent teeth in 12-year-olds (From Andreasen and Andreasen, 1994)

			Sex	
Author	*Year*	*Country*	*M*	*F*
Andreasen and Ravn	1972	Denmark	25.7	16.3
Clarkson *et al.*	1973	UK	11.6	9.6
Todd	1973	UK	22.0	12.0
Todd	1983	UK	29.0	16.0
Järvinen	1979	Finland	33.0	19.3
Baghdady *et al.*	1981	Iraq	19.5	16.1
Baghdady *et al.*	1981	Sudan	16.5	3.6
Garcia-Goday *et al.*	1985	Dominican Republic	18.0	12.0
Garcia-Goday *et al.*	1986	Dominican Republic	31.7	15.0
Holland	1988	Ireland	21.2	12.1
Hunter *et al.*	1990	UK	19.4	11.0
Forsberg and Tedestam	1990	Sweden	27.0	12.0

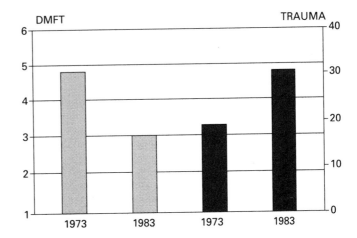

Fig. 6.4 Comparison of the prevalence of dental caries and dental trauma in England and Wales over a 10-year period. Modified from Todd and Dodd (1973, 1983)

Type of injuries sustained and treatment demands

The majority of injuries sustained in the primary dentition appear to be luxation injuries whereas crown fractures dominate in the permanent dentition (Andreasen and Ravn, 1972; Fig. 6.5). In the primary dentition the major therapeutic problem appears to be to diagnose and monitor healing of displaced primary incisors in order to prevent damage being transmitted to the permanent dentition (Andreasen and Andreasen,

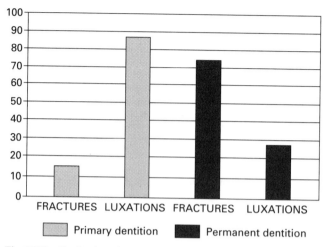

Fig. 6.5 The distribution of tooth fractures and tooth luxation in the primary and permanent dentition. From Andreasen and Ravn (1972), with permission.

1994). In the permanent dentition the most significant problem appears to be the restoration of crown fractured teeth which comprise about two-thirds of all injuries (Andreasen and Ravn, 1972; Fig. 6.5). The outcome of these treatments is usually satisfactory in relation to aesthetics, function, periodontal and pulpal health. A more serious challenge is found in the treatment of crown-root fractures, root fractures, tooth luxations and avulsions. Some of these injuries can be so harmful to the pulp and periodontium that in spite of intensive treatment the traumatized tooth is ultimately lost. In these cases a complicated treatment problem arises, namely how to restore a dentition with early loss of permanent anterior teeth (Andreasen and Andreasen, 1994). Presently tooth loss can be treated by fixed or removable prosthodontics, orthodontic space closure, implants or auto-transplantation of teeth. Whatever solution is chosen, a severe cost factor arises which in some countries ranges from US$250 to US$2000 (Andreasen, 1992). On top of that, sparse information exists on the long-term prognosis of these different treatment solutions (Andreasen, 1992).

Cost of dental traumas

It is surprising that in spite of the high frequency of traumatic dental injuries almost no data exist on the total cost of the immediate and late care of dental trauma patients. In a pilot study from Denmark in 1990 it was estimated that the immediate care of dental trauma patients (including cost of emergency treatment plus diagnosis and treatment of immediate complications such as pulp necrosis and root resorption) had a cost of US$3.6 million per million inhabitants (Andreasen and Andreasen, 1990). In a longitudinal study carried out in Sweden a cost of US$3.2 million was estimated per million (Glendor, 1995).

First-aid service to dental trauma patients

When a dental injury occurs the patient will normally seek professional help hours or sometimes days after the trauma. However, the demand for immediate treatment is heavily dependent upon information to the public, awareness of the possibility and necessity for care, as well as the actual facilities offered within the community.

In various countries it has been found that the majority of dental trauma patients have not received immediate or late care of their trauma (Järvinen, 1979; Todd, 1983). The immediate demand of a dental trauma appears to be diagnosis of the involved oral tissues (pulp, periodontium, alveolar bone, gingiva or mucosa). This phase implies a clinical examination and usually also a radiographic examination of the traumatized region. Based on this, a diagnosis of the traumatized tissues can be made and the immediate or late treatment demand can be ascertained.

In the *primary dentition* tooth luxations dominate and the general treatment principle based on clinical and experimental studies appears to be conservative–accepting the primary tooth in its displaced position and waiting for spontaneous realignment of the tooth. Exceptions to this rule are luxated teeth displaced into the permanent tooth follicles and luxated teeth presenting an obstacle to occlusion. In the former case the primary tooth should be removed, whereas in the latter case the displaced tooth is either repositioned or removed (Andreasen and Andreasen, 1994).

In the *permanent dentition* crown fractured teeth without a pulp exposure should be restored with composite (if no periodontal ligament (PDL) injury has occurred), temporarily covered with a hard-setting calcium hydroxide cement or if an intact fragment exists it can be bonded to the fracture surface. In crown fractures with pulp exposure, pulp capping or a pulpotomy can be performed with a high predictability of success. In crown-root fractures the definitive treatment is dependent upon the location of the fracture. Possible treatments include removal of coronal fragment and supragingival restoration, surgical exposure of fracture surface, surgical or orthodontic extrusion of an apical fragment and finally extraction of the tooth when the fracture is located too far below the gingival margin. In the case of root fracture, the treatment principle is repositioning of the coronal fragment and rigid splinting for 3 months. Luxation injuries with displacement represent a severe challenge to the pulp and periodontium. Treatment of luxated and displaced permanent teeth consists of repositioning and semirigid splinting for 2–8 weeks according to the extent of the periodontal damage. The optimal treatment of intruded permanent teeth is still unsettled; clinical experience indicates that spontaneous or ortho-dontic extrusion in some situations is to be preferred over immediate repositioning (Andreasen and Andreasen, 1994).

Treatment of the avulsed tooth has been the subject of numerous clinical and experimental investigations. A synopsis of these studies indicates that damage to the pulp and the periodontium elicited during the extra-alveolar phase is the most significant factor determining pulpal and periodontal healing. In the extra-alveolar period, drying damage to the PDL appears to be the most common cause of injury and this factor seems to operate after a few minutes. Also non-physiological storage (e.g. in sterilizing solutions) will lead to PDL and pulp damage, causing root resorption and pulp necrosis (Andreasen *et al.*, 1995a, 1995b, 1995c, 1995d). These findings indicate that immediate replantation should be carried out whenever possible followed by a short-term semirigid splinting. If such a procedure is carried out the majority of avulsed teeth can be saved on a permanent basis.

Public health implications

Organization of emergency care for dental trauma

As many injuries appear outside office hours, it is important that a dental emergency service is set up covering a given region. Ideally such a service should be available on a 24-hour basis. The location of such a service can be a hospital, dental school or a private office. It is essential that the staff offering trauma service are regularly exposed to trauma patients so that a high professional skill can be maintained.

In the examination of the traumatized patient it is important that an adequate clinical and radiographic examination is carried out. In that regard a preprinted emergency record for dental trauma patients will help to ensure that all pertinent questions are asked and relevant examinations carried out (Andreasen and Andreasen, 1985). Furthermore radiographic facilities must exist so that both intra- and extraoral exposures can be taken.

Ideally, the same dental staff should be available to provide both emergency and definitive treatment. This implies valuable constant feedback about the relation between the extent of the initial injury, the effect of emergency treatment and the final outcome. In most cases, however, such a set-up is not possible and the referral for definitive treatment to other professionals becomes necessary. In that situation it is necessary that sufficient information about the dental injury and emergency treatment is transferred to the next treatment-provider.

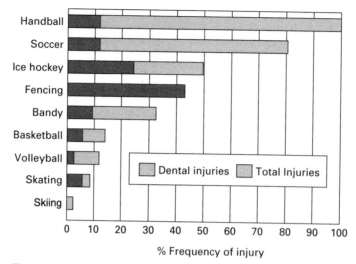

Fig. 6.6 The total number of sports injuries and the number of dental injuries per 10 000 players for the period 1981 to 1983 in Norway. Modified from Nysether (1987), with permission.

Prevention of dental injuries

The majority of dental traumas appear to be non-preventable; only sports injuries appear to offer the possibility of prevention by the use of mouthguards and sometimes helmets. The critical issue in regard to prevention appears to be the cost–benefit of such an intervention (Scheer, 1994). For a mouthguard to be effective it should be custom-made, which implies a rather high cost. This cost factor should be related to the potential risk of the individual type of sport and its ability to prevent or reduce damage to the dentition. Apart from boxing, rugby and American football there is rather limited information on the level of risk (Nysether, 1987). Based on present knowledge it seems relevant to use protection for heavy contact sports such as ice hockey, rugby, boxing and American football, whereas the use of mouthguards in popular sports such as handball and soccer can be questioned (Fig. 6.6).

Information about first-aid treatment to a trauma victim appears to be essential. Thus a recent study of the long-term prognosis of replanted and avulsed teeth showed that it is not the dentist but those closest to the scene of the accident who play the most important role in improving the chance of successful healing following dental injury (Andreasen and Andreasen, 1994), Therefore, it is necessary that information campaigns aimed at educating lay people of the correct first-aid treatment should bee carried out. Such campaigns have successfully been conducted in several countries, e.g. Denmark, Sweden, Norway, Australia, Brazil, Argentina and the USA. Several different trauma campaign brochures have been produced, all detailing the essential steps in emergency care. It is essential that the brochures or posters are distributed and displayed in strategic locations (e.g. sports clubs, ambulance services, to school physicians and nurses). Finally, it is important to consider that such campaigns need to be repeated at regular intervals.

References

Andreasen, J.O. (1992) Third international conference on dental trauma Copenhagen. *Endodontic and Dental Traumatology* **8**:69-70.

Andreasen, F.M. and Andreasen, J.O. (1985) Diagnosis of luxation injuries: the importance of standardized clinical, radiographic and photographic techniques in clinical investigations. *Endodontic and Dental Traumatology* **1**:160–169.

Andreasen, J.O. and Andreasen, F.M. (1990) Dental traumatology: quo vadis. *Endodontic and Dental Traumatology* **6**:160–169.

Andreasen, J.O. and Andreasen, F.M. (1994) *Textbook and Color Atlas of Traumatic Injuries to the Teeth.* Munksgaard, Copenhagen.

Andreasen, J.O. and Ravn, J.J. (1972) Epidemiology of traumatic dental injuries to primary and permanent teeth in a Danish population sample. *International Journal of Oral Surgery* 1: 235–239.

Andreasen, F.M., Noren, J.G., Andreasen, J.O., Engelhardtsen, S. and Lindh-Stromberg, U. (1995) Long-term survival of crown fragment bonding in the treatment of crown fractures. A multi-center clinical study of fragment retention. *Quintessence International*, (in press).

Andreasen, J.O., Borum, M., Jacobsen, H.L. and Andreasen, F.M. (1995a) Replantation of 400 traumatically avulsed permanent incisors. I. Diagnosis of healing complications. *Endodontic and Dental Traumatology* 11:51–58.

Andreasen, J.O., Borum, M., Jacobsen, H.L. and Andreasen, F.M. (1995b) Replantation of 400 avulsed permanent incisors. II. Factors related to pulp healing. *Endodontic and Dental Traumatology* 11:59–68.

Andreasen, J.O., Borum, M. and Andreasen, F.M. (1995c) Replantation of 400 avulsed permanent incisors. III. Factors related to root growth after replantation. *Endodontic and Dental Traumatology* 11:69–75.

Andreasen, J.O., Borum, M., Jacobsen, H.L. and Andreasen, F.M. (1995d) Replantation of 400 avulsed permanent incisors. IV. Factors relate to periodontal ligament healing. *Endodontic and Dental Traumatology* 11:76–89.

Baghdady, V.S., Ghose, L.J. and Enke, H. (1981) Traumatized anterior teeth in Iraqi and Sudanese children – a comparative study. *Journal of Dental Research*, 60: 677–680.

Clarkson, B.H., Longhurst, P. and Sheiham, A. (1973) The prevalence of injured anterior teeth in English school children and adults. *Journal of International Association of Dentistry in Children* 4: 21–4.

Forsberg, C. and Tedestam, G. (1990) Traumatic injuries to teeth in Swedish children living in an urban area. *Swedish Dentistry* 14: 115–122.

Garcia-Godoy, F., Morban-Laucher, F., Corominas, L.R., Franjul, R.A. and Noyola, M. (1983) Traumatic dental injuries in preschoolchildren from Santo Domingo. *Community Dental and Oral Epidemiology* 11: 127–130.

Garcia-Godoy, F., Morban-Laucher, F., Corominas, L.R., Franjul, R.A. and Noyola, M. (1983) Traumatic dental injuries in schoolchildren from Santo Domingo. *Community Dental and Oral Epidemiology* 13: 177–179.

Garcia-Godoy, F., Dipres, F.M., Lora, I.M. and Vidal, E.D. (1986) Traumatic dental injuries in children from private and public schools. *Community Dental Oral Epidemiology* 14: 287–290.

Glendor, U. (1995) Personal communication.

Holland, T., O'Mullane, D.O., Clarkson, J., O'Hickey, S.O. and Whelton, H. (1988) Trauma to permanent teeth of children aged 8, 12 and 15 years, in Ireland. *Paediatric Dentology* 4: 13–16.

Hunter, M.L., Hunter, B., Kingdon, A., Addy, M., Dummer, P.M.H. and Shaw, W.C. (1990) Traumatic injury to maxillary incisor teeth in a group of South Wales schoolchildren. *Endodontic and Dental Traumatology* 6: 260–264.

Järvinen, S. (1979) Fractured and avulsed permanent incisors in Finnish children. A retrospective study. *Acta Odontology Scandinavica* 37: 47–50.

Nysether, S. (1987) Dental injuries among Norwegian soccer players. *Community Dental and Oral Epidemiology* 15: 141–143.

Sanchez, A.V. and Garcia-Godoy, F. (1990) Traumatic dental injuries in 3- to 13-year-old boys in Monterrey, Mexico. *Endodontic and Dental Traumatology* 6: 63–65.

Scheer, B. (1994) Prevention of dental and oral injuries. In: *Textbook and Color Atlas of Traumatic Injuries to the Teeth* (J.O. Andreasen and F.M. Andreasen, eds), Munksgaard, Copenhagen, pp. 719–735.

Todd, J.. (1973) *Children's Dental Health in England and Wales*. Social Survey Division. Her Majesty's Stationery Office, London.

Todd, J.E. and Dodd, T. (1983) *Children's Dental Health in England and Wales*. Social Survey Division. Her Majesty's Stationery Office, London.

Public health aspects of developmental enamel defects

Terry W. Cutress and Grace W. Suckling

Introduction

While teeth are primarily concerned with the intake, preparation and ingestion of food, they are also a major facial attribute with implications for personality, social relationships and self-esteem. Irregularities and abnormalities of teeth in most communities are for most individuals a cause of embarrassment and distress, although in some societies normal teeth may be deliberately mutilated or adorned for cultural, ritual and cosmetic purposes. In many westernized countries, visible deficiencies in tooth quality have become increasingly important now that teeth are less likely to be disfigured or removed due to dental caries. Biologically, enamel defects have a particular fascination because they provide a durable record of local and systemic disturbances during tooth formation. Defects pose questions on fundamental developmental issues and have clinical, cosmetic and treatment relevance. They also provide a valuable record for studying stresses on past human populations. In this section, we consider developmental defects of enamel as they relate to public health.

Developmental defects, by definition, occur during tooth formation and are the consequence of disruption amelogenesis in the normal enamel development. Amelogenesis is a complex activity commencing with cell differentiation and organic matrix deposition in the early tooth germ and terminating with mature mineralized (97% w/w) dental enamel. During the prolonged period of 4 or more years of development the vital enamel organ is vulnerable to genetic, metabolic and physical factors. Alone or in combination, each may alter normal enamel formation to a greater or lesser degree, resulting in a wide spectrum of defects, affecting one, many or all teeth. The great diversity in appearance of defects explains the varied nomenclature and difficulties in obtaining a consensus on a standardized classification.

The relevance of enamel defects in public health depends on the prevalence of a disfiguring condition, the contributing aetiological factors, the need to monitor potential environmental factors affecting normal amelogenesis and the magnitude of community treatment needs. Defects arising from fluoride, trauma, systemic illness and tetracycline are certainly relevant, particularly as community action for prevention can sometimes be implemented. On the other hand, defects of genetic aetiology are uncommon and do not figure as public health issues unless an increased prevalence is noted.

History

The recorded history of tooth defects goes back over two centuries. During that time changes in the appearance of the enamel were associated with rickets, measles, scurvy, syphilis and some severe systemic illnesses. Before 1930, interest in enamel defects was confined to the quality of enamel and its subsequent susceptibility to dental caries. The discovery of relationships between the fluoride content of drinking water, the prevalence of dental caries and dental mottling resulted in a boom in epidemiological

research between 1930 and 1945. Dean's (1934) quantitative classification of the severity of fluorosis, established in the 1930s, has proved a robust epidemiological method but has tended to suppress progress in the understanding of non-fluoride defects. In the 1940s, Sarnat and Schour (1941, 1942) established a general classification of defective enamel linking the chronology of tooth development to the position of the defect on the tooth surface and known systemic illnesses (for review see, Suckling, 1989; Goodman and Rose, 1990).

The multidisciplinary interest in tooth defects produced a confusing diversity of nomenclature in clinical and scientific literature, making interpretation and interstudy comparisons difficult. For example, 'hypoplasia' is used by some to refer to all and others to one type of defect; 'mottled enamel' may or may not be presumed to relate to fluoride-induced defects. Other terms commonly used to describe defects were 'whitespots', 'internal hypoplasia', 'opacity', 'hypocalcification' and 'idiopathic enamel opacities'. Since the 1950s the significance of non-fluoride defects has increased with various proposals for descriptive indices. These and aetiologically based indices have been reviewed on various occasions (Cutress and Suckling, 1982; Clarkson, 1989; Murray *et al.*, 1991).

Terminology and classifications

Dental fluorosis has generated its own family of indices. While the classical Dean's index is still a commonly used index in public health studies, increasingly more researchers are choosing the more sensitive indices that overcome the shortcomings inherent in differentiating between the more severe conditions (Thylstrup and Fejerskov, 1978; Horowitz *et al.*, 1984). These have been extensively reviewed and discussed over the past 70 years (more recently by Horowitz, 1986; Clarkson, 1989; Cutress and Suckling, 1990). Diagnosis of fluorosis is presumed from a characteristic pattern of diffuse opacities observed in people living in communities exposed to different levels of naturally fluoridated water.

A weakness of fluoride classifications is the need to make a diagnosis based on the distribution pattern of opacities. Evidence is lacking that fluoride produces a unique pattern of defects (Cutress and Suckling, 1990). Of some concern is that a number of clinical cases of apparent moderate to severe fluorosis are diagnosed despite a subject having experienced only very low exposure to fluoride. Russell (1961) and others attempted to discriminate between fluoride and non-fluoride-induced opacities. This, however, is not always possible because, apart from some genetically linked defects, with few exceptions defects are not unique to any one disruptive factor. Suckling and colleagues (1976) proposed a descriptive classification suitable for all defects. Following field tests in various communities a terminology was further developed and later adopted by the Fédération Internationale Dentaire (FDI; FDI, 1982). Subsequently Suckling modified the Developmental Defects of Enamel index (DDE) which again was implemented through an FDI working group (FDI, 1992). In 1994, the World Health Organization adopted the basic DDE clinical criteria as their recommended survey procedure.

A common standard terminology based on accepted definitions would increase the value of clinical, public health and epidemiological reports on the prevalence and severity of enamel defects. While the DDE index is acceptable for general needs and monitoring purposes in public health, it does not satisfy all requirements for more specific-oriented research. In such cases, the criteria and procedures should be tailored to the study. For example, where the concern is only for fluorosis then one of the fluorosis indices would take priority. Almost all defects, however, can be classified on the basis of their macroscopic appearance into demarcated opacities, diffuse opacities and hypoplasia or a combination of these. The pathogenesis of the three types differs, but the appearance of all is influenced by the stage of ameloblast activity, duration and intensity of the factor responsible for temporary or permanent damage to the ameloblasts (Suckling, 1989). The three basic types are defined as follows:

- *Demarcated opacity* is a defect involving an alteration in the translucency of the enamel, variable in degree. It has a distinct and clear boundary with the adjacent normal enamel and can be white, cream, yellow or brown in colour. The defective enamel is of normal thickness and surface contour. The lesions vary in extent, position on the tooth surface

and distribution in the mouth. Some maintain a surface translucency while others are dull in appearance.
- *Diffuse opacity* is also a defect involving an alteration in the translucency of the enamel, variable in degree. There is no clear boundary with the adjacent normal enamel. The defective enamel is white in colour, of normal thickness and, at eruption, has a smooth surface. Diffuse defects can have a linear, patchy or confluent distribution. In some cases posteruptive changes (pitting, staining) may occur.
- *Hypoplasia* is a defect involving the surface of the enamel and is associated with a reduced localized thickness of enamel. It can occur in the form of: (a) pits–single or multiple, shallow or deep, scattered or in rows of pits arranged horizontally across the tooth surface; (b) grooves–single or multiple, narrow or wide (maximum 2 mm); (c) partial or complete absence of enamel over a considerable area of dentine. The enamel may be translucent or opaque.

Aetiology

There is no need here to refer to the hundred or more different aetiological factors which cause tooth defects. Pindborg (1982) and others have listed the many conditions, genetic, systemic and local, known to be associated. Exclusion of rare hereditary and metabolic factors greatly reduces the list. It is apparent that many observed defects cannot be assigned to a specific cause. They are more commonly non-specific phenomena and can be related to a variety of local and systemic disturbances, any of which, depending on severity and degree of tissue response, induces defective enamel and dentine (Kreshover, 1940). In the past the causes of enamel defects have been divided into genetic and environmental categories. This is convenient, but it should be borne in mind that it is also a rather simplistic approach.

Systemic/genetic

The typical and classical childhood illnesses, such as measles, chickenpox and mumps, respiratory and gastrointestinal episodes, are examples cited together with trauma and toxic substance-induced effects which interfere with normal amelogenesis. Some genetically determined defects may occur as one of many features of a disorder (e.g. coeliac disease) or it may be a single feature (e.g. amelogenesis imperfecta).

Trauma

Trauma to the deciduous predecessor is commonly associated with defects of permanent teeth. In particular this is observed in the maxillary incisor region. Andreasen and colleagues (1971) reported that 'external hypoplasia' resulted when trauma occurred at a fairly early age, while 'internal enamel hypoplasia' occurred with older children, when amelogenesis is more advanced. Enamel development remains vulnerable to disruptive influences even during the late stages of maturation.

Tetracycline

The unsightly appearance resulting from use of the antibiotic tetracycline is dependent on various factors–the dose, number of treatments, drug variant and the age of the child and thus the stage of tooth development. The discoloration is dependent on both enamel and dentine and is often associated with hypoplasia (King and Tsang, 1992). While guidelines and restrictions on antibiotic use have eliminated this defect as a public health concern in many countries, in others it remains a problem.

Pathogenesis

Earlier explanations of the pathogenesis of enamel defects and tooth development have been superseded by recent studies (Suckling, 1989; Suga, 1992). It is accepted that the severity and duration of action of the aetiological factors are important in determining the appearance of all lesions. The current consensus is that hypoplasia is produced by disturbances of synthesis and secretion of matrix substances which may occur during the matrix (secretory) formation stage; opacities, however, can either result from cells damaged during the secretory stage functioning deficiently during the maturation (mineralization) stage, or from disturbance of cell function initiated during the maturation stage.

Yellow demarcated opacities result from severe insult of short duration causing death of

the ameloblasts early in the maturation phase. More research is needed to clarify the interaction of factors resulting in white demarcated opacities.

Diffuse opacities result from a long-continued, low-grade disturbance to ameloblast activity in either the maturation and secretory phases or both. When an excessive intake of fluoride is limited to the maturation phase changes are restricted to the outer enamel. When excessive fluoride is available during the secretory phase changes also occur in the inner enamel, due to interference of matrix formation.

Hypoplastic defects are formed during the secretory phase of ameloblast activity. The duration of the disturbance causing the defect is short, and its severity determines the extent of the missing enamel and the translucency of any partially formed enamel. It should not be confused with posteruptive enamel loss. Goodman and Rose (1990) proposed a conceptual model for formation of hypoplastic defects which relates the amelogenesis disruption, aetiological factors and developmental age. Three prime aetiological factors were considered within the general categories of genetic, nutrition, illness.

Epidemiology

Various reviews (Cutress and Suckling, 1982; Smith, 1983; King and Wei, 1992) provide information on the prevalence of defects together with the indices used. The last-mentioned study lists more than 47 reports from 24 countries. Mouth prevalence for opacities ranged from 100% to 3%; tooth prevalence was much lower (and data less frequently provided), from 82% to virtually none. Much of the variation appeared to be explained by fluoride availability. Mouth prevalence for hypoplasia (16 studies) varied from 66% to none, and tooth prevalence from 18% to none. Preferred terminology was: opacities (22), fluorosis (10), mottling (9), hypoplasia (4), idiopathic (4).

Since 1989 a further 42 reports have been published indicating an accelerated interest in defects. The great majority were targeted to public health issues. Indices used were DDE index (12), Thylstrup and Fejerskov Index (TFI) (7), Tooth Surface Index of Fluorosis (TSIF) (5), Dean's (5) and others (4), with several studies comparing the suitability of different indices. A high level of interest (12 studies) is being shown in tooth defects by investigators in palaeoarchaeological research (see Goodman and Capasso, 1992) as a means of identifying stresses (nutrition, health) in ancient communities. Epidemiological monitoring of enamel defects has an important role in public health for minimizing and identifying factors which induce undesirable changes in the appearance of dental enamel.

References

Andreasen, J.O., Sundstrom, B. and Ravn, J.J. (1971) The effect of traumatic injuries to primary teeth on their permanent successors. *Scandinavian Journal of Dental Research* 79:219–294.

Capasso, L. and Goodman, A. Introduction. In, Recent contributions to the study of enamel developmental defects. *Journal of Paleopathology* 2, 11–15.

Clarkson, J. (1989) Review of terminology, classifications, and indices of developmental defects of enamel. *Advances in Dental Research* 3:104–109.

Cutress, T.W. and Suckling, G.W. (1982) The assessment of non-carious defects of enamel. *International Dental Journal* 32:117–122.

Cutress, T.W. and Suckling, G.W. (1990) Differential diagnosis of dental fluorosis. *Journal of Dental Research* 69:714–720.

Dean, H.T. (1934) Classification of mottled enamel diagnosis. *Journal of the American Dental Association* 21:1421–1426.

FDI technical report no. 15 (1982) An epidemiological index of developmental defects of dental enamel (DDE index). *International Dental Journal* 32:159–167.

FDI report (1992) A review of the developmental defects of enamel index (DDE index). *International Dental Journal* 42:411–426.

Goodman, A.H. and Capasso L.L. (1992) Recent contributions to the study of enamel developmental defects. *Journal of Paleopathology* 2.

Goodman, A.H. and Rose, J.C. (1990) Assessment of systemic physiological perturbations from dental enamel hypoplasias and associated histological structures. *Yearbook of Physical Anthropology* 33:59–110.

Horowitz, H.S. (1986) Indices for measuring dental fluorosis. *Journal of Public Health Dentistry* 46:179–183.

Horowitz, H.S., Driscoll, W.S., Meyers R.J., Heifetz, S.B. and Kingman, A. (1984) A new method for assessing the prevalence of fluorosis–the tooth surface index of fluorosis. *Journal of the American Dental Association* 109:37–41.

King, N.M. and Tsang, M.C.K. (1992) The presence of tetracycline in the dentine and enamel of extracted human teeth. *Journal of Paleopathology* 32:331–340.

King, N.M. and Wei, S.H.Y. (1992) A review of the prevalence of developmental enamel defects in permanent teeth. *Journal of Paleopathology* 32:341–357.

Kreshover, S.J. (1940) Histopathologic studies of abnormal enamel formation in human teeth. *American Journal of Orthodontics* 26:1083–1101.

Murray, J.J., Rugg-Gunn A.J. and Jenkins G.N. (1991) *Fluorides in Caries Prevention*, 3rd. edn, pp. 222–261. Wright, Oxford.

Pindborg, J.J. (1982) Aetiology of developmental enamel defects not related to fluorosis. *International Dental Journal* 32:123–134.

Russell, A.L. (1961) The differential diagnosis of fluoride and nonfluoride enamel opacities. *Journal of Public Health Dentistry* 21:143–146.

Sarnat, B.G. and Schour, I. (1941) Part I. Enamel hypoplasia (chronologic enamel aplasia) in relation to systemic disease: a chronologic, morphologic and etiologic classification. *Journal of the American Dental Association* 28, 1989–2000.

Sarnat, B.G. and Schour, I. (1942) Part II. Enamel hypoplasia (chronologic enamel aplasia) in relation to systemic disease: a chronologic, morphologic and etiologic classification. *Journal of the American Dental Association* 29, 67–75.

Smith, J.M. (1983) *The Epidemiology, Aetiology, and Histopathology of Developmental Defects in Human Teeth.* PhD thesis, University of London.

Suckling, G.W. (1989) Developmental defects of enamel–historical and present-day perspectives of their pathogenesis. *Advances in Dental Research* 3:87–94.

Suckling, G.W., Pearce E.I.F. and Cutress T.W. (1976) Developmental defects of enamel in New Zealand children. *New Zealand Dental Journal* 72:201–210.

Suga, S. (1992) Hypoplasia and hypomineralization of tooth enamel. *Journal of Paleopathology* 32:269–292.

Thylstrup, A. and Fejerskov, O. (1978) Clinical appearance of dental fluorosis in permanent teeth in relation to histologic changes. *Community Dental and Oral Epidemiology* 6:315–328.

Further reading

Proceedings of the symposium and workshop on developmental defects of enamel (1988) *Advances in Dental Research* 31:85–271.

Workshop on methods for assessing fluoride accumulation and effects in the body (1993) *Advances in Dental Research* 8:1–117.

Dentofacial irregularities

William C. Shaw

Prevalence of malocclusion

Estimates of the frequency of different traits of malocclusion are available from a number of different surveys, mainly north European and north American. Direct comparison between surveys is not generally possible as estimates vary according to the examining criteria adopted, levels of severity, sampling differences of age and gender, availability of study casts and radiographs (for detecting unerupted teeth), and the accuracy of the examiners. A brief synopsis of a number of surveys is presented in Table 6.4.

Determination of treatment need

More than 40 years ago a committee of the British Dental Association defined the aims of orthodontic treatment as being 'to produce improved function by the correction of irregularities and to create not only greater resistance to disease, but also to improve personal appearance, which later will contribute to the mental as well as to the physical well-being of the individual' (British Dental Association, 1954). Though the merit of these aims remains unquestionable, little progress has been made in defining exactly which occlusal irregularities require correction.

Traditionally orthodontists have taken a mainly utilitarian motive for their work, assuming that orthodontic treatment enhances dental health and function, and as such, provides greater assurance for the longevity of the dentition. A disappointing lack of evidence for these aspirations has, in recent years, led to the transcendence of a second motive or justification for orthodontic treatment–that it enhances

Table 6.4 Prevalence of common occlusal anomalies (%)

Intra-arch traits		Interarch traits	
Hypodontia		*Overjet*	
Permanent teeth (except third molars)	6	<0	3
Upper lateral incisors	1–2	+ve<5 mm	76
Premolars	1	5–7 mm	14
		>7 mm	8
Hyperdontia			
Supernumary teeth	0.1–4		
Ectopic eruption		*Overbite*	
One or more 16, 26	4	>5 mm incisal coverage	11–24
One or more 13, 23	2	>7 mm incisal coverage	3
Infraocclusion, deciduous molars	14	Traumatic	1
		Open bite	2–4
Cross-bite		*Dentoalveolar disproportion*	
Buccal		Deciduous	
Unilateral	10	Spacing (age)	90–95
Bilateral	2	Permanent	
Anterior	7	Spacing >2 mm	9
with displacement	75		
Lingual	7–8	Crowding	
		>2 mm	16–26
		>3 mm	25
		>6 mm	7
		>9 mm	3
Median diastema		*Miscellaneous*	
Before eruption 12, 22	95	Digit/dummy sucking	
After eruption 12, 22	25	Age 3 years	42
		Age 12 years	7

social and psychological well-being through improvements in appearance. Orthodontic 'ideal occlusion', apart from its rarity in modern humans, may have little biological validity and the human dentition in its contemporary, unworn condition may represent something of an anachronism. This would certainly help to explain the difficulty which researchers have consistently had in demonstrating important associations between malocclusion and dental health and function (Shaw *et al.*, 1991). Thus the disadvantage of malocclusion from the dental health and functional viewpoint seems rather modest. Early correction of prominent incisors reduces the risk of trauma, though the potential benefit becomes less with age. The risk of pathological sequelae of impaction have not been quantified but early avoidance of these problems is also desirable. Probably only extreme variations in alignment (large overjets, traumatic overbites and gross tooth displacements) represent true risks to dental health.

Minor intra- and interarch variations probably have little bearing on periodontal status, caries and mandibular function. In one study (Shaw, 1993) of 'surviving dentitions' in elderly individuals, the proportion of subjects with severe malocclusion was not less than that found in a group of children. In other words, the dentitions with malocclusions had not 'died out'.

On the psychological side, individuals with a conspicuous malocclusion will, even without treatment, continue to make their way through life, generally as well-adjusted and accomplished as others around them. However, personal feelings of dissatisfaction with their teeth and memories of teasing will remain with them, representing perhaps a general impairment of their quality of life.

Factors influencing the receipt of orthodontic treatment

Possession of a definite malocclusion is by no means the only factor that determines whether or not an individual will receive orthodontic treatment. Indeed, the presence of a malocclusion may hardly be necessary at all. Reference is often made to objective need, with a judgement based on an unbiased third-party assessment—usually the dentist's—and subjective need—the view of the individual with the malocclusion—but neither of these is simply related to the extent of the

variation. The eventual decision to embark upon orthodontic treatment derives from the views and attributes of both consumers (patient and parent) and providers (individual dentists, orthodontists and the health system generally).

Consumer factors

The desire to look better

Not surprisingly, this desire for improvement in appearance is a common motivation for seeking orthodontic treatment. In a study which assessed the attitude of a sample of 385 American and Welsh schoolchildren, the strongest perceived benefit of orthodontics was the opportunity for an improved appearance, and although improved dental health and function were also referred to, they appeared to be secondary in the individual's personal priorities (Tulloch *et al.*, 1984). Indeed, in another investigation, the majority of respondents actually reported that they would rather have straight teeth than healthy ones (Gochman, 1975). A large number of studies have confirmed the public's general agreement that the orthodontist's optimal occlusion looks best and that the desirability of treatment increases with the extent of deviation from this (Gochman, 1975; Tulloch *et al.*, 1984; Cons *et al.*, 1986). However, the perceived acceptable or normal range of variation may be fairly wide (Prahl-Andersen, 1978; Shaw, 1981).

Self (and parental) perception of malocclusion

In an investigation of the factors which may influence the desire for orthodontic treatment in a sample of 200 children (Shaw, 1981), a positive relationship between the objective severity of the visible irregularity and the desire for orthodontic treatment was confirmed. However, it was also evident that individual subjects acted inconsistently: 48% of those with moderate or severe visible irregularities, reported a high degree of satisfaction, but a similar proportion of those with minor irregularities or none at all, were dissatisfied. A possible explanation for this contradiction may lie partly in the imprecise way in which individuals regard their teeth before visiting an orthodontist; 83% of the above sample failed to describe their own anterior occlusal characteristics accurately and almost one-third of the children and parents failed to identify the child's dental photograph. The accuracy of self-report does however appear to improve with age; an investigation of young Norwegian adults revealed greater awareness (Espeland and Stenvik, 1991).

Whilst it has been shown that malocclusion appears to have little bearing upon self-esteem, effects have been shown to operate in the reverse direction, in that variations in self-esteem can influence personal judgements of the severity of malocclusion. In a study of American adults who were asked to identify facial profile outlines similar to their own, those with a high self-esteem selected better or more ideal profiles than they actually possessed (Pitt and Korabik, 1977). This conclusion was reinforced in a study in which children were asked to place their own dental attractiveness on a rating scale of dental attractiveness (Evans and Shaw, 1987). It appeared that those children who underrated their dental attractiveness (in comparison to an orthodontist) had, on average, a lower self-esteem than those who were accurate in their assessment.

General trust in the system

The remarkable basic faith that many consumers have in the health services they utilize was highlighted in a survey of the benefits that British patients and parents believed their orthodontic treatment would yield. For example, 75% of parents surveyed felt that orthodontic treatment was important for success in their child's future occupation and 92% believed that it would enhance dental health (Shaw *et al.*, 1980). It is unlikely that this represents the result of convincing 'sales talk', but rather that the dentist's referral for orthodontic care carries with it a strong implicit message that such treatment is both necessary and worthwhile and it is common experience amongst orthodontists that prospective patients often do not even know why they have been referred.

Gender and age

Surveys consistently reveal that more girls than boys receive orthodontic treatment in spite of the fact that the prevalence of malocclusion within the sexes is the same (Banks *et al.*, 1988). This trend is undoubtedly a reflection of sex role stereotyping, wherein society places greater emphasis on the possession of high physical attractiveness in the female. Awareness of malocclusion generally increases with age, reaching a peak around the mid-teens and, ironically, this concern often coincides with a growing reluctance to wear conspicuous orthodontic appliances.

Peer group norms

Reference to peers has been found to be a significant determinant of the uptake of orthodontic treatment. Most children with self-perceived anomalies want to be assimilated with other children through treatment. Their main dilemma is the anticipation of other children's responses to conspicuous appliances which will almost entirely depend on familiarity with appliances in the school and neighbourhood (Tulloch *et al.*, 1984). Common exposure to the sight of appliances may actually stimulate demand among those who wish to ensure that they have not missed out on an opportunity for self-improvement. Some reports indicate that appliances are worn as a 'badge of honour', or in certain settings, where this reflects a substantial economic investment by the family, as a status symbol (Baldwin, 1980).

Social class

Social class is also influential in the uptake of treatment. In a study of Welsh children, for whom any form of treatment would have been available at no cost, social class had no bearing upon the uptake of treatment when a high objective need for treatment was present (an anterior dentition which varied conspicuously from the ideal). However, in children with a low objective need, 19% of children in middle-class families went on to receive treatment, compared with 6% of those in the lower social groups (Kenealy *et al.*, 1989). It was suggested that this finding does not have its origin in actual class differences in the perception of malocclusion or treatment need. Instead it may be a reflection of the more regular pattern of dental attendance in the former group, their better organizational ability to avail themselves of any form of social service, and a facility to overcoming situational obstacles such as time off work, loss of earnings or transport difficulties. In an investigation into the uptake of dental and orthodontic treatment in two towns with differing dentist : population ratios, it was found that there was an increased uptake of treatment in the lower-social-class groups when the dentist: population ratio was favourable (O'Mullane and Robinson, 1977). This suggests that the potential demand for treatment by all social groups depends to a considerable extent upon the availability of dentists rather than inherent attitudes to treatment.

Provider factors

Dentist's awareness and attitudes

The general dentist's crucial role in the initiation of orthodontic treatment has been demonstrated in a survey of prospective patients in which 70% of referrals to orthodontists were initiated by the dentist (Shaw *et al.*, 1980). Nevertheless, remarkably little is known of the factors which influence the decision of the practitioner to initiate orthodontic treatment, either personally or by referral, and acuity and threshold appear to differ widely. Studies in the UK and in the Netherlands have shown that dentists and orthodontists are more critical than the general public about the acceptable range of dental irregularity (Shaw *et al.*, 1975; Prahl-Andersen, 1978).

Availability of services

Over the last two decades, most developed countries have seen a steady increase in the number of courses of orthodontic treatment provided annually. The capacity for orthodontics in any country's dental system reflects the number of dentists in the country; the proportion who undertake some orthodontics; the proportion who are in full-time specialist orthodontic practice; whether or not they employ dental assistants in an extended role; and the number of patients a single orthodontist is judged able to treat. The last statistic is also a significant determinant of treatment standards (Shaw, 1983). When all barriers to receiving care are removed, the uptake of orthodontic treatment may be as high as 60% (Helm, 1990). Table 6.5 shows the ratio of orthodontists to 12-year-olds for a number of developed countries.

Cost and method of dentist remuneration

The funding of orthodontic services is also remarkably different from one country to the next (Shaw, 1983), and in some, the family must meet the entire cost of treatment. More

Table 6.5 UK ratio of orthodontists to 12-year-old population

Norway	1:325	Finland	1:550
USA	1:352	Italy	1:787
Denmark	1:383	Greece	1:870
Sweden	1:416	Hungary	1:1542
Germany	1:427	Spain	1:1798
		UK	1:2389

commonly, treatment is either free or partly funded by state or private insurance, which reimburse the family's cost, often in proportion to the degree of severity of malocclusion. For instance, some form of treatment priority index is applied and full reimbursement is given for severe irregularities, less for moderate irregularities and none for minor irregularities. Thus, for children with minor irregularities or those living in a setting of purely private orthodontics, uptake of treatment will simply reflect the family's ability and willingness to pay. Levels of prescription of medical and dental care are known to be strongly influenced by the system of remuneration (Abel-Smith, 1976). In orthodontics, payment systems that calculate fees on the number of appliance components have been seen to encourage the use of multiple appliances, low general fee levels encourage large case loads, and low fixed-appliance fees may encourage treatment by simple methods (O'Brien *et al.*, 1989).

Orthodontics in the public health context

In many developed countries, orthodontic treatment is subsidized by public health resources or by state, personal or employment insurance schemes and mechanisms for ensuring appropriate targeting of resources and quality assurance are clearly desirable. Several indices have been developed for diagnostic classification, e.g. Angle's classification (British Standard, 1983); epidemiological data collection (Bjork *et al.*, 1964; Baume *et al.*, 1973); prioritizing treatment (described in more detail below); and evaluating treatment outcome (Richmond *et al.*, 1992a, 1992b).

Treatment need (treatment priority)

Several indices have been developed to attempt to categorize malocclusion into groups according to the level of treatment need. Examples of these are the Occlusal Index (Summers, 1971), the Handicapping Malocclusion Assessment Record (Salzmann, 1968) and the Treatment Priority Index (Grainger, 1967). These indices apply a score to each trait, which is then weighted to calculate an overall score. However, the selection of these weightings adds subjectivity to the assessments, no matter how objective the recording of the traits (Helm, 1977). Another method of allocation of treatment priority is the Swedish National Board for Health and Welfare Index (Linder-Aronson, 1974). Essentially this is a method of defining the severity or degree of traits that may constitute a threat to the longevity of the dentition. These traits are then allocated into grades which define the urgency of treatment need. However, the cut-off points between the grades are somewhat vague, and this may lead to loss of reproducibility, especially when the index is used by non-orthodontic personnel.

The *Index of Orthodontic Treatment Need (IOTN)* ranks malocclusion in terms of the significance of various occlusal traits for the individual's dental health and perceived aesthetic impairment, with the intention of identifying those individuals who would be most likely to benefit from orthodontic treatment. The index incorporates a dental health and aesthetic component (Brook and Shaw, 1989). The *Dental Health Component of IOTN* represents an attempt at synthesis of the current evidence for the deleterious effects of malocclusion and the potential benefits of orthodontic treatment, and is loosely based upon the Index of the Swedish Medical Board. Each occlusal trait thought to contribute to the longevity and satisfactory functioning of the dentition is defined and placed into five grades, with clear cut-off points between the grades (Table 6.6). In use, various features of the malocclusion are noted and measured, with a specially designed ruler. A fundamental premise of the index is the recognition that dental diseases are site-specific (for example, severe displacement of a particular tooth represents a particular disadvantage for that site) and the most severe trait identified is the basis for grading the individual's need for treatment on dental health grounds. Summing scores for a series of individual traits is not performed. Thus, multiple minor variations, each of which is unimportant with respect to dental health, cannot be added together to place an individual in a higher grade.

The *Aesthetic Component of IOTN* consists of a 10-point scale, illustrated by a series of numbered photographs, from an earlier study, which were rated for attractiveness by lay individuals and selected as being equidistantly spaced through the range of scores. A rating is allocated for overall dental attractiveness rather than specific morphological similarity to the photographs. The value arrived at gives an indication of the patient's treatment need on the grounds of aesthetic impairment, and by inference reflects the sociopsychological need for orthodontic treatment.

Recent public health studies in orthodontics

Estimation of treatment need

The dental health and the aesthetic components of IOTN were recorded for a sample of 333 children 11–12-years-old from a broad range of social backgrounds, attending schools in the north-west of England (Brook and Shaw, 1989). From the dental health component one-third of the children were categorized in the great (grade 4) and very great (grade 5) need for treatment grades; one-third were placed in grade 3 (which may be regarded as the borderline grade); and the remaining third were allocated to grades 2 and 1, representing little and no need for orthodontic treatment. In contrast, a sample of 222 patients referred to a regional consultant orthodontic department for advice or treatment was examined (Brook and Shaw, 1989). Not surprisingly, this referred sample comprised a large proportion of patients (74.4%) allocated to grades 4 and 5 and 19.7% to grade 3, with only 5.9% placed in grades 1 and 2.

Orthodontic treatment standards studies

In a study of treatment standards in the General Dental Services in England and Wales, where the majority of providers do not have a specialist qualification, 1010 pairs of before-and-after study casts submitted for payment to the central payment agency were randomly selected and analysed (Richmond *et al.*, 1993). Using a standardized measure of treatment outcome (Richmond *et al.*, 1992a, 1992b), 21% of cases were unimproved or worse as a result of orthodontic treatment. When outcome was related to choice of appliance, combined upper and lower fixed appliances produced the best

Table 6.6 The dental health component of the index of orthodontic treatment need (IOTN)

Grade 5 (Need treatment)

5.i   Impeded eruption of teeth (with the exception of third molars) due to crowding, displacement, the presence of supernumerary teeth, retained deciduous teeth and any pathological cause

5.h   Extensive hypodontia with restorative implications (more than one tooth missing in any quadrant) requiring prerestorative orthodontics

5.a   Increased overjet greater than 9 mm

5.m   Reverse overjet greater than 3.5 mm with reported masticatory and speech difficulties

5.p   Defects of cleft lip and palate

5.s   Submerged deciduous teeth

Grade 4 (Need treatment)

4.h   Less extensive hypodontia requiring prerestorative orthodontics or orthodontic space closure to obviate the need for a prosthesis

4.a   Increased overjet greater than 6 mm but less than or equal to 9 mm

4.b   Reverse overjet greater than 3.5 mm with no masticatory or speech difficulties

4.m   Reverse overjet greater than 1 mm but less than 3.5 mm with recorded masticatory and speech difficulties

4.c   Anterior or posterior cross-bites with greater than 2 mm discrepancy between retruded contact position and intercuspal position

4.l   Posterior lingual cross-bite with no functional occlusal contact in one or both buccal segments

4.d   Severe displacements of teeth greater than 4 mm

4.e   Extreme lateral or anterior open bites greater than 4 mm

4.f   Increased and complete overbite with gingival or palatal trauma

4.t   Partially erupted teeth, tipped and impacted against adjacent teeth

4.x   Presence of supernumerary teeth

Grade 3 (Borderline need)

3.a   Increased overjet greater than 3.5 mm but less than or equal to 6 mm with incompetent lips

3.b   Reverse overjet greater than 1 mm but less than or equal to 3.5 mm

3.c   Anterior or posterior cross-bites with greater than 1 mm but less than or equal to 2 mm discrepancy between retruded contact position and intercuspal position

3.d   Contact point displacement of teeth greater than 2 mm but less than or equal to 4 mm

3.e   Lateral or anterior open bite greater than 2 mm but less than or equal to 4 mm

3.f   Deep overbite complete on gingival or palatal tissues but no trauma

Grade 2 (Little)

2.1   Increased overjet greater than 3.5 mm but less than or equal to 6 mm with competent lips

2.b   Reverse overjet greater than 0 mm but less than or equal to 1 mm

2.c   Anterior or posterior cross-bite with less than or equal to 1 mm discrepancy between retruded contact position and intercuspal position

2.d   Contact point displacements of teeth greater than 1 mm but less than or equal to 2 mm

2.e   Anterior or posterior open bite greater than 1 mm but less than or equal to 2 mm

2.f   Increased overbite greater than or equal to 3.5 mm without gingival contact

2.g   Prenormal or postnormal occlusions with no other anomalies (includes up to half a unit discrepancy)

Grade 1 (None)

1.   Extremely minor malocclusions including contact point displacements less than 1 mm

standard of treatment. Cases with a borderline need for treatment (IOTN grade 3) were more liable to have unsuccessful treatment. A lack of improvement or worsening of the malocclusion occurred in 34% of cases.

The Regional Consultant Orthodontic Service provides treatment for 10% of British children. Treatment is provided by salaried orthodontic specialists with extensive training in the management of complex orthodontic problems. Seventeen regional centres were selected by a stratified random sampling procedure (O'Brien *et al.*, 1993). Each department was visited, and a sample of 100 consecutively started cases were

examined. The standard of treatment was high and only cases with a high level of need had received treatment. However, the results obtained by spring-type removable appliances were significantly inferior to those gained by fixed appliances.

A pilot study has been conducted to assess the standard of orthodontic treatment in Norway where care is provided almost exclusively by orthodontic specialists. A sample of 220 cases was collected and a high standard of treatment was found with only 5% of cases categorized as worse or no different (Richmond and Andrews, 1993).

Cleft lip and palate

Ascertainment and treatment of clefts of the lip and palate present a number of challenges in public health. Orofacial clefts occur in around 1 in 500 live Caucasian births, more frequently in oriental people, and less so in black people. However, the reliability of ascertainment is variable from one country to the next and is surrounded by many methodological concerns (Sayetta *et al.*, 1989).

Intercentre comparisons of treatment outcome have revealed striking differences in the quality of care between one centre and the next (Ross, 1987; Friede *et al.*, 1991; Roberts-Harry *et al.*, 1991; Shaw *et al.*, 1992; Enemark *et al.*, 1993). In one study the need for corrective secondary surgery in the late teens to compensate for poor surgery in infancy differed by a factor of 6 between the best and worst centres (Shaw *et al.*, 1992). Low-volume surgeons appear likely to produce unsatisfactory outcomes, whereas highly centralized and standardized services such as those available in some of the Nordic countries appear conducive to successful care. Interestingly, the clinical protocols of the latter also involve simplified protocols with reduced visits, expense and clinical burden. The poor results revealed in the UK by intercentre clinical audit recently led to a series of recommendations for cleft palate service purchasing; these emphasize the need for care to be provided by a highly experienced multidisciplinary team coordinated from a single regional centre.

Conclusions

Orthodontic services are an interesting aspect of dental public health. Malocclusion is not a disease but rather a set of dental variations that have, in the main, a limited influence upon oral health. Yet demand for services in most countries generally exceeds supply and presents difficult choices in the distribution of public health resources. The use of indices to target resources and secure an adequate risk–cost balance is desirable.

References

Abel-Smith, B. (1976) Tradesman or priest: the payment of the doctor. In: *Value for Money in Health Services: A Comparative Study*. Heinemann, London.

Baldwin, D.C. (1980) Appearance and aesthetics in oral health. *Community Dental and Oral Epidemiology* 8:244–256.

Banks P.A., Corkill, C.M., Bowden, D.E.J. *et al.* (1988) The consultant orthodontic service; 1985 survey. *British Dental Journal* 165:425–429.

Baume, L.J., Horowitz, H.S., Summers, C.J. *et al.* (1973) A method of examining occlusal traits developed by the FDI commission on classification and statistics for oral conditions (COGSTOC). *International Dental Journal* 23:530–537.

Bjork, A., Krebs, A. and Solow B. (1964) A method for the epidemiological registration of malocclusion. *Acta Odontologica Scandinavica* 22:27–41.

British Dental Association (1954) *Memorandum on Orthodontic Services*. British Dental Association, London.

British Standards Institution 1982 BS-4492. British Standards Glossary of Terms Relating to Dentistry–London, British Standards Institution.

Brook, P.H. and Shaw, W.C. (1989) The development of an orthodontic treatment priority index. *European Journal of Orthodontics* 11:309–320.

Cons, N.C., Jenny, J. and Kahout, F.J. (1986) *The Dental Aesthetic Index*. University of Iowa, Iowa.

Enemark, H., Friede, H., Paulin, G. *et al.* (1993) Lip and nose morphology in patients with unilateral cleft lip and palate from four Scandinavian centres. *Scandinavian Journal and Plastic and Reconstructive Hand Surgery* 27:41–47.

Espeland, L.V. and Stenvik, A. (1991) Orthodontically treated young adults: awareness of own dental arrangement. *European Journal of Orthodontics* 13:7–14.

Evans, R. and Shaw, W.C. (1987) Preliminary evaluation of an illustrated scale for rating dental attractiveness. *European Journal of Orthodontics* 9:314–318.

Friede, H., Enemark, H., Semb, G. *et al.* (1991) Craniofacial and occlusal characteristics in unilateral cleft lip and palate patients from four Scandinavian centres. *Scandinavian Journal and Plastic and Reconstructive Hand Surgery* 25:269–276.

Gochman, D.S. (1975) The measurement and development of dentally relevant motives. *Journal of Public Health Dentistry* 35:160–164.

Grainger R.M. (1967) *Orthodontic Treatment Priority Index*. Public health service publication no. 1000, series 2 no. 25. US Government Printing Office, Washington, DC.

Helm, S. (1977) Intra-examiner reliability of epidemiological registrations of malocclusion. *Acta Odontologica Scandinavica* 35:161–165.

Helm, S. (1990) *Reappraisal of the Criteria for Orthodontic Treatment*. PhD thesis, University of Oslo.

Kenealy, P., Frude, N. and Shaw, W.C. (1989) The influence of social class on the uptake of orthodontic treatment. *British Journal of Orthodontics* 16:107–111.

Linder-Aronson, S. (1974) Orthodontics in the Swedish public dental health system. *Transactions of the European Orthodontics Society*, pp. 233–240.

O'Brien, K.D., Shaw W.C., Roberts C.T. and Stephens C.D. (1989) Regional variation in the provision and cost of orthodontic treatment in England and Wales. *British Journal of Orthodontics* 16:67–74.

O'Brien, K.D., Shaw, W.C. and Roberts C.T. (1993) The effectiveness of the hospital orthodontic service of England and Wales. *British Journal of Orthodontics* 15:127–130.

O'Mullane, D.M. and Robinson, M.E. (1977) The distribution of dentists and the uptake of dental treatment by schoolchildren in England. *Community Dental and Oral Epidemiology* 5:156–159.

Pitt, E.J. and Korabik K. (1977) The relationship between self-concept and profile self-selection. *American Journal of Orthodontics* 72:459–460.

Prahl-Andersen, B. (1978) The need for orthodontic treatment. *Angle Orthodontics* 48:1–9.

Richmond, S. and Andrews, M. (1993) Orthodontic treatment standards in Norway. *European Journal of Orthodontics* 15:7–15.

Richmond, S., Shaw, W.C., Roberts, C.T. *et al.* (1992a) The development of the PAR index (peer assessment rating): reliability and validity. *European Journal of Orthodontics* 14:125–139.

Richmond, S., Shaw, W.C., Roberts, C.T. and Andrews, M. (1992b) The PAR index (peer assessment rating): methods to determine outcome of orthodontic treatment in terms of improvement and standards. *European Journal of Orthodontics* 14:180–197.

Richmond, S., Shaw, W.C., Stephens, C.D. *et al.* (1993) Orthodontics in the general dental services of England and Wales: a critical assessment of standards. *British Dental Journal* 174:315–329.

Roberts-Harry, D.P., Evans, R. and Hathorn, I.S. (1991) The effects of different surgical regimens on nasal symmetry and facial attractiveness in cleft lip and palate patients. *Cleft Palate Craniofacial Journal* 28:274–278.

Ross, R.B. (1987) Treatment variables affecting facial growth in complete unilateral cleft lip and palate. Part 1: Treatment affecting growth. *Cleft Palate Journal* 24:5–23.

Salzmann, J.A. (1968) Handicapping malocclusion assessment to establish treatment priority. *American Journal of Orthodontics* 54:749–765.

Sayetta, R.B., Weinrich, M.C. and Coston, G.N. (1989) Incidence and prevalence of cleft lip and palate: what we think we know. *Cleft Palate Journal* 26:242–247.

Shaw, W.C. (1981) Factors influencing the desire for orthodontic treatment. *European Journal of Orthodontics* 3:151–162.

Shaw, W.C. (1983) Improving British orthodontic services. *British Dental Journal* 155:131–135.

Shaw, W.C. (ed.) (1993) Risk Benefit Appraisal in Orthodontics. In *Orthodontics and Occlusal Management*, Butterworth-Heinemann, Oxford.

Shaw, W.C., Lewis, H.G. and Robertson, N.R.E. (1975) Perception of malocclusion. *British Dental Journal* 138:211–216.

Shaw, W.C., Gabe, M.J. and Jones, B.M. (1980) The expectations of orthodontic patients in South Wales and St Louis, Missouri. *British Journal of Orthodontics* 7:75–80.

Shaw, W.C., O Brien, K.D., Richmond, S. and Brook, P. (1991) Quality control in orthodontics: risk/benefit considerations. *British Dental Journal* 170:33–37.

Shaw, W.C., Asher-McDade, C., Brattstrom, V. *et al.* (1992a) Intercentre clinical audit for cleft lip and palate–a preliminary European investigation. In: *Recent Advances in Plastic Surgery*. (Jackson, I.T. and Sommerlad, B.C., eds), vol. 4, pp. 1–15. Churchill Livingstone, Edinburgh.

Shaw, W.C., Dahl, E., Asher-McDade, C. *et al.* (1992b) A six-center international study of treatment outcome in patients with clefts of the lip and palate: part 5. General discussion and conclusions. *Cleft Palate Craniofacial Journal* 29:413–418.

Summers, C.J. (1971) A system for identifying and scoring occlusal disorders. *American Journal of Orthodontics* 59:552–567.

Tulloch, J.F.C, Shaw, W.C. and Smith, A. (1984) A comparison of attitudes toward orthodontic treatment in British and American communities. *American Journal of Orthodontics* 85:253–259.

7

Community-based strategies for preventing dental caries

Brian A. Burt and Stephen A. Eklund

Prevention of oral diseases is a prime objective for the dental public health administrator. As in any area of public health, prevention can be approached through health education and health promotion, and through early case-finding and treatment. In addition, however, dentistry has a number of powerful and well-tested methods of primary prevention for caries, based on fluoride and sealants. The use of fluoride is a primary reason why oral health has improved so much in the developed world over the last generation or so, and when sealants are added to fluoride the potential exists virtually to eliminate caries.

The purpose of this chapter is to describe the main caries-preventive strategies from which the dental public health administrator can choose. We describe each strategy briefly, then assess the advantages and limitations of each.

Fluoride toothpastes

The goal of any use of fluoride is to keep a low level of fluoride constantly present in the oral environment, where it is available for re-mineralization of early lesions. Any strategy which produces that condition, therefore, is likely to be effective to some extent. Brushing with a fluoride toothpaste, a standard practice in many parts of the world, is an ideal way to maintain a level of fluoride in the oral cavity. Toothpaste is the most widely used fluoride vehicle in the world, and many consider it the most important single factor in the caries decline.

Early clinical trials in the 1950s used stannous fluoride as the active ingredient (Muhler *et al.*, 1955); later studies with stannous fluoride toothpastes reported caries reductions of 15–30% among children over periods of 2–3 years (Jordan and Peterson, 1959; Muhler, 1962; Horowitz *et al.*, 1966; James and Anderson, 1967; Slack *et al.*, 1967). Subsequent trials of other fluoride compounds, added to a number of different abrasive systems, have generally produced similar results. Toothpastes have now been successfully tested with stannous fluoride, sodium fluoride, sodium monofluorophosphate and amine fluoride as the active ingredient. Clinical trials of fluoride toothpastes in fluoridated areas have demonstrated an additive effect (Marthaler, 1974; Lind *et al.*, 1976), and there is evidence that fluoride toothpaste will prevent root caries in older adults (Jensen and Kohout, 1988).

By the 1990s, fluoride toothpastes accounted for 90% cent or more of the toothpaste market in most economically developed countries. Most products today contain sodium fluoride or sodium monofluorophosphate as the active ingredient, usually in concentrations of 1000–1100 mg F/g, though toothpastes with 1500 mg F/g have been successfully tested (Hanchowicz, 1984; Conti *et al.*, 1988; Fogels *et al.*, 1988) and are marketed in Europe and the USA. The cariostatic power of a toothpaste is proportional to the fluoride content (Stephen *et al.*, 1988), so those with 1500 mg F/g are more effective than those with lower concentrations

(Ripa, 1989). Trials have also been conducted with toothpastes of 2500 mg F/g or more (Lu *et al.*, 1987; Ripa *et al.*, 1988; Stephen *et al.*, 1988) though the European Community still maintains 1500 mg F/g as its upper limit for fluoride concentrations in toothpaste.

At the other end of the spectrum, concerns about the fluorosis risk from children swallowing toothpaste have led to lower-strength products being tested. Trials comparing toothpaste with 250 mg F/g fluoride against 1000 mg F/g products have yielded conflicting results (Forsman, 1974a; Koch *et al.*, 1982; Mitropoulos *et al.*, 1984). Findings from later studies of 500–550 mg F/g products, however, have suggested efficacy equivalent to the 1000 mg F/g toothpastes (Triol *et al.*, 1987; Winter *et al.*, 1989). Since children can swallow between 0.12 and 0.38 mg of toothpaste per brushing (Beltran and Szpunar, 1988), there is hope that lower-fluoride toothpastes may reduce the risk of fluorosis while substantially retaining caries-preventive benefits. Products with 400 mg F/g have been marketed for years in some countries as 'children's toothpastes,' but no clinical trials with these products have been conducted.

Advantages and limitations of fluoride toothpaste

Fluoride in toothpaste is taken up directly by demineralized enamel (Reintsema *et al.*, 1985; Stookey *et al.*, 1985), and it also increases the fluoride concentration in dental plaque (Duckworth *et al.*, 1989; Sidi, 1989), thus leaving a store of fluoride available for remineralization when pH drops (Schafer, 1989). Its principal advantage is that in much of the world tooth-brushing is a routine part of personal hygiene and grooming, and so people benefit from regular exposure to fluoride without having to change their daily routines.

Fluoride toothpaste is widely available and cheap in the economically developed world, and its developmental and distribution costs have been largely borne by private corporations. Public health administrators thereby enjoy the benefits of its use without having to add the costs on to their limited budgets. On the other hand, fluoride toothpaste remains too expensive for much of the developing world. The challenge to manufacturers and to public health, therefore, is how to make effective fluoride toothpastes available and affordable to most people in the developing world.

Water fluoridation

Fluoridation is the controlled adjustment of a fluoride compound to a public water supply in order to bring the fluoride concentration up to a level which effectively prevents caries. Fluoridation reaches everyone in a community, a feature which is both its greatest strength and its greatest problem in terms of social policy. Fluoridation is not a targeted approach to caries prevention–it reaches everybody.

The classic studies of H. Trendley Dean, during the 1930s in the USA, are described in detail in Chapter 14. It was Dean's work that led to the adoption of 1.0 mg/l as the fluoride concentration in drinking water which represented the best trade-off between substantial caries reduction and an acceptable level of the mildest forms of dental fluorosis. Following a series of epidemiological studies in the western part of the USA (Galagan and Lamson, 1953; Galagan and Vermillion, 1957), the concentration was modified to a range of 0.7–1.2 mg/l, depending on climate. These levels seem appropriate enough for economically developed nations of European heritage, and are still policy in the USA. Their validity for Asian and African conditions, however, is less clear. Hong Kong, for example, now fluoridates its water at 0.5 mg/l.

Following years of epidemiological studies in communities with naturally occurring fluoride in their drinking waters, four independent studies in controlled fluoridation began in the USA and Canada in 1945 and 1946. The two begun in 1945 were at Grand Rapids, Michigan, with nearby Muskegon as the control city (Dean *et al.*, 1950), and Newburgh, New York, with Kingston as the control city (Ast *et al.*, 1950a). In 1946 studies began at Evanston, Illinois, with Oak Park as control (Blayney and Tucker, 1948), and at Brantford, Ontario, with Sarnia as control. Naturally fluoridated Stratford, Ontario, was also included in this study (Hutton *et al.*, 1951). These studies all found positive reductions in caries experience; the results are summarized in Table 7.1. At the time of these studies, drinking water was virtually the only significant exposure to fluoride.

By 1984, there were 34 countries reporting fluoridation projects reaching some 246 million people, not including naturally occurring fluoride (Fédération Dentaire Internationale, 1987). Virtually 100% of the populations of Singapore and Hong Kong receive fluoridated

Table 7.1 Results of the first four controlled fluoridation studies in North America*

Community	Ages studied (years)	Year	Mean DMFT	Per cent improved	Mean M teeth	Per cent improved
Grand Rapids (F)	12–14	1944–45	9.58		0.84	
		1959	4.26	55.5	0.29	65.5
Evanston (F)	12–14	1946	9.03		0.19	
		1959	4.66	48.4	0.06	68.4
Brantford (F)	12–14	1959	3.23	56.7	0.22	70.7
Sarnia (no F)	12–14	1959	7.46		0.75	
Newburgh (F)	13–14	1960	3.73	70.1	0.10	89.1
Kingston (no F)	13–14	1960	12.46		0.92	

*Grand Rapids and Evanston used before-and-after analyses; Brantford and Newburgh employed Sarnia and Kingston, respectively, as concurrent controls.
DMFT = Decayed/missing/filled teeth; M teeth = missing teeth.
From Ast and Fitzgerald (1962), with permission.

water, as do over 50% of those in Australia, Malaysia, New Zealand and the USA. The UK has some 15% of its population receiving fluoridated water, and Birmingham has been fluoridated since 1964. At the other extreme, there is very little fluoridation in continental Europe. Ireland remains the only nation (Singapore excepted) to have a mandatory fluoridation law.

The outcomes from the many fluoridation studies conducted around the world have been remarkably uniform, despite variations in design and conduct (Chapter 14). For many years, the statement that fluoridation reduces dental caries experience by half was accepted with little question, and at a time when drinking water was the only significant source of fluoride that statement was true enough. Effectiveness of water fluoridation has not diminished over time, though the caries reductions directly attributable to water fluoridation have declined as other uses of fluoride have become more widespread (i.e. the benefits of water fluoridation have become 'diluted' by other uses of fluoride, though the overall fluoride benefits are thus increased). Current estimates are that fluoridation reduces coronal and root caries over a lifetime by 20–40% (Newbrun, 1989).

Advantages and limitations of water fluoridation

To be effective, or even feasible, water fluoridation has several preconditions. For a start, it requires a municipal water supply with one or more treatment plants and an operating staff. Water needs to be piped to the majority of homes in the community, and most people need to drink it (rather than water from individual wells, collected rainwater or commercially available bottled water). These preconditions, largely taken for granted in the economically developed world, imply a level of socioeconomic development which is only sometimes present in a developing nation. Without them, water fluoridation is not an option.

Fluoridation's greatest benefit is its relatively low cost, and the fact that it can reach an entire community. In the USA in 1989, fluoridation cost was estimated to average 51 cents/person per year (assuming an existing water system), though in any one community the annual cost ranged from 12 cents to $5.41 (Results, 1989). Per capita cost is usually inversely proportional to the population served, and total expenditures on equipment and material are naturally greater in larger communities. Additional personnel costs for fluoridation are virtually negligible in a large city's water treatment plant, though they can be significant in a small community.

In addition to being inexpensive (in an economically developed nation), water fluoridation is the most cost-effective method of bringing fluoride to a whole community. Health economists at the 1989 University of Michigan workshop (Results, 1989) concluded that water fluoridation was one of the few public health measures to demonstrate true cost-savings: it actually saved more money than it cost to operate. Fluoridation was estimated to cost $3.35 per carious surface saved, far beneath the fee for any restoration.

But fluoridation has been the subject of considerable political opposition in many parts of the world, and the financial and emotional cost of dealing with this opposition has to be considered by a public health administrator. Opposition can be centred on claims of risk to the environment or to human health–arguments which have a weak scientific base but powerful emotional appeal. Despite the complete absence of fluoridation in Norway, for example, a study in that country (Rise and Kraft, 1986) found a 20% rise in public opposition to fluoridated water between 1973 and 1983. This perplexing shift was thought to stem from a perception that dental health was improving anyway and that fluoridation was an unnecessary risk (Rise and Kraft, 1986). Some opposition in any community is based on the freedom-of-choice issue, where, as mentioned earlier, water fluoridation has its greatest problems as social policy. Fluoridation is dichotomous by nature; the community either fluoridates or it doesn't. Alone among the various uses of fluoride, this pits individual choice against political decisions made on behalf of the whole community.

Opponents have taken the legality of fluoridation to court on a number of occasions, though no American court of last resort has ever ruled against fluoridation for any reason. The most searching courtroom scrutiny of water fluoridation, especially in respect to its impact on human health, came from Glasgow in 1983 (McKechnie, 1985). Known as the Strathclyde case, this was the longest court case in British legal history. The presiding judge, Lord Jauncey, ruled that the evidence for fluoridation's safety was convincing (Opinion, 1983).

Fluoridated salt

Fluoridated salt uses the same principle as water fluoridation, namely that a small amount of fluoride in a commonly used dietary staple serves to inhibit dental caries with little conscious action on the individual s part. It was first used in 1955 in Switzerland, where water fluoridation is confined to the city of Basle. Switzerland is a prosperous and highly developed country with only one salt-processing and distribution company, so there have been few problems with control of the procedure. In more recent years, salt fluoridation has been adopted in France, Germany, Costa Rica, Jamaica and Mexico, and other countries are considering the measure.

The Swiss studies began with salt fluoridated to 90 mg F/kg, later increased to the current standard of 250 mg F/kg. Estimates of the most appropriate concentration have been made from studies of 24-hour urinary fluoride excretion (Ericsson, 1971; Obry-Musset *et al.*, 1992), and are related to quantities of salt consumed. The concentration of 250 mg F/kg is used by most countries which have recently adopted salt fluoridation, though the appropriateness of this level should be tested in light of variable national consumption.

Early evaluations of salt fluoridation in the canton of Zurich (90 mg F/kg at the time) found that children from families reporting the use of fluoridated salt had lower-than-usual caries prevalence (Marthaler and Schenardi, 1962). Interest by the World Health Organization led to field trials in Colombia in 1965, where substantial benefits were found among 12–14-year-olds who were 5–7 years old when the programmes started (Gillespie and Roviralta, 1985). Observational evidence of efficacy also came from Hungarian studies (Toth, 1984). In Switzerland, empirical evidence for the effectiveness of fluoridated salt has continued to be reported, especially from the cantons of Vaud and Glarus. In Vaud, caries experience in schoolchildren has been consistently lower than that from two adjacent control cantons (De Crousaz *et al.*, 1985), while from the introduction of fluoridated salt in Glarus in 1974 up to 1983, mean decayed, missing, filled teeth (DMFT) scores in 14-year-old children dropped 53% (Steiner *et al.*, 1986, 1989).

The evidence for the effectiveness of salt fluoridation is thus based on a limited number of observational studies; the nature of the procedure does not lend itself readily to randomized, double-blind clinical trials. As mentioned earlier, other uses of fluoride also make it difficult to ascribe specific effects to any one method of using fluoride. Even with these provisos, the evidence for the effectiveness of salt fluoridation is consistent.

Advantages and limitations of salt fluoridation

Fluoridated salt, when well-accepted by the public, has some parallels to water fluoridation in terms of wide coverage, little conscious action by the individual and low expense. It also requires systems of monitoring quality at the processing plants.

The political attractiveness of fluoridated salt,

as opposed to water fluoridation, is in the element of choice for consumers. In most places using fluoridated salt, it appears alongside non-fluoridated salt on the supermarket shelves. This makes fluoridated salt more palatable from the social policy viewpoint, but its community-wide caries-preventive impact is clearly related to the extent of public acceptance (in Switzerland, fluoridated salt claimed 75% of the national domestic salt market in 1987–91). The introduction of fluoridated salt, therefore, needs to be accompanied by public education and promotion. The Swiss canton of Vaud, interestingly enough, removes that choice by fluoridating all salt on the supermarket shelves as well as the salt delivered in bulk to restaurants, bakeries, food processors, hospitals and other institutions. Oral health should benefit as a result, though consumer choice is curtailed. (Actually, Vaud still permits 'natural' salt to be sold in specialty health food shops, but this market is small.) In France and Germany, which only accept fluoride uses which permit consumer choice, the fluoridated salt programme is limited to domestic salt, which is available alongside non-fluoridated salt. But in both Costa Rica and Jamaica all domestic and institutional salt, except that for bakeries, is fluoridated. Despite the extensive studies carried out in Colombia and Hungary, salt fluoridation has not become established in either country.

Salt fluoridation is not recommended in countries where there is extensive water fluoridation. Further research in salt fluoridation should be in its acceptance and effectiveness in the different countries now adopting the measure, and further refinement of country-specific concentrations with a variety of dietary practices. There is also little information on fluorosis resulting from salt fluoridation; that too requires documentation.

Dietary fluoride supplements

Fluoride supplements (tablets, lozenges, drops, liquids and fluoride–vitamin preparations) have been in use since the 1940s. They are usually made with fluoride quantities of 1.0, 0.5 or 0.25 mg. The original pills have been joined by chewable tablets and lozenges, the latter intended to be chewed or sucked before swallowing with the intent of getting both posteruptive and preeruptive effects. Dietary supplements usually contain neutral sodium fluoride (NaF) as the active ingredient, though other fluorides have been tested.

The first studies of fluoride supplements took place during the 1950s (Arnold et al., 1960). Subsequent studies, testing for pre-eruptive effects in infants and young children, reported that fluoride tablets taken daily resulted in a 50–80% caries reduction in the primary and the permanent dentitions (Binder et al., 1978). But many of these studies were seriously flawed. Problems included selection of participants for above-average motivation and compliance, self-selection into test and control groups or no concurrent controls, high attrition rates and lack of blindness among examiners. The association that practitioners have observed between conscientious use of fluoride supplements and freedom from caries cannot be taken as evidence of efficacy, for compliance is naturally higher among dentally aware people with other good oral health habits.

While the evidence for pre-eruptive benefits from fluoride supplements is weak, well-conducted clinical trials have shown that fluoride supplements are effective in school-age children. Studies in which the supplements were chewed, swished and swallowed under supervision have reported caries reductions of 20-28% over 3–6 years (DePaola and Lax, 1968; Driscoll et al., 1978). Reductions of 81.3% were reported from a Glasgow study in which children initially aged 5.5 years from lower socioeconomic groups sucked a 1.0 mg fluoride tablet, or a placebo, under supervision in schools every school day for 3 years (Stephen and Campbell, 1978).

Retrospective analyses of supplement use provide weaker evidence than do clinical trials because they can be biased by self-selection. Positive retrospective results have been reported (Marthaler, 1969; Fanning et al., 1980; Allmark et al., 1982; Widenheim et al., 1986; de Liefde and Herbison, 1989; Widenheim and Birkhed, 1991; D'Hoore and van Nieuwenhuysen, 1992), but self-selection bias was evident in all of these studies. There are also retrospective studies which found no difference in caries experience between those children who reported using fluoride supplements and those who did not (Thylstrup et al., 1979; Holm and Anderson, 1982; Friis-Hasche et al., 1984; Bagramian et al., 1989; Kalsbeek et al., 1992)

The efficacy of any preventive procedure, which is the first step in determining whether it should be used in a community preventive programme, should be based, as far as possible, on clinical trials which meet specific quality criteria. In the collective evidence on fluoride supplements, only a few studies meet these standards. The evidence from them is that supplements show posteruptive effectiveness in school-aged children when they are chewed or permitted to dissolve slowly in the mouth. But there is little good evidence for pre-eruptive effectiveness when fluoride supplements are given to infants and young children.

Advantages and limitations of fluoride dietary supplements

Tablets and lozenges are preferred in some school-based programmes because they are cleaner than mouthrinses and are less intrusive into the school routines. When used among children who are past the age of fluorosis concern (i.e. 7 years or older), supplements have posteruptive cariostatic benefits. Their use in an organized school-based programme also aids compliance, which is poor when tablets are simply made available to be picked up by parents. In many countries, fluoride supplements are only available on prescription, which obviously can restrict their use in community programmes even further.

The major concern now associated with supplements is that of dental fluorosis. While fluorosis can develop at any pre-eruptive stage under certain conditions, late secretion and early maturation have been identified as the developmental times when dental enamel is especially sensitive to ingested fluoride (Larsen *et al.*, 1985; Evans and Stamm, 1991; DenBesten and Thariani, 1992). While some reports found no association between supplement use and the development of fluorosis (Bagramian *et al.*, 1989; Stephen *et al.*, 1991), considerably more have reported the contrary (Aasenden and Peebles, 1974; Thylstrup *et al.*, 1979; Holm and Anderson, 1982; Suckling and Pearce, 1984; de Liefde and Herbison, 1985, 1989; Larsen *et al.*, 1989; Woltgens *et al.*, 1989; Woolfolk *et al.*, 1989; Riordan and Banks, 1991; D'Hoore and Van Nieuwenhuysen, 1992; Kalsbeek *et al.*, 1992). An excellent case-control study provides the strongest evidence from any one study for cause-and-effect (Pendrys and Katz, 1989). The weight of evidence is that fluoride supplements, when ingested prior to tooth eruption, are a risk factor for dental fluorosis.

Table 7.2 Fluoride supplement schedule (mg F/day) adopted by the Canadian Dental Association, 1992. Only to be applied with the fluoride concentration in drinking water <0.3 mg/l*

Age	Fluoride supplement (mg/day)
Birth–3 years	0
3–6 years	0.25
6+ years	1.0

*Supplements are not recommended when drinking water contains 0.3 mg F/l or more. Supplements are recommended only for high-risk children.

Table 7.3 Fluoride supplement schedule (mg F/day) recommended by the American Dental Association, 1994

	Fluoride concentration in drinking water (mg/l)		
Age	<0.3	0.3–0.6	>0.6
6 months–3 years	0.25	0	0
3–6 years	0.5	0.25	0
6–16 years	1.0	0.5	0

From American Dental Association 1994, personal communication.

Because it is now recognized that fluorosis risk is exacerbated by the intake of fluoride from multiple sources, there have been a number of recommendations for sharply reduced fluoride supplement schedules in recent years. A group from the European Community (EC) in 1991 recommended that a supplement of 0.5 mg F should be used only for at-risk individuals from the age of 3 years on, and that supplements had no place as a public health measure (Clarkson, 1992). Canada decided in 1992 to retain a supplement schedule only for use in high-risk children (acknowledging that the definition of high risk is elusive), and produced the restrictive schedule shown in Table 7.2. Like the EC recommendations, it does not advocate beginning supplements under the age of 3 years. In 1994, the American Dental Association recommended a reduced schedule for the USA: this schedule is shown in Table 7.3. Recommendations for reduced schedules have also been made for Australia (Riordan, 1993) and for Switzerland, where fluoridated salt is available across the nation (Marthaler, 1992). The end-result is that fluoride supplements have limited application in public health programmes, where their use should be restricted to children aged 7 years or older.

Fluoride mouthrinses

The idea of preventing caries by mouthrinsing with a dilute fluoride solution, in itself not new, became practical after a 1965 Swedish study reported nearly 50% reduction in caries increment over 2 years (Torell and Ericsson, 1965). Fluoride mouthrinses, usually with NaF as the active agent, are now widely used in school-based programmes as well as by individuals at home. A weekly or fortnightly schedule is most convenient in schools; this regimen uses 0.2% neutral NaF. Daily rinsing, not often used in public health but convenient for individual home use, usually employs neutral NaF at 0.05%, though 0.1% stannous fluoride is also marketed in the USA.

Efficacy studies, most of them from the time before the caries decline in the economically developed world was fully recognized, indicated that regular use of NaF mouthrinses reduced caries increments in children by about 20–35% over periods of 2–3 years (Horowitz *et al.*, 1971; Rugg-Gunn *et al.*, 1973; Forsman, 1974b; Birkeland and Torell, 1978; Ripa *et al.*, 1983). Benefits were also reported in the primary dentition (Ripa and Leske, 1979). Other successfully tested products include 0.1% stannous fluoride (Radike *et al.*, 1973; McConchie *et al.*, 1977); ammonium fluoride (DePaola *et al.*, 1977); and amine fluoride (Ringelberg *et al.*, 1979). NaF, however, is considered the most convenient product in public health programmes.

Advantages and limitations of fluoride mouthrinsing

A major attraction of fluoride mouthrinsing has been the seemingly low costs resulting from supervision by teachers, volunteer mothers or inexpensive hourly workers. Some claims of low costs have been exaggerated; it looks more expensive when the true costs of volunteer labour and promotion are included. Even so, the procedure would probably still be acceptably cost-effective if it prevented caries to the extent suggested by the early studies. But the results of the National Preventive Dentistry Demonstration Program, a project conducted in 10 US cities during the 1976–81 period to compare the costs and effectiveness of a series of preventive regimens, questioned the value of fluoride mouthrinsing in public health (Klein *et al.*, 1985).

In addition to costs being higher than expected, the effectiveness of weekly rinsing in the age of the caries decline was questionable. A comprehensive 1989 review concluded that fluoride mouthrinsing was a reasonable procedure to use in high-risk populations (Leverett, 1989), though it expressed reservations when caries experience was moderate to low. Fluoride mouthrinsing is not recommended in fluoridated communities because the low marginal benefits are unlikely to be worth the programme costs.

Fluoride mouthrinsing has proven to be a relatively easy programme to conduct in the school setting. It does require cups and associated supplies, as well as secure storage for the fluoride materials. It is an appropriate choice for high-risk communities, but is of doubtful benefit in places where caries experience is already low.

Fluoride varnishes

A fluoride varnish is a professionally applied adherent material. It is not intended to be as permanent as a fissure sealant; the original purpose was to hold fluoride in close contact with the tooth for a period of time. Varnishes permit the application of high fluoride concentrations in small amounts of material.

Early clinical trials of fluoride varnishes gave mixed results (Holm, 1979; Koch *et al.*, 1979; Murray *et al.*, 1977) and reviews in the 1980s also concluded that the clinical efficacy of varnishes was equivocal (Clark, 1982; Primosch, 1985). A large clinical trial in Quebec, which ran for nearly 5 years in communities with high caries experience, reported moderate efficacy (Clark *et al.*, 1987). As with most modern clinical trials in North America, the study was conducted in an environment of extensive fluoride exposure from toothpaste and other sources, which always makes the impact of any one fluoride procedure more difficult to discern. More recent studies in Europe have demonstrated the effectiveness of fluoride varnishes (de Bruyn and Arends, 1987; Helfenstein and Steiner, 1994).

Varnishes need to be reapplied at regular intervals to maintain their cariostatic effect (de Bruyn and Arends, 1987; Seppa, 1991), though application four times per year is no more effective than twice per year (Seppa and Tolonen, 1990). Another investigation of optimum application frequency found that applications three times a week, once per year, was more effective than the conventional twice-per-year regimen (Petersson *et al.*, 1991). This study also claimed that the three-per-week regimen was more cost-effective than twice per year, though the assumptions included make this finding worth further study. There is evidence that lower fluoride levels may not reduce the cariostatic effects of varnishes (de Bruyn *et al.*, 1988; Haugejorden and Nord 1991; Seppa *et al.*, 1994), another finding which invites further research.

Advantages and limitations of fluoride varnishes

While fluoride varnishes are effective, as a professionally applied procedure they are inherently more expensive than self-applied methods. They may well be cost-effective in Scandinavian countries with their highly developed school dental services, where dental professionals are seeing individual patients regularly. It is not yet clear whether varnishes would be most efficiently used in clinical programmes with high-caries populations, or whether their use is best reserved for individual patients on an *ad hoc* basis.

Supervised toothbrushing

Supervised toothbrushing was among the earlier public health programmes. It is now mainly of historical interest in the economically developed nations, where commercial advertising promotes oral hygiene. Supervised group brushing was once widely used in the school dental services in Norway and Sweden, where teeth were brushed under supervision every two months during the school year with neutral NaF solution at 0.5–1.0% fluoride (Torell and Ericsson, 1974).

In developing countries, however, toothbrushing habits may not be as well-established and toothbrushes and toothpaste can be relatively expensive. What are often called toothbrush drills may thus be relevant as a method of promoting oral hygiene habits, especially in localities where caries experience may be increasing. The decision on use of supervised toothbrushing should be based on cultural and economic factors as much as on caries status.

Other community-based fluoride procedures

Where community water fluoridation was not possible, school fluoridation was promoted in rural schools in the USA. The procedure was reported to reduce dental caries among schoolchildren by about 40% (Heifetz *et al.*, 1983), though none of the studies of the procedure used concurrent controls. Relative to community water fluoridation, the disadvantages of this method were that children did not receive the benefits until they were old enough to begin school, and they consumed the water only when school was in session. To compensate for this reduced exposure, a concentration of 4.5 times the optimum for the area was used. At its peak, school water fluoridation was introduced in 13 states, but problems with supervision have led to its decline. There is no record of school water fluoridation being used in countries outside the USA.

Milk fluoridation is the addition of a measured quantity of fluoride to bottled or packaged milk to be drunk by children. The rationale for adding fluoride to milk is that this procedure targets fluoride directly to children, and thus would be less expensive than fluoridating the drinking water. Having both fluoridated and non-fluoridated milk available also maintains consumer choice. However, the choice of milk as a vehicle for fluoride raises questions. The first concerns efficacy, in that fluoride is incompletely ionized in milk (Ericsson, 1958), which means that little posteruptive effect can take place. There are also practical concerns, such as the considerable number of children who do not drink milk for one reason or another. There have been only a few studies testing the efficacy of fluoridated milk, and some of them are seriously flawed. Few public health programmes using fluoridated milk have become established, though there are reports of such programmes in Bulgaria and another in St Helens, near Liverpool (Jones *et al.*, 1992). However, it is hard to recommend further research into milk fluoridation in view of the large number of fluoride vehicles available today and the restricted posteruptive effects from fluoride in milk.

Pit and fissure sealants

A fissure sealant is a plastic material used to occlude the pits and fissures on occlusal, buccal and lingual surfaces of teeth. The purpose is to prevent caries by providing a physical barrier to cariogenic bacteria in those crevices.

The idea of occluding pits and fissures, in this case by minimal operative preparation of sound fissures and restoration with amalgam, dates from the 1920s (Hyatt, 1923). There were also attempts in the pre-fluoride era to paint various chemicals on to teeth to prevent caries, but none proved successful (Ast *et al.*, 1950b; Klein and Knutson, 1942). Even after fluoride entered dental practice, interest in a specific preventive agent for pit-and-fissure caries persisted, but it proved difficult to find a material that adhered successfully to enamel in the oral environment. The breakthrough came in 1955 with the development of the acid-etch technique (Buonocore, 1955).

Modern sealants were developed as primary prevention for sound fissures, but the question soon arose about whether caries could progress beneath a sealant. A number of studies have since shown that when sealant is placed over an incipient lesion, where cavitation has not yet occurred, caries does not progress so long as the sealant remains intact (Going, 1984; Handelman *et al.*, 1986, 1987; Mertz-Fairhurst *et al.*, 1986; Swift, 1988).

By the end of the 1970s there was clear evidence from numerous clinical trials in different populations that sealants were highly efficacious when applied correctly (Ripa, 1980). Studies since then with second- and third-generation sealants have almost all been highly favourable; reviews of what is now an extensive literature have all reached highly favourable conclusions (Ripa, 1983, 1993; Stephen and Strang, 1985; Weintraub, 1989).

Advantages and limitations of sealants

The teeth with greatest potential to benefit from sealants are the permanent molars, and virtually all of the efficacy and cost-effectiveness data come from studies involving permanent molars in children. The potential value of sealants in primary molars is limited by the relatively higher frequency of approximal caries in these teeth, combined with their predictable exfoliation. Low caries levels in bicuspids also limit the value of sealants in these teeth (Eklund, 1986).

Sealant programmes seem a logical public caries-preventive strategy for children, though the decline in caries does present a dilemma. On the one hand, sealants provide virtually 100% protection from caries when they adhere properly to a tooth surface. On that basis it is tempting to argue that they should be applied to all teeth. At the same time, however, caries has declined substantially, so that the potential benefit from wholesale sealant application is decreasing. With an essentially fixed cost per tooth and per child, as the level of disease declines, the benefit per unit of expenditure must also decline (Eklund, 1986; Weintraub, 1989). The need for periodic maintenance of sealants for maximum effectiveness also means that their placement on low-risk teeth is unlikely to be cost-effective (Chestnutt *et al.*, 1994). Nevertheless, the full nature of the trade-off between wholesale application in groups of children versus selective use has not been fully explored. For example, while the wholesale use of sealants may be inefficient when children are appointed and treated one at a time, they may not be when entire classrooms of children can be treated in one sitting by auxiliary personnel. These cost-effectiveness concerns have lead to a search for ways of targeting sealants and other preventive services to those most likely to develop disease. For example, Leverett and colleagues (1983) found a benefit-to-cost ratio of only $0.3:1$ when sealants were used in caries-inactive subjects, but a ratio of $1.02:1$ when used in caries-active children. This suggests that applying sealants only to those teeth with early lesions is likely to be efficient, but that a blanket sealing of all potentially at-risk teeth will not be.

The use of sealant only on incipient lesions is, in effect, using it as an early restoration rather than as primary prevention–an approach which may require a different mind-set in prevention-oriented dentists (Nuttall *et al.*, 1994). It also further blurs the distinction between sealants as primary preventive agents and their various uses in minimal-preparation restorations. As caries experience continues to decline, the future of sealants is likely to be concentrated on the early lesion rather than the totally sound tooth.

Summary

The administrator in dental public health has a variety of strategies to choose from in preventing caries. The choices must always be made first on the demonstrated efficacy of the procedures, but they must also factor in the fundamental areas of health planning: educational levels, economic development, nature of the disease problems, populations to be reached and resources available. Careful choices and sound programme evaluation will lead to the most effective prevention at the community level. One also must be mindful of the fact that there is unlikely to be a universal best approach. What is cost-effective and appropriate at one time and place may not necessarily be so at another.

References

Aasenden, R. and Peebles, T.C. (1974) Effects of fluoride supplementation from birth on deciduous and permanent teeth. *Archives of Oral Biology* 1: 321–326.

Allmark, C., Green, H.P., Linney, A.D. *et al.* (1982) A community study of fluoride tablets for school children in Portsmouth. Results after six years. *British Dental Journal* 153: 426–430.

American Dental Association (1994) New fluoride schedule adopted. *ADA News*, May 16: 12.14.

Arnold, F.A. Jr, McClure, F.J. and White, C.L. (1960) Sodium fluoride tablets for children. *Dental Progress* 1: 8–12.

Ast, D.B. and Fitzgerald, B. (1962) Effectiveness of water fluoridation. *Journal of the American Dental Association* 65: 581–588.

Ast, D.B., Finn, S.B. and McCaffrey, I. (1950a) The Newburgh-Kingston caries-fluorine study. I. Dental findings after three years of water fluoridation. *American Journal of Public health* 40: 716–724.

Ast, D.B., Bushel, A. and Chase, H.C. (1950b) A clinical study of caries prophylaxis with zinc chloride and potassium ferrocyanide. *Journal of American Dental Association* 41: 442.

Bagramian, R.A., Narendran, S. and Ward, M. (1989) Relationship of dental caries and fluorosis to fluoride supplement history in a non-fluoridated sample of schoolchildren. *Advances in Dental Research* 3: 161–167.

Beltran, E.D. and Szpunar, S.M. (1988) Fluoride in toothpastes for children: suggestion for change. *Pediatric Dentistry* 10: 185–188.

Binder, K., Driscoll, W.S. and Schutzmannsky, G. (1978) Caries-preventive fluoride tablet programs. *Caries Research* 12 (suppl. 1): 22–30.

Birkeland, J.M. and Torell, P. (1978) Caries-preventive fluoride mouthrinses. *Caries Research* 12 (suppl. 1): 38–51.

Blayney, J.R. and Tucker, W.H. (1948) The Evanston dental caries study. *Journal of Dental Research* 27: 279–286.

Buonocore, M.G. (1955) A simple method of increasing the adhesion of acrylic filling materials to enamel surfaces. *Journal of Dental Research* 34: 849–853.

Chestnutt, I.G., Schafer, F., Jacobson, A.P. and Stephen, K.W. (1994) The prevalence and effectiveness of fissure sealants in Scottish adolescents. *British Dental Journal* 177: 125–129.

Clark, D.C. (1982) A review on fluoride varnishes: an alternative topical fluoride treatment. *Community Dental and Oral Epidemiology* 10: 117–123.

Clark, D.C., Stamm, J.W., Tessier, C. and Robert, G. (1987) The final results of the Sherbrooke-Lac Megantic fluoride varnish study. *Journal of Canadian Dental Association* 53: 919–922.

Clarkson, J. (1992). A European view of fluoride supplementation. *British Dental Journal* 172: 357.

Conti, A.J., Lotzkar, S., Daley, R. *et al.* (1988) A 3-year clinical trial to compare efficacy of dentifrices containing 1.14% and 0.76% sodium monofluorophosphate. *Community Dental and Oral Epidemiology* 16: 135–138.

Dean, H.T., Arnold, F.A. Jr., Jay, P. and Knutson, J.W. (1950) Studies on mass control of dental caries through fluoridation of the public water supply. *Public Health Report* 65: 1403–1408.

de Bruyn, H. and Arends J. (1987) Fluoride varnishes–a review. *Journal de Biologie Buccale* 15: 71–82.

de Bruyn, H., Buskes, J.A., Jongbloed, W. and Arends, J. (1988) Fluoride uptake and inhibition of intra-oral demineralization, following the application of varnishes with different concentrations of fluoride. *Journal de Biologie Buccale*, 16: 81–87.

De Crousaz, P., Marthaler, T.M., Weisner, V. *et al.* (1985) Caries prevalence of children after 12 years of salt fluoridation in a canton of Switzerland. *Helvetica Odontolgica Acta* 29: 21–31.

de Liefde, B. and Herbison, G.P. (1985) Prevalence of developmental defects of enamel and dental caries in New Zealand children receiving differing fluoride supplementation. *Community Dental and Oral Epidemiology* 13: 164–167.

de Liefde, B. and Herbison, G.P. (1989). The prevalence of development defects of enamel and dental caries in New Zealand children receiving differing fluoride supplementation, in 1982 and 1985. *New Zealand Dental Journal* 85: 2–8.

DenBesten, P.K. and Thariani, H. (1992) Biological mechanisms of fluorosis and level and timing of systemic exposure to fluoride with respect to fluorosis. *Journal of Dental Research* 71: 1238–1243.

D'Hoore, W. and Van Nieuwenhuysen, J.P. (1992) Benefits and risks of fluoride supplementation: caries prevention versus dental fluorosis. *European Journal of Pediatrics* 151: 613–616.

DePaola, P.F. and Lax, M. (1968) The caries-inhibiting effect of acidulated phosphate-fluoride chewable tablets: a two-year double-blind study. *Journal of the American Dental Association* 76: 554–557.

DePaola, P.F., Soparkar, P., Foley, S. *et al.* (1977) Effect of high-concentration ammonium and sodium fluoride rinses in dental caries in schoolchildren. *Community Dental and Oral Epidemiology* 5: 7–14.

Driscoll, W.S., Heifetz, S.B. and Korts, D.C. (1978) Effect of chewable fluoride tablets on dental caries in schoolchildren: results after six years of use. *Journal of the American Dental Association* 97: 820–824.

Duckworth, R.M., Morgan, S.N. and Burchell, C.K. (1989) Fluoride in plaque following use of dentifrices containing sodium monofluorophosphate. *Journal of Dental Research* 68: 130–133.

Eklund, S.A. (1986) Factors affecting the cost of fissure sealants: a dental insurer's perspective. *Journal of Public Health Dentistry* 46: 133–140.

Ericsson, Y. (1958) State of fluorine in milk and its absorption and retention when administered in milk. Investigations with radio-active fluorine. *Acta Odontological Scandinavia* 16: 51–72.

Ericsson, Y. (1971) Urinary estimation of optimal fluoride dosage with domestic salt. *Acta Odontological Scandinavia* 29: 43–51.

Evans, R.W. and Stamm, J.W. (1991) An epidemiologic estimate of the critical period during which human maxillary central incisors are most susceptible to fluorosis. *Journal of Public Health Dentistry* 51: 251–259.

Fanning, E.A., Cellier, K.M. and Somerville, C.M. (1980) South Australian kindergarten children: effects of fluoride tablets and fluoridated water on dental caries in primary teeth. *Australian Dentistry Journal* 25: 259–263.

Fédération Dentaire Internationale (1987). *Basic Fact Sheets*. Fédération Dentaire Internationale, London.

Fogels, H.R., Meade, J.J., Griffith, J. *et al.* (1988) A clinical investigation of a high-level fluoride dentifrice. *Journal of Dentistry in Children* 55: 210–215.

Forsman, B. (1974a) Studies on the effect of dentifrices with low fluoride content. *Community Dental and Oral Epidemiology* 2: 166–175.

Forsman, B. (1974b) The caries preventing effect of mouthrinsing with 0.025 percent sodium fluoride solution in Swedish children. *Community Dental and Oral Epidemiology* 2: 58–65.

Friis-Hasche, E., Bergmann, J., Wenzel, A. *et al.* (1984) Dental health status and attitudes to dental care in families participating in a Danish fluoride tablet program. *Community Dental and Oral Epidemiology* 12: 303–307.

Galagan, D.J. and Lamson, G.G. Jr (1953) Climate and endemic dental fluorosis. *Public Health Reports* 68: 497–508.

Galagan, D.J. and Vermillion, J.R. (1957) Determining optimum fluoride concentrations. *Public Health Report* 72: 491–493.

Gillespie, G.M. and Roviralta, G. (eds) (1985) *Salt Fluoridation*. Scientific publication no. 501. Pan American Health Organization (WHO-AMRO), Washington, DC.

Going, R.E. (1984) Sealant effect on incipient caries, enamel maturation, and future caries susceptibility. *Journal of Dental Education* 48: 35–41.

Hanachowicz, L. (1984) Caries prevention using a 1.2% sodium monofluorophosphate dentifrice in an aluminium oxide trihydrate base. *Community Dental and Oral Epidemiology* 12: 10–16.

Handelman, S.L., Leverett, D.H., Espeland, M.A. and Curzon, J.A. (1986) Clinical radiographic evaluation of sealed carious and sound tooth surfaces. *Journal of the American Dental Association* 113: 751–754.

Handelman, S.L., Leverett, D.H., Espeland, M. and Curzon, J. (1987) Retention of sealants over carious and sound tooth surfaces. *Community Dental and Oral Epidemiology* 15: 1–5.

Haugejorden, O., and Nord, A. (1991) Caries incidence after topical application of varnishes containing different concentrations of sodium fluoride: 3-year results. *Scandinavian Journal of Dental Research* 99: 295–300.

Heifetz, S.B., Horowitz, H.S. and Brunelle, J.A. (1983) Effect of school water fluoridation on dental caries: results in Seagrove, NC, after 12 years. *Journal of the American Dental Association* 106: 334–337.

Helfenstein, U., and Steiner, M. (1994) Fluoride varnishes (Duraphat): a meta-analysis. *Community Dental and Oral Epidemiolooly* 22: 1–5.

Holm, A.K. (1979) Effect of fluoride varnish (Duraphat) in preschool children. *Community Dental and Oral Epidemiology* 7: 241–245.

Holm, A.K. and Andersson, R. (1982) Enamel mineralization disturbances in 12-year-old children with known early exposure to fluorides. *Community Dental and Oral Epidemiology* 10: 335–339.

Horowitz, H.S., Law, F.E., Thompson, M.B. and Chamberlin, S.R. (1966) Evaluation of a stannous fluoride dentifrice for use in dental public health programs. I. Basic findings. *Journal of the American Dentistry Association* 72: 408–422.

Horowitz, H.S., Creighton, W.E. and McClendon, B.J. (1971) The effect on human dental caries of weekly oral rinsing with a sodium fluoride mouthwash; a final report. *Archives of Oral Biology* 16: 609–616.

Hutton, W.L., Linscott, B.W. and Williams, D.B. (1951) The Brantford fluorine experiment. Interim report after five years of water fluoridation. *Canadian Journal of Public Health* 42: 81–87.

Hyatt, T.P. (1923) Prophylactic odontotomy. *Dental Cosmos* 65: 234–241.

James, P.M.C. and Anderson, R.J. (1967) Clinical testing of a stannous fluoride–calcium pyrophosphate dentifrice in Buckinghamshire school children. *British Dental Journal* 123: 33–39.

Jensen, M.E. and Kohout, F. (1988) The effect of a fluoridated dentifrice on root and coronal caries in an older adult population. *Journal of the American Dentistry Association* 117: 829–832.

Jones, S., Crawford, A.C., Jenner, A.M. *et al.* (1992) The possibility of school milk as a vehicle for fluoride: epidemiological, organisational and legal considerations. *Community Dental Health* 9: 335–342.

Jordan, W.A. and Peterson, J.K. (1959) Caries inhibiting value of a dentifrice containing stannous fluoride: final report of a two-year study. *Journal American Dentistry Association* 58: 42–44.

Kalsbeek, H., Verrips, E. and Dirks, O.B. (1992) Use of fluoride tablets and effect on prevalence of dental caries and dental fluorosis. *Community Dental and Oral Epidemiology* **20**: 241–245.

Klein, H. and Knutson, J.W. (1942) Studies on dental caries. Effect of ammoniacal silver nitrate on caries in the first permanent molars. *Journal of the American Dental Association* **29**: 1420–1426.

Klein, S.P., Bohannan, H.M., Bell, R.M. *et al.* (1985) The cost and effectiveness of school-based preventive dental care. *American Journal of Public Health* **75**: 382–391.

Koch, G., Petersson, L.G. and Ryden, H. (1979) Effect of fluoride varnish (Duraphat) treatment every six months compared with weekly mouthrinses with 0.2 percent NaF solution on dental caries. *Swedish Dental Journal* **3**: 39–44.

Koch, G., Petersson, L.G., Kling, E. and Kling, L. (1982) Effect of 250 and 1000 ppm fluoride dentifrice on caries. A three-year clinical study. *Swedish Dental Journal* **6**: 233–238.

Larsen, M.J., Richards, A. and Fejerskov, O. (1985) Development of dental fluorosis according to age at start of fluoride administration. *Caries Research* **19**: 519–527.

Larsen, M.J., Kirkegaard, E., Poulsen, S. and Fejerskov, O. (1989) Dental fluorosis among participants in a non-supervised fluoride tablet program. *Community Dental and Oral Epidemiology* **17**: 204–206.

Leverett, D.H. (1989) Effectiveness of mouthrinsing with fluoride solutions in preventing coronal and root caries. *Journal of Public Health Dentistry* **49**: 310–316.

Leverett, D.H., Handelman, S.L., Brenner, C.M. and Iker, H.P. (1983) Use of sealants in the prevention and early treatment of carious lesions: cost analysis. *Journal of the American Dental Association* **106**: 42.

Lind, O.P., Von der Fehr, F.R., Joost Larsen, M. and Moller, I.J. (1976) Anticaries effect of a 2% Na$_2$PO$_3$F-dentifrice in a Danish fluoride area. *Community Dental and Oral Epidemiology* **4**: 7–14.

Lu, K.H., Ruhlman, C.D., Chung, K.L. *et al.* (1987) A three-year clinical comparison of a sodium monofluoro-phosphate dentifrice with sodium fluoride dentifrices on dental caries in children. *Journal of Dentistry in Children* **54**: 241–244.

McConchie, J.M., Richardson, A.S. Hole, L.W. *et al.* (1977). Caries-preventive effect of two concentrations of stannous fluoride mouthrinse. *Community Dental and Oral Epidemiology* **5**: 278–283.

McKechnie, R. (1985) The Stratchclyde fluoridation case. *Community Dental Health* **2**: 63–68.

Marthaler, T.M. (1969) Caries inhibiting effect of fluoride tablets. *Helvetica Odontologica Acta* **13**: 1–13.

Marthaler, T.M. (1974). Caries inhibition by an amine fluoride dentifrice: results after 6 years in children with low caries activity. *Helvetica Odontologica Acta* **18**: 35–44.

Marthaler, T.M. (1992) Age-adjusted limits of fluoride intake to minimize the prevalence of fluorosis. *Journal de Biologie Buccale* **20**: 121–127.

Marthaler, T.M. and Schenardi, C. (1962) Inhibition of caries in children after 5½ years' use of fluoridated table salt. *Helvetica Odontological Acta* **6**: 1–6.

Mertz-Fairhurst, E.J., Schuster, G.S. and Fairhurst, C.W. (1986) Arresting caries by sealants: results of a clinical

study. *Journal of the American Dental Association* **112**: 194–197.

Mitropoulos, C.M., Holloway, P.J., Davies, T.G. and Worthington, H.V. (1984) Relative efficacy of dentifrices containing 250 or 1000 ppm F- in preventing dental caries–report of a 32-month clinical trial. *Community Dental Health* **1**: 193–200.

Muhler, J.C. (1962) Effect of a stannous fluoride dentifrice on caries reduction in children during a three-year study period. *Journal of the American Dental Association* **64**: 216–224.

Muhler, J.C., Radike, A.W., Nebergall, W.H. and Day, H.G. (1955) Comparison between the anticariogenic effects of dentifrices containing stannous fluoride and sodium fluoride. *Journal of the American Dental Association* **51**: 556–559.

Murray, J.J., Winter, G.B. and Hurst, C.P. (1977) Duraphat fluoride varnish: a 2-year clinical trial in 5-year-old children. *British Dental Journal* **143**: 11–17.

Newbrun, E. (1989) Effectiveness of water fluoridation. *Journal of Public Health Dentistry* **49**: 279–289.

Nuttall, N.M., Fyffe, H.E. and Pitts, N.B. (1994) Caries management strategies used by a group of Scottish dentists. *British Dentistry Journal* **176**: 373–378.

Obry-Musset, A.M., Bettembourg, D., Cahen, P.M. *et al.* (1992) Urinary fluoride excretion in children using potassium fluoride containing salt or sodium fluoride supplements. *Caries Research* **26**: 367–370.

Opinion of Lord Jauncey in causa Mrs. Catherine McColl (A.P.) against Strathclyde Regional Council. The Court of Session, 1983.

Pendrys, D.G. and Katz, R.V. (1989) Risk of enamel fluorosis associated with fluoride supplementation, infant formula, and fluoride dentifrice use. *American Journal of Epidemiology* **130**: 1199–1208.

Petersson, L.G., Arthursson, L., Ostberg, C. *et al.* (1991) Caries-inhibiting effects of different modes of Duraphat varnish reapplication: a 3-year radiographic study. *Caries Research* **25**: 70–73.

Primosch, R.E. (1985) A report on the efficacy of fluoridated varnishes in dental caries prevention. *Clinical Preventive Dentistry* **7**: 12–22.

Radike, A.W., Gish, C.W., Peterson, J.K. *et al.* (1973) Clinical evaluation of stannous fluoride as an anticaries mouthrinse. *Journal of the American Dental Association* **86**: 404–408.

Reintsema, H., Schuthof, J. and Arends, J. (1985) An *in vivo* investigation of the fluoride uptake in partially de-mineralized human enamel from several different dentifrices. *Journal of Dental Research* **64**: 19–23.

Results of the workshop (1989) *Journal of Public Health Dentistry* **49** 331–337.

Ringelberg, M.L., Webster, D.B., Dixon, D.O. and LeZotte, D.C. (1979) The caries-preventive effect of amine fluorides and inorganic fluorides in a mouthrinse or dentifrice after 30 months of use. *Journal of the American Dental Association* **98**: 202–208.

Riordan, P.J. (1993) Fluoride supplements in caries prevention: a literature review and proposal for a new dosage schedule. *Journal of Public Health Dentistry* **53**: 174–189.

Riordan, P.J. and Banks, J.A. (1991) Dental fluorosis and fluoride exposure in Western Australia. *Journal of Dental Research* **70**: 1022–1028.

Ripa, L.W. (1980) Occlusal sealants: rationale and review of clinical trials. *International Dental Journal* **30**: 127–139.

Ripa, L.W. (1983) Occlusal sealants: an overview of clinical studies. *Journal of Public health Dentistry* **43**: 216–225.

Ripa, L.W. (1989) Clinical studies of high-potency fluoride dentifrices: a review. *Journal of the American Dental Association* **118**: 85–91.

Ripa, L.W. (1993) Sealants revisited: an update of the effectiveness of pit-and-fissure sealants. *Caries Research* **27** (suppl): 77-82.

Ripa, L.W. and Leske, G.S. (1979) Two years' effect on the primary dentition of mouthrinsing with a 0.2% neutral NaF solution. *Community Dental and Oral Epidemiology* **7**: 151–153.

Ripa, L.W., Leske, G.S., Sposato, A.L. and Rebich, T. Jr (1983) Supervised weekly rinsing with a 0.2% neutral NaF solution: results after 5 years. *Community Dental and Oral Epidemiology* **11**: 1–6.

Ripa, L.W., Leske, G.S., Forte, F and Varma, A. (1988) Caries inhibition of mixed $NaF-Na_2PO_3F$ dentifrices containing 1000 and 2500 ppm F: 3-year results. *Journal of the American Dental Association* **116**: 69-73.

Rise, J. and Kraft, P. (1986) Opinions about water fluoridation in Norwegian adults. *Community Dental Health* **3**: 313–320.

Rugg-Gunn, A.J., Holloway, P.J. and Davies, T.G.H. (1973) Caries prevention by daily fluoride mouthrinsing. *British Dental Journal* **135**: 353–360.

Schafer, F. (1989) Evaluation of the anticaries benefit of fluoride toothpastes using an enamel insert model. *Caries Research* **23**: 81–86.

Seppa, L. (1991) Studies of fluoride varnishes in Finland. *Proceedings of the Finnish Dental Society* **87**: 541–547.

Seppa, L. and Tolonen, T. (1990) Caries preventive effect of fluoride varnish applications performed two or four times a year. *Scandinavian Journal of Dental Research* **98**: 102–105.

Seppa, L., Pollanen, L. and Hausen, H. (1994) Caries-preventive effect of fluoride varnish with different fluoride concentrations. *Caries Research* **28**: 64–67.

Sidi, A.D. (1989) Effect of brushing with fluoride toothpastes on the fluoride, calcium, and inorganic phosphorus concentrations in approximal plaque of young adults. *Caries Research* **23**: 268–271.

Slack, G.L., Berman, D.S., Martin, W.J. and Hardie, J.M. (1967) Clinical testing of a stannous fluoride-calcium pyrophosphate dentifrice in Essex school girls. *British Dental Journal* **123**: 26–32.

Steiner, M., Marthaler, T.M., Wiesner, V. and Menghini, G. (1986) Kariesbefall bei Schulkindern des Kantons Glarus, 9 Jahre nach Einfuhrung des hoher fluoridierten Salzes (250 mg F/kg). *Schweizerische Monatsschrift Zahnmedizin* **96**: 688–699.

Steiner, M., Menghini, G. and Marthaler, T.M. (1989)

Kariesbefall bei schulkindern des Kantons Glarus, 13 jahre nach einfuhrung des hoher fluoridierten salzes. *Schweizerische Monatsschrift Zahnmedizin* **99**: 897–906.

Stephen, K.W. and Campbell, D. (1978) Caries reduction and cost benefit after 3 years of sucking fluoride tablets daily at school. A double-blind trial. *British Dental Journal* **144**: 202–206.

Stephen, K.W. and Strang, R. (1985) Fissure sealants: a review. *Community Dental Health* **2**: 149–156.

Stephen, K.W., Creanor, S.L., Russell, J.I. *et al.* (1988) A 3-year oral health dose-response study of sodium monofluorophosphate dentifrices with and without zinc citrate: anti-caries results. *Community Dental and Oral Epidemiology* **16**: 321–325.

Stephen, K.W., McCall, D.R. and Gilmour, W.H. (1991) Incisor enamel mottling prevalence in child cohorts which had or had not taken fluoride supplements from 0–12 years of age. *Proceedings of the Finnish Dental Society* **87**: 595–605.

Stookey, G.K., Schemehorn, B.R., Cheetham, B.L. *et al.* (1985) *In situ* fluoride uptake from fluoride dentifrices by carious enamel. *Journal of Dental Research* **64**: 900–903.

Suckling, G.W. and Pearce, E.I. (1984) Developmental defects of enamel in a group of New Zealand children: their prevalence and some associated etiological factors. *Community Dental and Oral Epidemiology* **12**: 177–184.

Swift, E.J Jr (1988) The effect of sealants on dental caries: a review. *Journal of the American Dental Association* **116**: 700–704.

Thylstrup, A., Fejerskov, O., Bruun, C. and Kann, J. (1979) Enamel changes and dental caries in 7-year-old children given fluoride tablets from shortly after birth. *Caries Research* **13**: 265–276.

Torell, P. and Ericsson, Y. (1965) Two-year clinical tests with different methods of local caries-preventive fluorine application in Swedish school-children. *Acta Odontological Scandinavica* **23**: 287–322.

Torell, P. and Ericsson, Y. (1974) The potential benefits to be derived from fluoride mouth rinses. In *International Workshop on Fluorides and Dental Caries Reductions.* (Forrester, DJ and Schultz E.M., eds). pp. 113–166. University of Maryland, Baltimore MD.

Toth, K. (1984) *Caries Prevention by Domestic Salt Fluoridation.* Akademiai Kiado, Budapest.

Triol, C.W., Mandanas, B.Y., Juliano, G.F. *et al.* (1987). A clinical study of children comparing anticaries effect of two fluoride dentifrices. A 31-month study. *Clinical Preventive Dentistry* **9**: 22–24.

Weintraub, J.A. (1989) The effectiveness of pit and fissure sealants. *Journal of Public Health Dentistry* **49**: 317–330.

Widenheim, J. and Birkhed, D. (1991) Caries-preventive effect on primary and permanent teeth and cost-effectiveness of an NaF tablet preschool program. *Community Dental Oral Epidemiology* **19**: 88–92.

Widenheim, J., Birkhed, D., Granath, L. and Lindgren, G. (1986) Preeruptive effect of NaF tablets on caries in children from 12 to 17 years of age. *Community Dental and Oral Epidemiology* **14**: 1–4.

Winter, G.B., Holt, R.D. and Williams, B.F. (1989) Clinical trial of a low-fluoride toothpaste for young children. *International Dental Journal* **39**: 227-235.

Woltgens, J.H., Etty, E.J. and Nieuwland, W.M. (1989) Prevalence of mottled enamel in permanent dentition of children participating in a fluoride programme at the Amsterdam dental school. *Journal de Biologie Buccale* **17**: 15–20.

Woolfolk, M.W., Faja, B.W. and Bagramian, R.A. (1989). Relation of sources of systemic fluoride to prevalence of dental fluorosis. *Journal of Public Health Dentistry* **49**: 78–82.

8

Trends in oral health

John J. Murray and Nigel B. Pitts

Introduction

In the last 25 years there have been dramatic changes in both the pattern and distribution of dental caries in children in the UK and many other developed countries. There are unique data available from the decennial national surveys of the UK and these are used to present an overview of trends as these are common to a range of countries. International data are summarized to extend the discussion, with further detail being available in Chapter 17. Substantial improvements have occurred in the oral health of adults, partly because of changes in attitudes on the part of patients and the dental profession and also because the overall decline in caries in children is now having an effect on the oral health of adults. At the same time the pace of change in the way in which dental services are provided has quickened and a number of far-reaching reforms have been introduced in many countries and more are being contemplated. The need to monitor trends in oral health, especially the prevalence and distribution of dental caries, should be self-evident. Without good data there is little point in setting out goals or strategies, either internationally (World Health Organization (WHO) Global Goals for Oral Health) or nationally (e.g. Protocol for Health Gain (Wales), Oral Health Strategy for England, Oral Health Strategy for Scotland) because to determine whether progress is being made towards set objectives, it is essential to measure change accurately. However, it is very important

also that the quality of the caries data which is used locally, regionally and nationally to evaluate changes in caries prevalence is safeguarded and factors which may have an impact on the measurement of dental caries are considered carefully. Such factors include changes in the morphology of carious lesions, the use of fissure sealants and tooth-coloured restorative materials and changes in the delivery of dental care.

This chapter is divided into two main sections. The first part will consider trends in oral health, principally in the UK, over the last 25 years, together with international comparisons. The second part will consider changes in the distribution of caries within a population, and then discuss trends in caries diagnosis, treatment and the delivery of dental care which impact on the monitoring of oral health. It is suggested that over the next 25 years changes will continue to occur. The magnitude and direction of these trends will need to be monitored and evaluated even more carefully than in the past, in order to understand the increasingly complex factors that will affect oral health. This text builds on the understanding of dental caries already provided in Chapter 6. Our focus on caries is intentional as, despite shifts in the prevalence and distribution of this disease, the provision of care for caries and its sequelae which is appropriate for different population groups remains as a pivotal problem in many countries. Important changes in other aspects of oral health are outlined elsewhere: changes in periodontal diseases and oral cancer and our understanding of these conditions are outlined in Chapter 6 while changes in oral health provision are covered in Chapter 16.

The primary dentition

Dental caries in the pre-school child

There has been comparatively little population-based information available for this age group but the recently published dental survey conducted in the UK and linked to the National Diet and Nutrition Survey: children aged $1\frac{1}{2}$–$4\frac{1}{2}$ years (Hinds and Gregory, 1995) has remedied that situation. A total of 1685 children participated in the dental component. Seventeen per cent of the children had some experience of decay and the proportion increased from 4% of $1\frac{1}{2}$–$2\frac{1}{2}$-year-olds to 30% of $3\frac{1}{2}$–$4\frac{1}{2}$-year-olds. Decay was related to the social class of the head of household and to the level of educational attainment of the mother, whereby children of mothers with the highest attainments had least decay. The background to this common finding of social inequities in health is described in detail in Chapter 3 of this book. Similarly, the survey reported that Scottish children and those in the north of England had more decay than those in other more affluent parts of England and Wales. A key finding was that the younger children were when they started having their teeth brushed, or brushing their own teeth and the more frequently the teeth were brushed, the lower the proportion having dentinal decay. By and large, toothbrushing is undertaken with toothpaste and since the vast majority of toothpaste is fluoridated, toothbrushing directly reflects frequency of fluoride application and this is the most likely explanation for the reported benefit of early and frequent use. Age of commencement of toothbrushing is social class-related with more high-social-class parents reporting early commencement and twice-a-day frequency (Milsom and Mitropoulos, 1990; Mitropoulos, 1993).

Dental caries in 5-year-old children, 1973–93

The first coordinated national survey of children's dental health in England and Wales was carried out in 1973 (Todd, 1975); subsequent decennial surveys included Scotland and Northern Ireland. These surveys are commissioned by the UK Departments of Health and undertaken by the governmental Office of Population, Censuses and Surveys (OPCS). The dental examinations are conducted by salaried dentists working in the Community Dental Service who are trained to use the same diagnostic criteria in their assessment of oral health. In common with all the population surveys described, untreated decay was diagnosed at the level of involvement of dentine, with enamel caries not recorded. The implications of this measurement technique are discussed later in this chapter.

In 1973, 30% of 5-year-old children were diagnosed as being caries-free; the mean decayed, missing, filled deciduous teeth (dmft) was 4.0 (Table 8.1).

Between 1973 and 1983 the mean dmft had halved (from 4.0 to 2.1) and the proportion caries-free had almost doubled (from 30% to 50%). However, very little improvement had occurred between 1983 and 1993 in mean dmft values (Todd and Dodd, 1985; O'Brien, 1994). About 70% of the decay remains untreated over the 20-year period and no encouraging trend is discernible. Some concern has been expressed (Palmer and Pitts, 1994) that the gradual decline in caries in 5-year-old children may have bottomed out and that since then modest increases have occurred (Fig. 8.1).

Dental caries in 6–13-year-olds

The 1993 national survey in the UK addressed the question of trends in decay experience in the primary dentition by considering the total number of teeth which were diagnosed as filled or actively decayed on examination. (Teeth which were extracted because of decay or which were decayed when they exfoliated were excluded because the examining dentists were not asked to make any assumptions about the

Table 8.1 Dental caries in 5-year-old children in the UK

	1973*	1983	1993
Proportion 'caries-free'	30	50	55
Mean dmf	4.0	2.1	2.0
Average number of untreated teeth		1.3	1.4
Proportion with some filled teeth		23	15
Filled teeth as a proportion of dmf		28	18

*England and Wales only.
dmf = decayed, missing, filled.
Data from Todd (1975); Todd and Dodd (1985); O'Brien (1994).

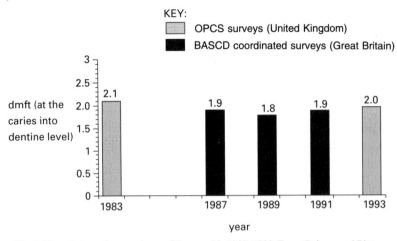

Fig. 8.1 Trends in caries experience of 5-year-olds 1983–1993. From Palmer and Pitts (1994), with permission. OPCS = Office of Population, Censuses and Surveys; dmft = decayed, missing, filled deciduous teeth. BASCD = British Association for the Study of Community Dentistry.

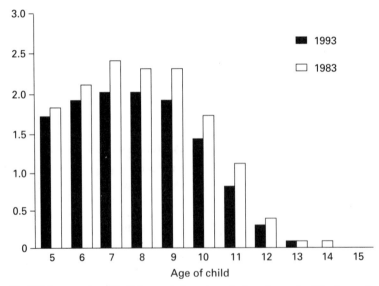

Fig. 8.2 Mean number of teeth known to have decay in the primary dentition by age in the UK in 1983 and 1993. Modified from O'Brien (1994), with permission.

decay experience of missing primary teeth.) Obviously the number of decayed or filled primary teeth present in the mouth starts to *decrease* after the age of 7 years because of exfoliation; bearing this in mind, the data for 6–13-year-olds (Fig. 8.2) suggest that there may have been a slight overall decrease in caries in primary teeth in 1993, compared with 1983. This is confirmed by an estimate of total decay experience (d + m + f) in the primary teeth of 6–8-year-old children (Table 8.2; O'Brien, 1994).

Table 8.2 Estimated number of primary teeth with decay experience among 6–8-year-olds in the UK 1983–93

Age (years)	Mean dmf	
	1983	1993
6	2.7	2.3
7	3.4	2.7
8	4.2	2.9

dmf = decayed, missing, filled.
From O'Brien (1994), with permission.

The permanent dentition

Changes in DMF values in 6–15-year-olds

The 1973 survey reported that the mean DMF of 15-year-old children in England and Wales was 8.4. Data for the UK showed that the DMF had fallen to 5.9 in 1983 and 2.5 in 1993 (Table 8.3). The number of children who were said to be caried-free had risen substantially between 1983 and 1993 from 7% to 37%. These dramatic improvements in the dental health of children are clearly portrayed in Figures 8.3 and 8.4.

Table 8.3 Dental caries in 15-year-old children in the UK

	1973*	1983	1993
Proportion 'caries-free'		7	37
Mean DMF	8.4	5.9	2.5
Number of untreated teeth		1.0	0.7
Proportion with some filled teeth		85	52
Filled teeth as a proportion of DMF		70	65

*England and Wales only.
DMF = decayed, missing, filled.
Data from Todd (1975); Todd and Dodd (1985); O'Brien (1994).

However, recent reductions in the relative proportion of decayed teeth which receive fillings are worrying. In Scotland, for example, 14-year-olds showed a fall in the Care Index (filled teeth as a proportion of DMF) from 73% in 1991 to 52% in 1995 (Pitts *et al.*, 1995a). The impact that variations in the dental health care delivery systems can have on oral health are discussed further later in this chapter and in Chapters 16 and 17.

Changes in dental health of young adults

The first national survey of adult dental health in England and Wales in 1968 (Gray *et al.*, 1970) found that two factors, attendance pattern and region of the country, were the most important variables in the dental health of dentate adults. Adults aged 16–34 years who were domiciled in London and the south-east, and who claimed to attend the dentist regularly, had more fillings, fewer extractions and fewer untreated carious lesions than adults of similar age living in the north of England who claimed to attend only when in trouble. Ten years later, the 1978 survey (Todd and Walker, 1980) showed that the differences between these two subgroups had hardly changed. What was obvious was that

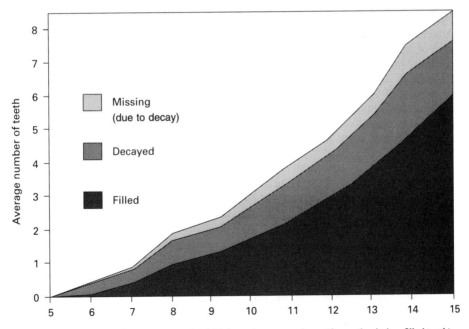

Fig. 8.3 Average number of permanent teeth which have decay experience (decayed, missing, filled teeth) by age in England and Wales in 1973. Modified from Todd (1975), with permission.

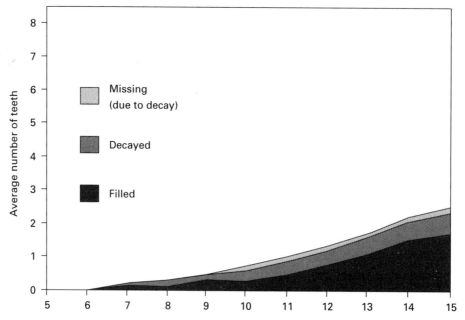

Fig. 8.4 Average number of permanent teeth which have decay experience (decayed, missing, filled teeth) by age in the UK in 1993. Data from O'Brien (1994).

the 'north irregulars' had substantially more sound untreated teeth than 'London regulars', according to the diagnostic criteria used by the survey examiners.

The impact of the decline in caries in children in the UK, first noticed in the early 1970s, on the dental health of adults, can be seen by comparing the condition of individual teeth for adults aged 16–24 and 25–34 years, as found in the 1988 adult dental health survey (Todd and Lader, 1991). The pattern of tooth loss, or untreated caries, is not very different, but the number of fillings, particularly in molars, premolars and upper canines and incisors, is markedly lower for 16–24-year-olds (Fig. 8.5).

When decay was very prevalent in the community, the only way to achieve long-term reliance on natural teeth was by way of restorative dentistry. In such times, the presence of a large number of filled teeth was an asset and indicated that care and attention had been paid to dental health. With increasing knowledge about the limited durability of restorative dentistry coupled with the much lower level of dental caries in the younger generation, it is now possible to consider goals related to low disease levels as well as goals related to the restoration of decayed teeth. This approach is supported by

the interview data collected in these national surveys in that in 1978, only 67% of dentate adults expected to keep their natural teeth for life, compared to 87% by 1988. In the 1988 Adult Dental Health Report (Todd and Lader, 1991) the proportion of people with 18 or more sound untreated teeth was taken as an indication of low disease. The improvement in the number of 16–24-year-olds (Table 8.4) who have a considerable number of such teeth has been dramatic over the last 20 years (44% in 1968, 53% in 1978, 83% in 1988).

The 16–24-year-olds in 1968 were the 35–44-year-olds in 1988. The deterioration over time for this indicator of low disease has been from 44% to 23% in 20 years, or approximately 10 percentage points for every 10 years. If this rate of deterioration were to be maintained, then in 1998, 75% of 25–34-year-olds will have 18 or more sound and untreated teeth. The results suggest that the dental health of 16–24-year-olds in 1988 will not deteriorate as quickly as in the past. This, in turn, should reinforce more positive attitudes to the preservation of teeth in older adults in the future.

The index of 12 or more filled teeth was used as a measure of evidence of considerable restorative treatment. In 1968, 32% of 16–24-

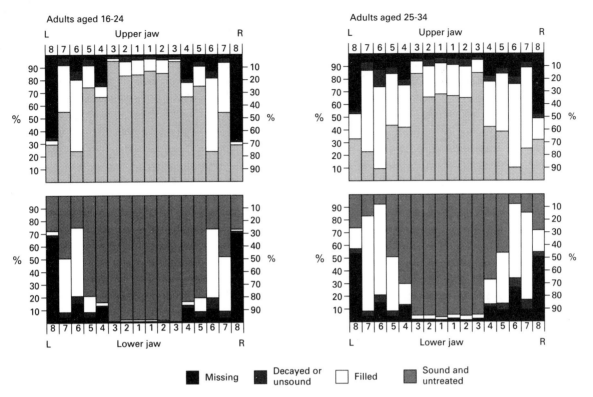

Fig. 8.5 The distribution of tooth conditions around the mouth for dentate adults in different age groups in 1988 in the UK. From Todd and Lader (1991), with permission.

Table 8.4 The proportion of dentate adults with 18 or more sound and untreated teeth in England and Wales 1968–88

Age (years)	Proportion of dentate adults with 18 or more sound (and untreated) teeth		
	1968 (%)	1978 (%)	1988 (%)
16–24	44	53	83
25–34	23	28	42
35–44	19	20	23

From Todd and Lader (1991), with permission.

Table 8.5 The proportion of dentate adults with 12 or more filled teeth by age in England and Wales 1968–88

Age (years)	England and Wales Proportion of dentate adults with 12 or more filled teeth		
	1968 (%)	1978 (%)	1988 (%)
16–24	32	23	7
25–34	36	40	40
35–44	24	34	49
45–54	15	21	41
55 and over	9	9	19
All ages	25	27	31

Data from Todd and Walker (1980); Todd and Lader (1991).

year-olds had 12 or more filled teeth (Table 8.5). Ten years on in 1978, 40% of this cohort now aged 25–34 years had 12 or more filled teeth, rising to 49% in 1988. Similarly, those aged 16–24 in 1978 moved from 23% (with 12 or more filled teeth) to 40% in 1988. However, only 7% of 16–24-year-olds in 1988 were in this category. It will be interesting to see whether the young adults of 1988 can maintain their position in terms of this parameter in 10 years' time.

Speculating on the possible benefits of prevention and the move away from large numbers of fillings should not blind us to the fact that restorative treatment is still necessary for a large proportion of people. Among dentate adults in the UK in 1988, 44% had at least one

it was decayed at the survey level of
, or had an unsound filling. The
ar age group had the lowest proportion
:ayed or unsound teeth at 62%.
Therefore, even under survey conditions, more
than a third of young adults required restorative
dental care in the UK in 1988.

Aspects of access and uptake of care are
presented in Chapter 17 and should be
considered with the improved understanding
of the movement towards healthy lifestyles
(Chapters 12 and 15), which should support
improving oral health. However, the reduction
in caries documented here has been uneven
across the population and a health divide in oral
health is apparent and discussed in more detail
later in this chapter.

International comparisons

The WHO Global Data Bank provided information on trends in dental caries (DMFT)
values) of 12-year-old children from 1967 to
1981. DMFT values in 12-year-olds were
considered at the First International Conference
on Changing Caries Prevalence. Data from nine
countries all showed that a decline in DMFT
values from the countries varied considerably in
the early 1970s–from 10.1 in Norway to 3.8 in
the USA. Second, even in 1983, considerable
intercountry differences were still observed–from
4.7 in Denmark to 2.6 in the USA (Renson *et al.*,
1985).

The presentations at the Second International
Conference on Changing Caries Prevalence
showed that intercountry differences seemed to
have narrowed further by the 1990s. The results
provided, for studies carried out in 1987–93, for
5-, 12- and 15-year-old children have been
tabulated (Murray, 1994). (The WHO databank
now holds an impressive range of results from
a wide spread of countries. As, however,
some results relate to national surveys with
representative samples, while others relate only
to local pathfinder survey, caution is required in
making simplistic intercountry comparisons
using the raw databank figures.)

DMFT values for 5-year-olds in 1990–93

Information on 5–6-year-old children came from
12 countries (Murray, 1994). As with the
earlier data, the sample sizes taken and the

methodology employed varied considerably and
this must be taken into account when comparing
results. For example, the data for England and
Wales came from the latest national survey
carried out in 1993, when over 17 000 children
aged 5–15 years from 500 schools were
examined. Other studies, although labelled for
example Canada or Belgium, were local surveys
and did not claim to be truly representative of
that country. Nevertheless, the range for dmft
values from 11 countries was from 1.3 (Canada)
to 2.1 (Norway; Table 8.6). The proportion
caries-free varied from 55 to 72% (Murray,
1994). Data from one country, Iceland, fell
outside this range (mean dmft 2.9, 40%
caries-free). (The countries are listed in the order
of the presentations at the Conference.)

DMFT values for 12-year-olds in 1990–93

Information on 12-year-old children was provided
from 14 countries (Table 8.7). The mean DMF
varied from 1.1 (Switzerland and England and
Wales) to 2.7 (Belgium). All countries were well
below the WHO goal of a mean DMF value of
less than 3 by the year 2000. The per cent
caries-free varied from 25% (Belgium) to 60%
(the Netherlands) with many studies showing
that about 50% of 12-year-olds were caries-free
at the dentinal level of diagnosis.

DMFT values for 15-year-olds in 1990–93

Seven studies provided data for 15-year-old
children (Table 8.8). In six studies the mean
DMF varied from 2.1 to 3.6. In four studies,

Table 8.6 Data from 12 countries providing dmft values for
5–6-year-old children in 1987–93

Country	Year	Mean DMF	% Caries-free
England and Wales	1993	1.8	55
Denmark	1992	1.5	61
Finland	1991	1.4	60
Iceland	1988	2.9	40
Norway	1992	1.4	63
Sweden	1991		72
Belgium	1990	1.05	59
Netherlands	1993	1.3	55
Switzerland	1992	1.55	
USA	1987	2.0	50
Canada	1990	1.3	65
Australia	1992	2.0	

DMF = Decaysed, missing, filled.
From Murray (1994), with permission.

Table 8.7 Data from 14 countries providing decayed, missing, filled teeth (DMFT) values for 12-year-old children

Country	Year	Mean DMF	% Caries-free
England and Wales	1993	1.1	50
Denmark	1991	1.3	49
Finland	1991	1.2	30
Iceland	1991	2.5	23
Norway	1991	2.2	36
Sweden	1991	1.6	43
Belgium	1990	2.7	25
Germany	1993	2.5	
Netherlands			60
Eire GHB	1992	1.5	
Eire WHBF	1992	1.6	
Eire WHB non F	1992	2.1	
Switzerland	1992	1.1	
Canada	1990	1.5	
Australia	1992	1.2	55
China (Beijing)	1993	1.3	50

From Murray (1994), with permission.

Table 8.8 Data from seven studies providing decayed, missing, filled teeth (DMFT) values for 15-year-old children

Country	Year	Mean DMF	% Caries-free
England and Wales	1993	2.1	40
Denmark	1991	3.1	25
Finland	1991	3.1	23
Iceland	1991	5.3	9
Sweden	1991	3.6	70
Switzerland	1992	2.2	
China (Beijing)	1981	2.1	29

From Murray (1994), with permission.

caries-free was 23-40%, but the study from Sweden reported that 70% of 15-year-olds were caries-free, even though this country had the second highest mean DMF at 3.6. This suggests that a considerable amount of caries is concentrated in 30% of their population. Iceland was exceptional in that only 9% of 15-year-olds were caries-free with a mean DMF of 5.3.

DMFT values for adult dentate populations

One other aspect which was covered in the second conference was the standard of dental health of the adult dentate population. More variation was evident here, particularly in the age groups reported on (28-year-olds in Finland up to 45–54-year-olds in the Netherlands and Germany). Nevertheless, apart from 35-year-olds in Norway, who had a mean DMF of 25,

all the other results reported were clustered between 16.7 and 19.0 (Table 8.9).

In round figures, the average dentate 40-year-old, from nine countries around the world, has a mean DMFT value of 18, but the average 15-year-old, in 1991–93, had a mean DMFT value of less than 3. The question for the future is, will the present 15-year-old deteriorate by 15 DMFT in 25 years, or will the low caries experience of present-day teenagers ensure a much healthier dentate population when they reach middle age?

Dental health of the elderly

Edentulousness

Probably the most remembered statistic from the 1968 Adult Dental Health Survey in England and Wales (Gray *et al.*, 1970) is that 37% of adults aged 16 years and over were edentulous. The figure fell to 29% in 1978 (Todd and Walker, 1980) and 20% in 1988 (Todd and Lader, 1991). Obviously this headline figure was heavily dependent on age and by the treatment received by adults in the past (Fig. 8.6), but substantial differences in edentulousness were found between males and females, and among different social class groups, as has been presented in Chapter 3 of this book. The largest difference was found between social classes, with 31% of adults in households headed by unskilled workers being edentulous compared to only 14% of households headed by those in skilled non-manual occupations.

The prevalence of edentulousness in the elderly was described first in the UK by Richards

Table 8.9 Mean decayed, missing, filled teeth (DMFT) values for adult dentate populations from nine countries

Country	Year	Age (years)	Mean DMF
England and Wales	1988	35–44	19.0
Denmark	1990	30–39	17.8
Finland	1986	28	16.7
Norway	1993	35	25.0
Sweden	1985	30	17.5
Netherlands	1986	35–44	17.4
Netherlands		45–54	18.4
Germany	1989	35–44	16.7
Germany		45–54	18.4
Australia	1987/88	35–44	18.8
New Zealand	1988	35–44	18.3

From Murray (1994), with permission.

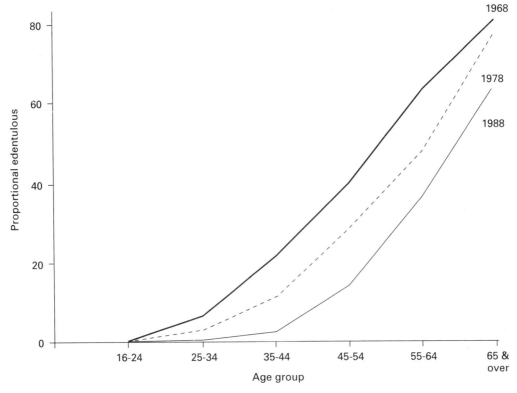

Fig. 8.6 The proportion of edentulous adults in England and Wales 1968–88 by age. From Todd and Lader (1991), with permission.

and co-workers (1965b; 1968). In Salisbury, 85% of over-60-year-olds were edentulous compared to 78% in Darlington in 1962. By 1992, there had been a remarkable improvement in the dental status. The prevalence in Darlington was now 57%, but only 33% in Salisbury (Steele *et al.*, 1996). Clearly, the change in Salisbury had been much greater, having either started earlier or proceeded more rapidly.

The dentate elderly

Focusing only on the proportion of the population who are dentate does not give an accurate picture of the dental needs of the adult population. Nearly a quarter of the dentate elderly in the recent study in Salisbury, Darlington and Richmondshire (Steele *et al.*, 1996) were edentulous in one arch. Pilot and Miyazaki (1991) addressed the needs of the senior citizen in the following way. 'For a senior citizen, a socially acceptable, functioning natural dentition is not a set of 32 teeth, caries free

in perfect alignment with nice gingivae to the cemento-enamel junction, but something expressed as "enough good teeth to smile and to chew"'. An extensive exposition of the development of sociodental indicators, aimed at supplementing those of the normative measures used in this chapter, is given in Chapter 4 of this book. One normative measure which would complement Pilot and Miyazaki's proposal has been described by Kayser as a 'shortened dental arch' of at least 20 teeth, with no gaps and no need for a removable prosthesis (Kayser, 1981). The 1988 UK survey (Todd and Lader, 1991) considered this aspect of oral health by determining the proportion of dentate adults with 21 or more standing teeth (Table 8.10).

The improvement in the number of dentate adults with 21 or more natural teeth between 1978 and 1988 is marked, but if the 1988 data are taken one stage further, to determine the proportion with a 'shortened dental arch' (Gordon *et al.*, 1994), then it can be seen how much further improvement in oral health is required before the majority of the population enjoy natural 'teeth for life' (Table 8.11).

Root caries

So far, only coronal caries has been considered. As teeth are retained longer, then the development of root caries can become a public health problem. The 1988 UK Adult Dental Health Survey (Todd and Lader, 1991) included an assessment of root surfaces for the first time in this series. Two-thirds of dentate adults had some root surfaces that were exposed. Root surface problems were highly correlated with age. Nearly 80% of young dentate adults aged 16–24 years had no exposed root surfaces, but only 5% of those aged 45 years or more had no exposed surfaces. The average number of teeth that had some exposed root surface was 5.3, but most of these–on average 3.7–were exposed with

no further problem. Therefore, 1.6 teeth, on average, had worn, filled or decayed surfaces according to the survey criteria. Most of the root surfaces that were damaged were worn but had no disease. Those aged 65 years or over had 1.9 decayed or filled root surfaces (Table 8.12).

The recent survey of the elderly in Richmondshire, Darlington and Salisbury (Steele *et al.*, 1996) gave similar but somewhat higher figures on the extent of root caries and concluded that those aged 75 and over had 2.6–3.0 root surfaces decayed or filled. In terms of *numerical* treatment (but not necessarily *complexity* of treatment), the number of root surfaces decayed or filled in the elderly now exceeds the number of decayed primary teeth in 5-year-old children in the UK. This illustrates the extent of the dramatic changes in oral health status that have taken place over the past 20 years.

The distribution of caries

Changes in the distribution of caries in populations

Prior to the dramatic reductions in caries prevalence seen in many developed countries in recent years (Renson *et al.*, 1985), the distribution of caries in populations was often considered to approach normality. However, the changes in caries have also extended to its distribution. There is said to have been a polarization of disease towards the extremes. This means that, rather than having a numerical majority of individuals clustered around a mean caries level, there are now large numbers at both the

Table 8.10 The percentage of dentate adults in the UK with 21 or more standing teeth, by age, in 1978 and 1988

Age (years)	1978 (%)	1988 (%)
16–24	97	100
25–34	89	96
35–44	75	86
45–54	50	72
55–64	29	48
65–74	29	25
75 and over		16
All dentate adults	73	80

From Todd and Lader (1991), with permission.

Table 8.11 Some characteristics of dentate adults in the 1988 Adult National Survey (Todd and Lader, 1991) plus a supplementary analysis of the percentage of dentate adults with four good quadrants (equivalent to a shortened dental arch)

Age range (years)	No. in group	Subsample		
		21 or more standing teeth (%)	21 or more standing teeth and no spaces (%)	Percentage with four 'good quadrants'
16–24	493	100	83	90
25–34	508	96	66	75
35–44	511	90	41	54
45–54	365	72	19	29
55–64	239	48	8	16
65+	181	23	3	2
Total	2297	81	46	54

Table 8.12 Numbers of teeth with roots that are exposed, worn, filled or decayed by age, in 1988 UK dentate adults

| Age (years) | No. in group | Mean number of teeth | | | |
		Exposed only	Worn only	Filled	Decayed
16–24	706	0.6	0.1		
25–34	678	2.6	0.3	0.2	0.1
35–44	618	4.6	0.8	0.6	0.2
45–54	417	6.2	1.4	0.8	0.4
55–64	311	6.5	1.7	1.2	0.7
65 and over	241	5.4	2.4	1.2	0.7
All dentate adults	2970	3.7	0.8	0.5	0.2

From Todd and Lader (1991), with permission.

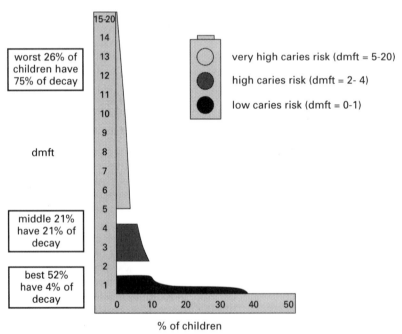

Fig. 8.7 Uneven distribution of dentinal caries experience among Scottish 5-year-olds, 1991. Data from Scottish Health Boards' Dental Epidemiological Programme, 1991/1992 (Pitts *et al.*, 1992).

low caries and the high caries ends of the distribution. This change has important consequences for the interpretation of mean figures; it can no longer be assumed that the mean will be representative of different groups within a population.

This situation can be illustrated using data from a representative national sample of more than 5000 Scottish 5-year-olds taken from the Scottish Health Boards Dental Epidemiological Programme (Pitts *et al.*, 1992). In Figure 8.7 the distribution has been plotted with the percentage

of children on the horizontal axis and a traffic light analogy has been employed to illustrate the varying levels of caries risk present in three subgroups.

Using arbitrary cut-offs, it is evident that over half of the children (52%) are in a relatively low-risk group and that these account for only 4% of the dentinal caries seen in this population of 5-year-olds. The high-risk group comprise 21% of the population and have 21% of the caries experience. Although the very-high-risk group (dmft of 5–20 at age 5 years) make up only a quarter (26%) of the children, they harbour three-quarters of the disease present (75%). These data illustrate the phenomenon in one setting, yet, at the Second International Conference on Changing Caries Prevalence (Murray, 1994), there was widespread agreement that this change in caries distribution has taken place in many developed countries. It has been termed the 80–20 phenomenon, where 20% of children have 80% of the disease, and the background and consequences are discussed in Chapter 6 of this book.

One impact of this new shape of caries distribution is that strategies that can preferentially influence the minority who have most of the disease now have the potential to achieve major effects on the overall mean values which are often used as targets. The change in the distribution also means that the potential benefits of the population strategy for prevention which often assumes a near bell-shaped distribution of disease (Sheiham and Joffe, 1991) are more limited while a high-risk preventive strategy becomes more effective. For example, it has led some northern European countries to question the cost-effectiveness of school-based fluoride rinsing programmes covering the whole school population when only a minority now experience the disease. On the other hand, there are still many regions in the north of England, in Scotland and in southern Europe which would benefit from fluoridation of water supplies–a truly population approach. Therefore, a consideration of combining the two strategies, population approach and high-risk approach, is likely to be beneficial in many communities.

In spite of considerable study, risk assessment at the individual level still remains a challenging and inexact task. Further work is needed (and is ongoing in many countries) in order to permit more accurate determination of the high-risk individuals who now have most of the disease. On a community basis, groups at higher risk have been identified. The most consistent indicators have been those related to material and social deprivation and are described in further detail in Chapters 3 and 6. Other groups where deprivation can be compounded by language include recent immigrant groups. This phenomenon has been reported in many European countries and studies in the UK (Bedi and Elton (1993) and the Netherlands (Verrips *et al.*, 1993) indicate that maternal lack of fluency in the language of the host country acts as a barrier to the attainment of oral health in both children and adults. Recent data from the Netherlands indicate that where succeeding generations integrate into the host country, differences in prevalence of dental caries are effectively eliminated (Kalsbeek *et al.*, 1995). In Sweden and Switzerland, immigrant groups with high caries levels are requiring types of intensive preventive and operative care not needed for some years by indigenous members of these societies.

Trends in economic status and access to health care delivery systems are additional dimensions that need to be understood, illustrating how deprivation can be compounded in subgroups with high caries levels. A further complication of the skewed distribution is that the well-motivated regular dental attenders who often make up the numerical majority of a general dentist's patients will be quite different from those in the high disease tail, many of whom attend infrequently. Thus the dentists' perceptions of a normal patient (derived from the regular attenders) are becoming more widely separated from population-derived estimates of dental health status.

The consequences of the changed and now markedly skewed distribution of caries should be appreciated by all involved in planning or assessing dental services. Considerations of costs, benefits and effectiveness of preventive programmes are covered in detail in Chapter 10. Changes in caries distribution should be monitored, along with trends in caries prevalence, dental attendance and access to services, if we are to be able to provide appropriate services for the future and if we are to understand what is happening currently to all sections of the community.

Changes associated with caries diagnosis

Changes in lesion morphology and caries activity

Consequent on the reductions in caries prevalence recorded in many developed countries, the lesions that do progress often do so at a much slower rate (Pitts and Kidd, 1992). The widespread availability of fluoride in the oral environment has resulted in a change in the shape of caries lesions, as described in Chapter 6. For example, occlusal lesions now cavitate at a later stage such that dentinal lesions which would previously have been seen as an open cavity are now either seen only as a subtle discoloration in the apparently intact enamel or, in other cases, are not seen at all. This phenomenon of hidden dentinal occlusal caries was described in the 1980s by general dental practitioners and has since been demonstrated in clinical trial subjects, in hospital dental practice and in population screening activities (Ismail *et al.*, 1992; Kidd *et al.*, 1993). These occult lesions can often be detected radiographically in dentine, but are not unambiguously identifiable as caries by clinical examination, even with the aid of a dental light and compressed air. Recent reports from Scotland found, on average, one hidden dentinal occlusal lesion per child amongst regularly attending adolescents (Pitts and Deery, 1994), whereas a group of high-caries-risk individuals of the same age were found to have more than two such lesions per child radiographically (Pitts *et al.*, 1995b).

The problem also exists for the approximal surfaces (Pitts, 1991; Pitts and Kidd, 1992) where the relationship between lesion depth and the presence or absence of cavitation also seems to have changed (Pitts and Rimmer, 1992). Whereas cavitation was assumed when the radiolucency reached the area of the enamel–dentine junction, it now appears that many lesions of this depth are not cavitated. A further complication is the suggestion that, with more available fluoride, shadows representing approximal lesions on bitewing radiographs are becoming more heterogeneous and radiopaque, rather than uniformly and darkly radiolucent (Pitts, 1992).

It should be appreciated that, although the recent reductions in caries prevalence are unarguable, the changes in caries morphology and activity make the lesions that are now present more difficult to detect either clinically or radiographically. As radiographs are not used for epidemiological examinations in most countries, the change in presentation of disease could increase the inherent and systematic underscoring of both approximal and occlusal lesions associated with a survey-type examination. However, at present there is little epidemiological evidence that slowly progressing caries lesions are appearing in the young adult cohorts of populations. This somewhat contentious issue is giving rise to some anxiety and debate in several Scandinavian countries and needs continuing vigilance. The question

posed above remains: will the present 15-year-old cohort deteriorate over the next 25 years, or will the low caries experience of present-day teenagers ensure a very much healthier dentate population when they in turn reach middle age?

Changes in caries diagnosis and measurement

There are currently a series of evaluations underway assessing the performance of both new and exciting diagnostic tools in detecting and measuring contemporary carious lesions in the 1990s. These studies are providing different results when compared to assessments of the same diagnostic methods undertaken using material collected in the 1960s and 1970s, when lesion morphology was typified by rapid cavitation. Now different types of carious lesions are detected at varying diagnostic thresholds (Pitts and Fyffe, 1988). Although the caries process is a continuum, it may be visualized in the form of an iceberg, as shown in Figure 8.8.

At the top of the iceberg are the clinically detectable lesions which are in dentine. Diagnosing at this level (the so-called D3 threshold, accepted as an international standard in epidemiology) excludes all other sizes of lesion. Next there are clinically detectable cavities which appear to be limited to the enamel. Inclusion of these lesions constitutes the D2 threshold. The next group of lesions are enamel lesions with apparently intact surfaces, the whitespot and brownspot lesions. Adding these to the count brings one to the D1 level of clinical examination. Even deeper below the water line of the imaginary iceberg are the lesions (both enamel and dentine) which can be detected only by using some sort of diagnostic aid such as bitewing radiography or fibreoptic transillumination. At the most sensitive level there are a further group of subclinical lesions which may only be discernible with histological techniques. These lesions are continually progressing and regressing; they represent both an opportunity for preventive treatments and the starting point from which larger lesions can start if the environment favours continuing demineralization.

There is a serious but underrecognized problem concerning different interpretations and usage of some key terms in the measurement of caries which constitute a trap for the unwary. As dental caries is measured in a number of different, but superficially similar ways, confusion and inappropriate usage of epidemiological and

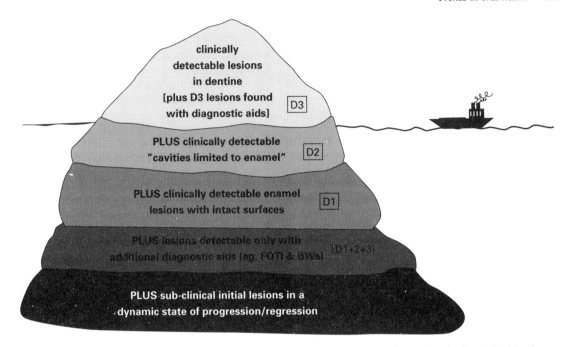

clinically
detectable lesions
in dentine
[plus D3 lesions found
with diagnostic aids]

D3

PLUS clinically detectable
"cavities limited to enamel"

D2

PLUS clinically detectable enamel
lesions with intact surfaces

D1

PLUS lesions detectable only with
additional diagnostic aids (eg. FOTI & BWs)

[D1+2+3]

PLUS sub-clinical initial lesions in a
dynamic state of progression/regression

Fig. 8.8 The iceberg of caries experience: differing diagnostic thresholds. FOTI = Fibreoptic transillumination; BW = bitewing.

service data can result. A specific example centres on the term caries-free. If all layers of the iceberg in Figure 8.8 are recognized as truly carious, then the meaning of caries-free is obvious. If, however, in an epidemiological setting the accepted convention of excluding D1 and D2 lesions is adhered to, it may not be readily apparent to a general dentist, or politician, that someone caries-free at the D3 (dentinal) diagnostic threshold can have a number of whitespot lesions or small cavities limited to the enamel. Similarly, those groups who regularly rely on diagnostic aids as an adjunct to their clinical examinations must appreciate that others making assessments for different reasons in different environments will not be using these aids and will therefore not achieve comparable results.

Changing caries measurement methods in epidemiology

The traditional level of measurement in dental epidemiology has been frank cavitation into dentine (that is, a visible carious hole in the tooth). Recording at this comparatively gross level, where treatment need is unequivocal, is essential if survey results are to be compared

with other countries and with surveys conducted previously. However, the fundamental difference between recording at the dentine (D3) level (used in the UK Surveys discussed earlier) and the more sensitive (D1) level used by clinicians should be appreciated (Pitts and Fyffe, 1988). Even in regularly attending 12-year-olds, the mean number of DMFT can range from 1.0 at the D3 survey level to 11.8 at the D1 clinician level (Pitts *et al.*, 1993). A further complication is that, as open cavitation has become more of a rarity, epidemiological criteria have had to evolve to reflect this change in the presentation of disease (Pitts, 1993a). The inaccuracies inherent in making simple predictions about the level of provision of subsequent dental treatment on the sole basis of epidemiological data collected at the dentine (D3) level have been demonstrated (Nuttall and Davies, 1988). This problem is less of an issue in northern European countries where over 90% of children may be in dental programmes providing comprehensive care. In these countries, epidemiological data to monitor trends in dental caries experience largely comprise a count of the fillings placed by the salaried dentists providing that care. In this way, the diagnostic decisions on the presence or absence of disease lie with the clinician, not the epidemiologist.

In some countries there is still a continuing debate as to the use of an *exclusively visual* as opposed to a *visuotactile* method of diagnosis for survey examinations (Pitts, 1993b). There is a growing movement of consensus towards the visual approach. Lussi (1993) has shown the tactile element to be of no added diagnostic benefit. However, sharp probing carries a theoretical risk of damaging the surface of reversible whitespot lesions in such a way that will promote subsequent lesion progression. There are indications that the WHO will join the shift away from the use of tactile criteria and sharp probes in the near future, but this will remain a contentious area for debate for some time, particularly in the USA.

Safeguarding appropriate quality in epidemiology

As both the pattern of disease encountered and the types of care provided in communities are changing rapidly, it is imperative to evaluate trends over time in order to understand better the oral health status and needs within a community. To do this, reliable, high-quality data are required at local, regional and national levels. In countries where the level of coverage achieved by state schemes is more modest than that seen, for example, in Scandinavia, many dentinal lesions remain untreated and a census approach to oral health monitoring is not feasible. In these environments assessments of DMF still have to be made and as the overall prevalence of caries and fillings declines, examination of proportionately more unrestored sound or equivocal surfaces makes the use of reproducible criteria even more important than it used to be.

To measure changes over time in a changing environment, periodic reviews of methodology and quality standards are needed (Pitts, 1993a). This process should be non-threatening, although this can be difficult as the area of methodology tends to be rather emotive and individuals who have been collecting data in a particular way for many years may be loath to consider any type of change. There is a need to balance the important principle of collecting exactly the same information over time with sensible reactions to intermediary changes in the disease process which may lead to spurious inferences if methodology does not evolve to

compensate. Some methods which were entirely appropriate in the 1960s may not deliver what was intended when used to record the different type of decay found in the 1990s. What is needed are balanced compromise decisions which aim to ensure that valid assessments of trends over time can be made.

There are great variations in the amount and quality of epidemiological data available in different countries. In some Scandinavian countries, Denmark in particular, comprehensive information systems track the dental status of each child each year. In the UK great strides have been made in the last 20 years in the systematic collection of data from representative samples of the population (Downer, 1992); similarly, national surveys in Ireland, the USA and France have provided essential insights into dental status, but the ability to track trends in disease varies. At the other end of the spectrum there are many countries for whom few representative data are available; frequently a WHO pathfinder survey of populations in a single area is all that is available.

In the UK, most surveys are undertaken by community dental officers, salaried public health dentists who have a role in the provision of primary dental care to priority groups. They act as examiners in the decennial surveys conducted by the OPCS and also carry out the National Health Service dental epidemiological programme coordinated by BASCD, the British Association for the Study of Community Dentistry. This complementary activity reports each year on the dental status of representative samples of 5-, 12- or 14-year-olds from each region of England as well as from Wales, Scotland and, more recently, Northern Ireland (Pitts, 1993a). These surveys use standardized criteria and methodology to provide regular dmf/DMF data from more local populations which can aid in the evaluation of trends at both local and national levels.

In order to achieve this there has been an ongoing process of evolution and development of the methodology (Pitts, 1993a, 1995; Palmer, 1995; Pine, 1995). Although there have been some tensions in keeping all of the semi-autonomous regions and countries in step with each other by agreeing to an evolving standardized core of methodology and time-tabling, agreement has been achieved and maintained. For example, harmonized standards have been agreed for the type of examining light suitable for use which will also conform to UK legislation in this area, and for the posture of children undergoing examinations (supine).

The refinements introduced have included evolution of the wording of the diagnostic criteria which relate to the definition of dentine caries in order to accommodate the changed presentation of disease discussed earlier (Pitts, 1993b). Open frank cavitation greater than a predetermined size is no longer a requirement for the scoring of dentinal caries; unambiguous visual changes associated with dentine caries are now sufficient. In debating written criteria it has become apparent that there are many inescapable ambiguities in written paragraphs seeking to describe a particular stage of disease. In order to promote consistent interpretation of the agreed criteria across the UK a BASCD trainers' pack has now been introduced which comprises written criteria supplemented by a standard set of clinical slides and acetates highlighting key points (Mitropoulos *et al.*, 1992). Using this pack and cascading down the standardized training through a series of regional benchmark examiners who are responsible for local training has been found to improve the quality and comparability of the programme (Pitts, 1995). The BASCD coordinated programme has recently agreed standardized methodologies for calibration methods and the standards used to decide who can participate as an examiner (Pine *et al.*, 1995a). A further document covers a standardized approach to sampling to ensure that results are truly representative of the districts, regions and countries from which they are drawn (Pine *et al.*, 1995b).

All of these methodological aspects of dental epidemiology have to be addressed on a continuing basis if the quality of the data collected is to be safeguarded to ensure that valid monitoring of changes in disease status over time can be made. Such assessments are increasingly called for following the setting of local and national targets. WHO's global goals are but one example at the country level.

The rapid pace of organizational change and consequent reorganization of dental delivery systems in many countries (particularly those currently happening in eastern Europe) also increase the need for assessment of trends in oral health. In many cases it is beneficial to have a neutral body to provide objective and valid criteria for the assessment of oral health and this

is why the WHO guidelines have been so important in the past. It is to be hoped that the forthcoming updated edition of WHO's *Basic Methods* for oral health surveys will carry forward this role.

Changes in dental treatment

Changes in the use of pit-and-fissure sealants and sealant restorations

In many countries the use of pit-and-fissure sealants has increased in recent years as more dentists use this method of protecting surfaces which are at particular risk to dental caries. In the UK in 1983, on average a maximum of 6% of children had any sealed teeth (sealants and/or sealant restorations), although in Scotland, 16% of 11-year-olds had received sealants (O'Brien, 1994). In 1993, around one-third of English and Welsh 15-year-olds had sealants (34% and 31%) compared with around half of children in Scotland (52%) and Northern Ireland (47%). In 1994/95, the Scottish figure had increased, with some 67% of Scottish 14-year-olds having one or more sealants or sealant restorations (Pitts *et al.*, 1995a). There are indications also that sealant use is increasing in the USA and in other populations.

What effect will this have on monitoring trends in disease? It is clear that many occlusal surfaces which in the past would have been classified as sound, decayed or filled according to survey criteria are now in an indeterminate sealed status which does not contribute to the traditional DMF index. With the changing pattern of care it may be that modifications to or alternatives to the DMF index are required (Davies, 1991). As sealants become more prevalent, then the impact of teeth which were formerly restored with amalgam but which are now therapeutically treated with sealants becomes larger.

In a field setting there is no reliable way of differentiating between a preventive sealant, placed in the clinical absence of caries, and a sealant restoration deliberately placed as a preventive method of managing dental caries while preserving as much tooth structure as possible. Even in ideal circumstances this is a difficult task (Deery *et al.*, 1995). The increasing difficulty of reliably detecting the presence or absence of occlusal caries referred to earlier is a further complication as there may already be caries in a tooth which is assumed to be sound and is treated with a supposedly purely preventive sealant.

The impact of changes in restorative materials on monitoring trends

The developments in dental biomaterials in recent years have provided dentists with an ever-widening range of choices when they elect to restore missing tooth tissue. In response to professional and patient demand, most newer materials are tooth-coloured and great strides have been made in the aesthetic appearance of restorations. Well-finished composite fillings are often very difficult to distinguish from enamel, particularly in field survey settings where moisture control and lighting are not at the level available in a dental surgery. The impact of this change is that examiners have to be explicitly trained to look for tooth-coloured fillings as opposed to relying on the visual appearance of amalgam restorations to make the filling self-evident. Therefore, there is an increasing risk that the level of restorative intervention will be underestimated in surveys. With a range of environmental and other campaigns attempting to limit the use of dental amalgam in the future, this problem is set to increase.

Changes in treatment philosophy and decision-making

Dental services in the developed countries have moved through an extractive phase–dealing with the removal of large numbers of teeth and the provision of dentures–via a *restorative phase*– when at a time of higher caries activity the detection of decay was followed promptly by the excision of the lesions and placement of a filling–to a *preventive phase*–in which primary and secondary prevention are the focus and restorations are provided once preventive treatment has been initiated and once a certain threshold of lesion severity has been exceeded. There is an increasing desire to avoid the placement of premature or unnecessary restorations as a treatment for small lesions that could be managed more conservatively.

It should be appreciated that the extent to which dental services have moved in this direction varies between countries and, within a particular dental care system, there will be variations between dentists as to how far they subscribe to a preventive treatment philosophy

(Nuttall and Pitts, 1990). These phases are described for dental care in the UK in Chapter 17. There is no doubt, however, that in the UK many general dentists profess to use a preventive approach to the management of caries (Nuttall *et al.*, 1994).

In developing countries there are initiatives to promote the use of a limited intervention preventive approach when restorative intervention is indicated. An example is the current ART initiative of WHO, which is advocating the atraumatic restorative treatment technique. This is based upon the removal of carious tissue with hand instruments and the filling of cavities with adhesive materials such as glass ionomers. The technique is currently undergoing evaluations in a variety of different settings (see Chapter 2).

The impact of these changes in treatment philosophy on attempts to monitor changes in dental health over time is that some level of systematic change in the DMF can be anticipated even if the prevalence of disease stays the same. For equivocal lesions dentists move from an 'if in doubt, fill with amalgam' philosophy (which would yield an F score) to an 'if in doubt, prevent and monitor the outcome' philosophy (a similar lesion would now be kept under review and the surface scored as caries-free). The tendency will thus be for a reduction in the observed DMF. The magnitude of this reduction is unclear, but it will be smaller than the overall dramatic decline in prevalence seen in children.

The effect of changes in the delivery of dental care on monitoring trends

The principles of delivery of oral health care and specific examples are outlined in Chapters 16 and 17 and will not be addressed here. However, within the context of trends in oral health, we will set out some examples from the UK which demonstrate simultaneous interactions between changes in disease and changes in the delivery of dental care which serve to complicate the analysis of trends in disease.

In 1990 a hybrid capitation system was introduced in the UK for the payment of general dentists treating children up to age 18 years. The focus was a preventive one in which clinical freedom and a preventive approach were encouraged (replacing an earlier item of service system). Unfortunately the funding side of the package was part of a remuneration negotiation process with the profession that was, at times, acrimonious and the package did not have universal support at introduction. With hindsight it could also be said that the change in treatment philosophy sought required a greater emphasis on continuing professional education than was appreciated at the time.

Recent epidemiological evidence has suggested that, since 1990, the decline seen previously in overall caries in 5-year-olds has ceased and that there are disturbing changes in the component parts of the DMF index. Trends here suggest that the provision of fillings has declined markedly, whilst untreated dentinal decay has risen. The proportion of the caries experience made up of fillings (the Care Index) has been showing a deterioration in the primary teeth of 5-year-olds for some time (Pitts and Palmer, 1995) and a similar pattern is now being seen for permanent teeth in 12-year-olds (Pitts and Palmer, 1994) and 14-year-olds (Pitts *et al.*, 1995a).

Although the changes are striking and apparently linked to the changed remuneration system, it must be appreciated that other rapid changes were also underway during the same period. The role of the Community Dental Service in the UK has been changing following a decision announced in 1989 to move away from the routine care of children and to take on other tasks for the provision of care to special-needs groups as well as developing roles in health promotion and dental epidemiology. With the polarization of caries into high- and low-risk groups, it may well be that many of the high-caries children previously treated by the Community Dental Service failed to make the transition to family dental practices and have not been receiving care. Although a relatively small group in overall terms, they can exert a disproportionate effect on mean dmft/DMFT.

At around the same time there were also significant changes in guidelines relating to the use of general anaesthesia in general dental practices. The net effect of these new more stringent guidelines was to discourage the provision of general anaesthesia in a general practice setting and redirect patients towards hospital or community facilities. These centres became very busy and, in some cases, were sited at a greater distance from patients. Therefore, at any one time there were more children in the community awaiting extraction of carious teeth than had been the case in previous years. Thus a further complication to changes in the dmf of 5-year-olds is that some of the decayed unrestored teeth which are now being recorded might, under the previous system, have been extracted under general anaesthetic.

These examples should serve to illustrate why detailed knowledge about changes in the delivery of dental services is needed to interpret changes in the results of epidemiological assessments of trends in oral health.

Importance of recognizing local variations in oral health

A further danger in interpreting such data is the wide local variations which exist in the levels of oral health. If country means and changes in them are used for planning local services, inappropriate decisions may well result. To use the UK as an example, there have been consistent reports in the decennial surveys demonstrating significant and systematic differences between England, Wales, Scotland and Northern Ireland (O'Brien, 1994). However, if a larger sample is taken at a more regional level then further variations become evident. Figure 8.9 is a bar chart showing trends in caries experience in 5-year-olds examined across the UK between 1985/86 and 1993/94 in the British Association for the Study of Community Dentistry Epidemiology Programme.

It can be seen that there are considerable differences in mean dmft between 'N. Western' in England and the fluoridated 'W. Midlands' also in England. There is a general pattern of lower levels of disease in the south with higher levels in the north. It is also apparent that while in recent years further declines have been seen in some areas at the low caries end of the chart, increases in mean dmft have been recorded in some other areas towards the high caries end. This level of detail still does not provide the whole answer–a single mean is given for Scotland, for example, which administratively is made up of 15 separate health boards. Caries prevalence in Scotland is monitored by the Scottish Health Boards' Dental Epidemiological Programme, a joint venture between all 15 health boards (mediated through the CADOs group) and Chief Scientist Office's Dental Health Services Research Unit in Dundee (Pitts and Davies, 1992). The mean levels in the different

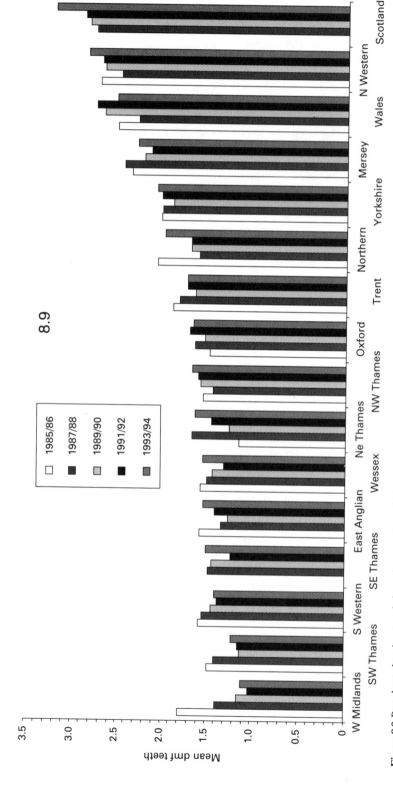

Figure 8.9 Bar chart showing trends in caries experience in 5-year-olds examined across the UK between 1985/86 and 1993/94 in the British Association for the Study of Community Dentistry Dental Epidemiology Programme.

boards span a wide range; some approach the low levels seen in the south of England while others are amongst the highest seen anywhere in the UK. It is clear that to be able to interpret changes in oral health fully, smaller area statistics are needed, complemented by local sociodemographic information.

Conclusions

In considering trends in oral health, we have reviewed the changes in caries prevalence across all age groups where banks of sufficient data exist to undertake this task. It is clear that in order to make sense of these past changes, we need an understanding of a variety of overt and subtle factors underlying them. Changes in the distribution, morphology and activity of caries, together with changes in caries management techniques, health funding and access to dental care are all operating at the same time. This will mean that a variety of different, locally tailored solutions will have to be introduced and assessed to inform decision-making about the types of dental services which will be required to secure the oral health of different sections of communities in the future. Undoubtedly, changes in oral health will continue to occur. The magnitude and direction of these trends will need to be evaluated even more carefully than in the past, in order to understand the increasingly complex and interrelated factors affecting trends in oral health.

References

Bedi, R. and Elton, R.A. (1993) Dental caries experience and oral cleanliness of Asian and white Caucasian children aged 5 and 6 years attending primary schools in Glasgow and Trafford, UK. *Community Dental Health* **9**:17–23.

Davies, J.A. (1991) Should we continue to use DMF to measure caries experience in children? *Community Dental Health* **8**:209.

Deery, C., Fyffe, H.E., Nugent, Z. *et al.* (1995) The effect of placing a clear pit and fissure sealant on the validity and reproducibility of occlusal caries diagnosis. *Caries Research* **29**: 377–381.

Downer, M.C. (1992) The quality of caries data from national and BASCD surveys. *Community Dental Health* **9**:107–108.

Gordon, P.H., Murray, J.J.M. and Todd, J.E. (1994) The shortened dental arch: supplementary analyses from the 1988 adult dental health survey. *Community Dental Health* **11**:87–90.

Gray, P.G., Todd, J.E., Slack, G.L. and Bulman, J.S. (1970) *Government Social Survey–Adult Dental Health in England and Wales in 1968*. HMSO, London.

Hinds, K. and Gregory, J. (1995) *National Diet and Nutrition Survey: Children aged 1½ to 4½ years. Volume 2: Report of the Dental Survey*. HMSO, London.

Ismail, A.I., Brodeur, J-M., Gagnon, P. *et al.* (1992) Prevalence of non-cavitated and cavitated carious lesions in a random sample of 7–9 year old schoolchildren in Montreal, Quebec. *Community Dental and Oral Epidemiology* **20**:25–255.

Kalsbeek, H., Eijkman, M.A.J. and Verrips, G.H. (1995) Change in caries prevalence in children with a Turkish or Moroccan origin in The Netherlands. *Caries Research* **29**:300.

Kayser, A.F. (1981) Shortened dental arches and oral function. *Journal of Oral Rehabilitation* **8**:457–462.

Kidd, E.A.M., Ricketts, D.N.J. and Pitts, N.B. (1993) Occlusal caries diagnosis: a changing challenge for clinicians and epidemiologists. *Journal of Dentistry* **21**:323–331.

Lussi, A. (1993) Comparison of different methods for the diagnosis of fissure caries without cavitation. *Caries Research* **27**:409–416.

Milsom, K. and Mitropoulos, C.M. (1990) Enamel defects in 8-year-old children in fluoridated and non-fluoridated parts of Cheshire. *Caries Research* **24**:286–289.

Mitropoulos, C.M. (1993) The contrast in dental caries experience amongst children in the north west of England. *Community Dental Health* **10**:9–18.

Mitropoulos, C.M., Pitts, N.B. and Deery, C. (1992) *BASCD Trainers' Pack for Caries Prevalence Studies*. Dental Health Services Research Unit, University of Dundee.

Murray, J.J. (1994) Comments on results reported at the second international conference 'changes in caries prevalence'. *International Dental Journal* **44**:457–458.

Nuttall, N.M. and Davies, J.A. (1988) The capability of the 1983 Children's Dental Health Survey in Scotland to predict fillings and extractions subsequently undertaken. *Community Dental Health* **5**:355–362.

Nuttall, N.M. and Pitts, N.B. (1990) Restorative treatment thresholds reported to be used by dentists in Scotland. *British Dental Journal* **169**:119–126.

Nuttall, N.M., Fyffe, H.E. and Pitts, N.B. (1994) Caries management strategies used by a group of Scottish dentists. *British Dental Journal* **176**:373–378.

O'Brien, M. (1994) *Children's Dental Health in the UK, 1993*. HMSO, London.

Palmer, J. (1995) 1994 Epidemiology Co-ordinators' Meeting and Developments. *Community Dental Health* **12**:119.

Palmer, J.D. and Pitts, N.B. (1994) Child dental health–is it still good news? *British Dental Journal* **177**:235–237.

Pilot, T. and Miyazaki, H. (1991) Periodental conditions in Europe. *Journal of Clinical Periodontology* **18**:353–357.

Pine, C.M. (1995) BASCD guidance on sampling and calibration. *Community Dental Health* **12**:120.

Pine, C.M., Pitts, N.B. and Nugent, Z. (1995a) *BASCD*

Guidance on the Statistical Aspects of Training and Calibration of Examiners for Survey of Child Dental Health. Dental Health Services Research Unit, University of Dundee.

Pine, C.M., Pitts, N.B. and Nugent, Z. (1995b) *BASCD Guidance on Sampling for Surveys of Child Dental Health.* Dental Health Services Research Unit, University of Dundee.

Pitts, N.B. (1991) The diagnosis for dental caries: 2. The detection of approximal, root surface and recurrent lesions. *Dental Update* **18**:436–442.

Pitts, N.B. (1992) The diagnosis of dental caries: 3. Rationale and overview of present and potential future techniques. *Dental Update* **19**:32–42.

Pitts, N.B. (1993a) Safeguarding the quality of epidemiological caries data at a time of changing disease patterns and evolving dental services. *Community Dental Health* **10**:1–9.

Pitts, N.B. (1993b) Current methods and criteria for caries diagnosis in Europe. *Journal of Dental Education* **57**:409–414.

Pitts, N.B. (1995) The 1994 BASCD training and calibration exercise. *Community Dental Health* **12**:119–120.

Pitts, N.B. and Davies, J.A. (1992) The Scottish Health Boards' dental epidemiological programme: initial surveys of 5- and 12-year-olds. *British Dental Journal* **172**:408–413.

Pitts, N.B. and Deery, C. (1994) Prevalence of 'hidden' occlusal dentine caries in regularly attending Scottish adolescents. *Journal of Dental Research* **73**:802.

Pitts, N.B. and Fyffe, H.E. (1988) The effect of varying diagnostic thresholds upon clinical caries data for a low prevalence group. *Journal of Dental Research* **67**:592–596.

Pitts, N.B. and Kidd, E.A.M. (1992) Some of the factors to be considered in the prescription and timing of bitewing radiography. *Journal of Dentistry* **20**:74–84.

Pitts, N.B. and Palmer, J. (1994) The dental caries experience of 5-, 12- and 14-year-old children in Great Britain. Surveys co-ordinated by the British Association for the Study of Community Dentistry in 1991/92, 1992/93 and 1990–91. *Community Dental Health* **11**:42–52.

Pitts, N.B. and Palmer, J. (1995) The dental caries experience of 5-year-old children in Great Britain. Surveys co-ordinated by the British Association for the Study of Community Dentistry in 1993/94. *Community Dental Health* **12**:52–58.

Pitts, N.B. and Rimmer, P.A. (1992) An *in vivo* comparison of radiographic and directly assessed clinical caries status of posterior approximal surfaces in primary and permanent teeth. *Caries Research* **26**:146–152.

Pitts, N.B., Deery, C. and Fyffe, H.E. (1993) Children's caries prevalence: comparing estimations used by

epidemiologists and practitioners. *Journal of Dental Research* **72**:142.

Pitts, N.B., Nugent, Z., Fyffe, H.E. and Smith, P. (1992) *The Scottish Health Boards' Dental Epidemiological Programme. Report of the 1991/92 Survey of 5 year old Children.* University of Dundee, Dundee.

Pitts, N.B., Fyffe, H.E. and Nugent, Z. (1995a) *The Scottish Health Boards' Dental Epidemiological Programme. Report of the 1994/95 Survey of 14 year old Children.* University of Dundee, Dundee.

Pitts, N.B., Pine, C., Forgie, A.H. and Nugent, Z. (1995b) The contribution of bitewing radiography to detecting hidden dentinal caries in high-caries-risk Scottish adolescents. *Caries Research* **29**:293.

Renson, C.E., Crielaers, P.J.A., Ibikunle, S.A.J. *et al.* (1985) Changing patterns of oral health and implications for oral health manpower. Part 1. *International Dental Journal* **35**:235–251.

Richards, N.D., Willcocks, A.J., Bulman, J.S. and Slack, G.L. (1965a) A survey of the dental health and attitudes towards dentistry in two communities. Part 1: sociological data. *British Dental Journal* **118**:199–205.

Richards, N.D., Willcocks, A.J., Bulman, J.S. and Slack, G.L. (1965b) A survey of the dental health and attitudes towards dentistry in two communities. Part 2: dental data. *British Dental Journal* **124**:549–554.

Sheiham, A. and Joffe, M. (1991) Public dental health strategies for identifying and controlling dental caries in high and low risk populations. In: *Risk Markers for Oral Diseases. Volume 1. Dental Caries Markers of High and Low Risk Groups and Individuals.* (Johnson, N.W., ed.), pp. 455–482.

Steele, J.G., Walls, A.W.G., Ayattollahi, S.M.T. and Murray, J.J. (1996) Major clinical findings for a dental survey of elderly people in three different English communities. *British Dental Journal* **180**: 17–23.

Todd, J. (1975) *Children's Dental Health in England and Wales 1973.* HMSO, London.

Todd, J.E. and Dodd, T. (1985) *Children's dental health in the UK, 1983.* HMSO, London.

Todd, J.E. and Lader, D. (1991) *Adult Dental Health, 1988, UK.* HMSO, London.

Todd, J.E. and Walker, A.M. (1980) *Adult Dental Health, Volume 1, England and Wales, 1968–1978.* HMSO, London.

Verrips, G.H., Kalsbeek, H. and Eikjman, M.A. (1993) Ethnicity and maternal education as risk indicators for dental caries and the role of dental behaviour. *Community Dentistry and Oral Epidemiology* **21**:209–214.

9

Statistics in community oral health

Albert Kingman

Introduction

Studies in community oral health involve gathering data on human populations. These studies are characterized as association studies in which one or more response variables (disease status, clinical signs or symptoms, personal habits or behaviours, economic costs or incentives) are investigated as they vary with a set of explanatory factors. Associations between an explanatory factor of particular interest, such as the exposure to some condition, thought to be beneficial or potentially hazardous, and the response variables are studied, usually in the presence of related explanatory factors called confounders. The observed variables may be inherently qualitative or quantitative in nature, and measured using a categorical or continuous measurement scale. The exposure factors may or may not be able to be controlled or manipulated. In longitudinal studies some variables may be time-dependent while others remain constant.

An observational study investigating how utilization rates of dental services vary among specific geographical districts is one example of a community oral health study. So too is a prospective randomized clinical trial in which a fee for service schedule is compared with a capitation plan for cost-effectiveness for the comprehensive provision of dental prevention and care for children. Thus, a diversity of statistical designs and analytical strategies are needed to describe, analyse and interpret findings from such studies. An indepth discussion of these factors is presented in Chapter 5 of

this book. Those less familiar with study design aspects and their relation to statistical considerations in community oral health are advised to read Chapter 5 before this chapter.

Design issues

Purpose of the study

A sample of research questions involving community oral health issues might include the following:

1 Is it cost-effective to apply dental sealants to first molars of children between the ages of 5 and 10
2 How are the prevalence and severity of gingivitis related to the level of oral hygiene practised among teenaged populations?
3 Is there a documentable increase in the prevalence of dental fluorosis among young children who ingest dentifrice while brushing their teeth?
4 Is there a noticeable loss in decay-preventive effectiveness experienced by using a 500 p.p.m. sodium fluoride (NaF) dentifrice rather than one with 1000 p.p.m. NaF?
5 How is the prevalence of oral cancer associated with smoking and alcohol consumption?
6 Is there a difference in the quality of oral health attributable to the level of annual expenditures incurred for dental care?
7 What are the relative costs of restoring small pit-and-fissure lesions with a composite

material rather than amalgam over a 5-year period? For a 25-year period?

The type of study suggested by each of the seven questions above seems readily apparent at first glance, but closer scrutiny suggests that, although several study designs may be employed, not all designs will answer the same question. One of the first, and most frequently asked questions by investigators when designing a study is: How many subjects will be needed in each group? My favourite response, borrowed from the late Professor Gertrude Cox, is to reply, in Socratic style, with a question: How many bricks does it take to build a wall? The point is quickly communicated and a meaningful dialogue is established between the investigator and statistician. This interaction usually produces a more focused delineation as to the primary purpose of the investigation, including the identification of what can and cannot be done. An analytical plan is ultimately developed in which the study design and approach to data acquisition to be used are identified, as well as the anticipated statistical methods which will be used to analyse the data.

Suppose we consider the issue of cost-effectiveness of using dental sealants in children. A definition of terms is needed before any meaningful design can be selected. How will cost-effectiveness be defined? This involves the identification of what expenditures and time will be considered as costs and what indicators of effectiveness will be used. To illustrate, the costs may be quite different if public health dental personnel place sealants on first molars in school health clinics than if dentists are reimbursed to place them while in their private dental offices. Questions related to the expected longevity of such sealants and the planned frequency of reseals must also be addressed. For effectiveness, will the retention rate of placed sealants be the measure of effectiveness, the development of dental caries, or will there be other measures as well? Over what time period will these costs and effect measures be taken? One can see that different answers may be obtained to this question, depending on how the study is designed and how one interprets the question. A useful aphorism states: It is more beneficial to obtain an approximate answer to a specific research question than a precise answer to a vague one.

Issues in variable selection

Variable selection becomes a delicate matter whenever one investigates a safety issue. For example, if one were interested in determining whether or not there are potential side-effects of placing tetracycline-treated fibres in periodontal pockets, what variables should be of primary concern? Can one correctly anticipate the wide range of potential effects of such a drug, both in the short term, but more importantly, in the long term? It is axiomatic that one can never prove safety. One can demonstrate a potential hazard exists, provided it is of sufficient magnitude. The real danger occurs when safety is routinely concluded from the non-significance of statistical test procedures. Too often studies have insufficient sensitivity to identify the very risk they were designed to detect. It should be remembered that the absence of evidence does not necessarily imply the evidence of absence.

Variable selection can be difficult because more than one yardstick exists. The optimal criterion for measuring a variable may not be known. For example, suppose one were investigating the effect of fluoride concentration in a community water supply on the prevalence and severity of dental fluorosis in the associated exposed population groups. Some would argue that one should score the teeth for the presence of all enamel opacities. Subsequently, one determines whether these opacities are associated with fluoride. Second, several indices exist for scoring dental fluorosis, but each is based on distinct measurement units, focuses on or emphasizes different aspects of clinical signs and symptoms and varies in the number of assessments made per subject. Thus, the form of the appropriate variable to measure is not always obvious. The choice of index may well depend on the purpose of the study. In some instances it may be desirable to use more than one index.

Potential confounders or covariates measured should be selected because they are associated with the primary response variables and also with the explanatory variables under study. Demographic variables such as age, gender and ethnic category or socioeconomic status are often important determinants of oral health responses. However, the inclusion of too many variables can cause problems in the statistical analyses.

Whatever the final choice for variable

inclusion, the minimal criteria are that the primary variables be valid and reproducible. This means that the measurement ought to reflect the characteristic or condition one is trying to assess. Validity is a difficult property to demonstrate because the true value of a measurement may be unknown. However, the primary measurements should be reproducible. An investigator ought to obtain the same values for repeated evaluations on the same subject. The primary variables ought also to be reproducible by other investigators as well.

Appropriate study populations

The characteristics of an appropriate study population will depend on the purpose of the study protocol. As an example, for the cost-effectiveness question on sealants one would wish to find a population in which there is sufficient dental caries occurring, yet not so much as to render it meaningless in terms of extrapolation to real populations. The answer one obtains from a sealant study will be highly correlated with the dental caries levels found in the study population. Therefore, the study ought to be conducted in a population similar to the target population for which the question is asked, utilizing the types of dental personnel they have available and under a care structure thought to be practical for that population.

As a second example, if one thought that the difference between the decay-preventive effectiveness level of a 500 p.p.m. NaF and a 1000 p.p.m. NaF dentifrice were trivial in magnitude, the importance of observing small differences between the caries incidences of these two products would be stronger if they were obtained from a high-caries study population than from a low-caries study population. However, it would be difficult to conclude that these dentifrices were equally effective in a high caries population based on small benefits obtained from a low-caries study population.

In survey research a different concern regarding appropriate study populations can occur. Suppose the study objective is to evaluate specific aspects of oral health of adults within a particular country. One standard sampling approach is based on a household probability sample. However, a sampling frame (list) of the households within that country would have to be available to use this approach. For example, this approach is used in the UK National Surveys described in Chapter 8. However, in many countries such a sampling frame is not available. A different procedure would have to be used. One could randomly select specific geographic areas and then examine every household in that area. A less rigorous method could utilize a convenience sample, where persons readily available are examined. In some instances these convenience samples may be the only option available. The choice of sampling strategy will produce quite different study populations whose oral health status may or may not be representative of the adult population living in that country. For such sampling plans caveats regarding potential bias should be mentioned and discussed.

Sampling strategies and probabilistic methods of assigning subjects to groups

The laws of chance, more formally termed the laws of probability, are the true basis for valid statistical inference. In well-designed studies great care is taken to ensure that randomization methods are utilized, whenever possible. When conducting large epidemiological surveys, complex multistage probability sampling strategies are typically necessary. Complex survey sampling requires that great care be taken in its execution. This involves attention being given to detail, enormous amounts of tedium spent on perusing the characteristics of sampling frames, examining them for their extent of coverage of the population of interest, their expected overall accuracy level and specifying methods for handling the types of non-response. Once an acceptable sampling frame is identified and procured, the process of sample selection is begun. Random sampling can be invoked at many levels in the same survey. For example, in the National Institute of Dental Research (NIDR) National Oral Health Surveys of Children simple random sampling, stratified random sampling and systematic random sampling coexisted within a multistage sampling procedure (National Caries Program, 1982; DEODP, 1989). Precise definitions are developed as to what constitutes a response at all stages of the sampling process. Statistical weights are then determined and applied to the observed data to estimate characteristics in the target population of interest.

In comparative longitudinal studies, especially clinical trials, random assignment of participants to the specific study groups is essential. Double-blinding relative to study group identity is always the goal (ideally, triple-blinding would be even better–also blinding the statistician). In a double-blind study neither the study participant nor the examiner or investigator knows the study group identity of any participant. This goal is not always possible to achieve. For example, if one were to compare a scaling and root planing intervention strategy for periodontal disease with an intervention involving only a chemotherapeutic mouthrinse, blindness to the patient is clearly lost. In such studies, however, it may be possible to retain the blinding of the examiners who are involved in the evaluation of the effects of therapy. Whenever possible, such single blinding is preferred to minimize examiner biases.

Sometimes simple random assignment of study participants to treatment groups is not very efficient, even though double-blinding is possible. For example, suppose one were to compare the longevity and quality of two types (A and B) of single root dental implants. A study involving 40 patients is designed where 20 patients are randomly assigned to receive type A or type B implant. The 40 participants will be entered sequentially and assigned case numbers 1 through 40. A random permutation is consulted with the following group assignments:

Group A

1,	10,	34,	36,	8
32,	5,	2,	22,	21
31,	25,	26,	39,	24
16,	28,	17,	19,	38

The remaining 20 persons belong to group B. The patient numbers are then ordered and entered into the study according to the following schedule:

Group A					*Group B*				
1,	2,	5,	8,	10	3,	4,	6,	7,	9
16,	17,	19,	21,	22	11,	12,	13,	14,	15
24,	25,	26,	28,	31	18,	20,	23,	27,	29
32,	34,	36,	38,	39	30,	33,	35,	37,	40

So far everything appears to be consistent with one's expectations regarding random permutations. However, suppose this study had to be aborted after 15 patients were entered. The results now show that

Group A					*Group B*				
1,	2,	5,	8,	10	3,	4,	6,	7,	9
					11,	12,	13,	14,	15

reflecting a 2 to 1 imbalance between groups. This can be avoided by utilizing a blocking procedure (Fleiss, 1986). Here one would select a group of 4 or 6 patients (called a block) and randomly assign an equal number of patients within the block to each treatment group. This is repeated for each block, ensuring that the degree of imbalance at any point in chronological time is minimal. Several such blocking procedures can be used to improve efficiency. Some thought given to the possibility of early termination at the design stage can often minimize the impact of unscheduled changes in protocol.

The calculus of sample size determination

The process of sample size determination illustrates many of the aspects of experimental design, such as the importance of having a clear study objective, some knowledge concerning the behaviour of the types of variables that are being assessed, and in comparative studies, how large differences (in means, percentages, etc.) between groups must be that are worth detecting. Ideally, before undertaking a study, the experimenter should discuss the protocol with a statistician and obtain expert help in not only determining sample size but also identifying the effect of potential confounders and selecting the appropriate analysis. Much time and effort can be wasted when a statistician is not an integral member of a study team. The process of sample size estimation undertaken by the statistician and which should be understood in principle by the study clinician and public health planner is illustrated below for both population parameter estimation problems and for statistical hypothesis testing, separately.

For estimation problems

The goal of many studies, especially surveys, is to obtain estimates of the mean (μ) or the proportion (π) of the population having a specific condition or characteristic. One first needs to identify a statistic with optimal properties that can be used to estimate the unknown parameter. Most often a statistic exists which is unbiased and has minimum variance. Next, one has to specify the precision that is required of the parameter estimator used.

Categorical responses

Suppose one wished to know what percentage of 12–16-year-olds in a community use smokeless tobacco products. For a simple random sample design (to keep the calculations manageable here) the proportion of adolescents (call it p) observed in the sample is a statistic having optimal properties for estimating the true proportion (call it π). For any sample size (n) the standard error of the sampled proportion p is written as

$$s.e.(p) = \sqrt{\frac{\pi(1-\pi)}{n}}$$

The corresponding $100(1-\alpha)\%$ confidence interval for π can then be written as

$$[p - z_{\alpha/2}s.e.(p), \ p + z_{\alpha/2}s.e.(p)]$$

The investigator can then determine a reasonable sample size by specifying the precision level desired. For example, one might require that the proportion be estimated within a margin of error of $\pm 4\%$ (Scheaffer *et al.*, 1990). This requirement sets the width of the confidence interval estimate of π, because the 4% desired margin of error bound implies that:

$$0.04 = 1.96 \ s.e.(p)$$

where the 1.96 corresponds to the z value for a 95% confidence interval. After squaring both sides this becomes:

$$0.0016 = 3.84\pi(1-\pi)/n$$

or

$$n = [3.84/0.0016]\pi(1-\pi)$$
$$= 2400\pi(1-\pi) \leqslant 2400(0.25) = 600$$

since, even though the quantity π is unknown, it is easily shown that the quantity $\pi(1-\pi) \leqslant 0.25$ for all values of π. Therefore, a sample size of 600 will ensure that the margin of error does not exceed $\pm 4\%$. This is a conservative estimate in that it will suffice for any value of π. If one has prior or supplemental information regarding possible values for π (suppose one knows π cannot be larger than 25% for this aged

population), then the maximum for the quantity $\pi(1-\pi)$ can be refined to be

$$\pi(1-\pi) = 0.25(0.75) = 0.1875$$

and a sample of $n = 2400 \ (0.1875) = 450$ will suffice. (It is implicitly assumed here that the respondents tell the truth regarding smokeless tobacco use. If one suspects that this will not occur, there are other techniques for gathering such sensitive information. The randomized response methodology can be used, but this methodology will require larger numbers of subjects to achieve the same precision of the estimator.) It should be noted that in these examples the sample sizes reflect the number of persons from whom data are obtained, and do not account for possible non-response rates that could occur in the actual study. If one anticipated a 15% non-response rate then the number of 12–16-year-olds that should be sampled would be larger than 600. In fact, one would inflate the calculated number of subjects to be sampled (n) by selecting N, where

$$N = \frac{n}{1 - NR} = \frac{600}{0.85} = 706$$

Here NR represents the proportion of non-response in sampled population.

Continuous responses

For a continuous variable one would be interested in estimating the true mean value, call it μ, for the population. Here the variable is assumed to have mean μ and variance σ^2 in the population. Let $\bar{x}$ and s represent the sample mean and standard deviation for a random sample of n persons. Under general conditions the sample mean $\bar{x}$ has optimal properties, with $E(\bar{x}) = \mu$ and $var(\bar{x}) = \sigma^2/n$. The associated $100(1-\alpha)\%$ confidence interval for μ is given by:

$$[\bar{x} - t_{\alpha/2}s/\sqrt{n}, \ \bar{x} + t_{\alpha/2}s/\sqrt{n}]$$

where $t_{\alpha/2}$ represents the value of a t-statistic with $(n-1)$ df. If one requires the estimate of μ to have a margin of error of $\pm d$ units, then the width of the confidence interval can be no larger than $2d$ units. This means that:

$$d = t_{\alpha/2}\frac{s}{\sqrt{n}}$$

A little algebra produces the following result for n,

$$n = [t_{\alpha/2} s/d]^2$$

To solve this equation for n can be more difficult. One can assume that the sample size needed is large enough to assume the t-statistic is $t_{\alpha/2} = 2.0$, and can specify a value for d, but one would need to have an estimate of s. Sometimes an estimate is available from a previous study or other published sources. For example, if one wished to estimate the mean number of restorations in 12-year-olds for a specific population with an error rate of ± 0.5 surfaces, many published data exist regarding decayed, missing, filled (DMF) surface scores for 12-year-olds. Assuming an estimate were $s = 3.0$ surfaces, one obtains:

$$n = [t_{\alpha/2} s/d]^2 = [(2.0) \cdot 3.0/0.5]^2 \approx (12)^2 = 144$$

But often a good estimate s is not available. One alternative would be to use a crude estimator such as $s = \text{range}/4$, where the range is the range of values for x in the population. One could also specify d in terms of the true standard deviation σ. That is, write $d = c\sigma$, for some c. Then:

$$n = [z_{\alpha/2} \sigma/c\sigma]^2 = [z_{\alpha/2} 1/c]^2$$

and after a value for c is specified, no estimate for the standard deviation is needed to determine n. Suppose one required that the estimate of μ be within $\pm 0.1\sigma$, making the total width of the interval no larger than $0.2\sigma [d = 0.1\sigma]$. Here $c = 0.1$. Then the formula above for n becomes:

$$n = [z_{\alpha/2} 1/0.1]^2 = 100(3.84) = 384$$

for $z_{\alpha/2} = 1.96$. Note here that the actual magnitude of $d = c\sigma$ can vary considerably because it is a function of the standard deviation σ. Again the actual number of subjects who need to be recruited would be larger depending on the expected magnitude of non-response, as before.

For making statistical comparisons (hypothesis testing)

Categorical responses

Suppose one were to study the effects of repeated ingestion of fluoride dentifrice by small children residing in a non-fluoridated community on the levels of dental fluorosis in these subjects. Let us assume there is a group of 10–12-year-old children who are known to have ingested small amounts of fluoride dentifrice repeatedly as small children. Can one design a study in which an increase of 10% or more in the prevalence of dental fluorosis, if present, is demonstrated? The needed sample size for a comparative study can be given by the following formula (Fleiss, 1981; Selvin, 1989);

$$n \geqslant \left[\frac{z_{\alpha/2} \sqrt{2\pi(1-\pi)} - z_{1-\beta} \sqrt{\pi_c(1-\pi_c) + \pi_t(1-\pi_t)}}{\Delta} \right]^2$$

where π is the value for the common proportion under the null hypothesis of no difference in groups, π_c and π_t are the proportions in the control and treatment groups, respectively, and $\Delta = |\pi_c - \pi_t|$ is the minimum value for a difference in the proportions worth detecting. The value for α is usually taken as 0.05, and represents the false-positive rate. The false-negative rate, denoted by β, is often set at 0.10 or 0.20.

To illustrate the process, suppose there are a sufficient number of children who were exposed (ingested dentifrice) and unexposed (did not ingest dentifrice) available in a non-fluoridated community. To determine an appropriate sample size of exposed and unexposed subjects to study, one needs to specify values for the five parameters in the formula. It will be assumed that the fluorosis diagnoses will be assessed by Dean's index. Under normal conditions for a non-fluoridated community it is expected that 20% of the 10–12-year-old children will have some fluorosis ($\pi_c = 0.20$). The size of the increase in fluorosis prevalence considered as important is given as 10% ($\Delta = 0.10$). This also determines $\pi_t = 0.30$, because $\pi_t = \Delta + \pi_c$, reflecting the prevalence in the exposed group (ingested fluoride dentifrice). Let us assume that the comparison will be made at the 5% level, $\alpha = 0.05$. The probability of failing to detect a 10% increase in fluorosis, if it occurs, will be set at 20%. A 20% false-negative rate ($\beta = 0.20$) implies $1 - \beta = 0.80$. Correct interpretation of this means that if several studies were conducted with this sample size, 80% of the time an actual 10% or greater increase in fluorosis would be correctly identified.

The calculations can now be performed by substitution into the formula:

$$n \geqslant \left[\frac{z_{\alpha/2} \sqrt{2\pi(1-\pi)} - z_{1-\beta} \sqrt{\pi_c(1-\pi_c) + \pi_t(1-\pi_t)}}{\Delta} \right]^2$$

$$= \frac{1.96\sqrt{2(0.20)(0.80)} - }{\left[\frac{(-0.842)\sqrt{(0.20)(0.80)+(0.30)(0.70)}}{0.10} \right]^2}$$

$$= \left[\frac{1.96(0.566)+0.842(0.608)}{0.10} \right]^2 = \left[\frac{1.6213}{0.10} \right]^2 = 262$$

Thus, roughly 260 subjects per group would be needed. The calculations seem tedious, but the process is illustrated to reinforce the importance of understanding all aspects of the study design. Many statistical textbooks and software programs are available to perform the needed calculations. Again one ought to recruit more subjects to accommodate any anticipated attrition by using the formula:

$$N = \frac{n}{1 - NR}$$

Here NR represents the proportion of non-response in sampled population.

Continuous responses

The two independent sample t-test will be used to illustrate the procedure for sample size determination. Suppose one wished to compare the caries incidence scores in a randomized 3-year clinical trial for 12-year-olds who regularly brush their teeth twice a day with a 1000 p.p.m. NaF dentifrice with those who regularly brush with a 500 p.p.m. NaF dentifrice. It is expected that the mean 3-year caries incidence will be about 3 DMF surfaces with a standard deviation of 3 DMF surfaces. How many subjects would have to be included in the trial to ensure that a difference of 0.5 DMF surfaces would be correctly identified 80% of the time?

The formula for sample size determination for the two independent sample t-test is given by:

$$n \geqslant 2 \frac{s^2(t_{\alpha/2}-t_{1-\beta})^2}{\Delta^2}$$

The problem here is that the $t_{\alpha/2}$ and $t_{1-\beta}$ values depend on n as well. One can solve for n iteratively by substituting and resolving. However, if one writes the formula as:

$$C(n, \alpha, \beta) = \frac{(t_{\alpha/2}-t_{1-\beta})^2}{n} \leqslant \frac{\Delta^2}{2s^2}$$

only the left-hand side depends on n. Tables for $C(n, \alpha, \beta)$ can easily be derived (Kingman,

Table 9.1 Selected values for the function $C(n, \alpha, \beta)$: two-tailed test

	$\alpha = 0.05$				
n	*0.50*	*0.60*	*0.70*	*0.80*	*0.90*
50	0.0808	0.1026	0.1288	0.1635	0.2191
100	0.0394	0.0501	0.0631	0.0801	0.1073
150	0.0260	0.0331	0.0417	0.0530	0.0710
200	0.0194	0.0247	0.0311	0.0396	0.0530
250	0.0155	0.0197	0.0249	0.0316	0.0423
300	0.0129	0.0164	0.0207	0.0263	0.0352
350	0.0110	0.0140	0.0177	0.0225	0.0301
400	0.0096	0.0123	0.0155	0.0197	0.0263
450	0.0085	0.0109	0.0137	0.0175	0.0234
500	0.0077	0.0098	0.0124	0.0157	0.0211
550	0.0070	0.0089	0.0112	0.0143	0.0191
600	0.0064	0.0081	0.0103	0.0131	0.0175

1978) or simple software can be generated to assist the investigator in obtaining the needed values for n. In Table 9.1 a partial listing for the quantity $C(n, \alpha, \beta)$ for the two-tailed test procedure is produced to illustrate the process. In our example the usual value for $\alpha = 0.05$ will be assumed. The clinical difference worth detecting, denoted by Δ, is 0.5 DMF surfaces. The estimate of the variation in caries incidences is given as 3.0 DMF surfaces. The right-hand side of equation is then $\Delta^2/2s^2(0.5)^2/2(3.0)^2 = 0.25/18 = 0.0139$. From Table 9.1, reading down in the 80% column, the value 0.0139 falls between those corresponding to $n = 550$ and $n = 600$. Interpolation shows value for $n \approx 570$ will suffice. The interpretation is that for the vast majority of clinical trials (80%), comparing a 500 p.p.m. NaF with a 1000 p.p.m. NaF dentifrice with 570 subjects per group, a difference in caries incidence of 0.5 surfaces or greater will be detected, if it were present under the conditions assumed for the study population. *Reminder*: 570 is the group size that would be needed at the end of the study, not the beginning. Any attrition would have to be compensated for by inflating the original number of subjects recruited for the study. Attrition rates in longitudinal studies can be substantial, often ranging between 5 and 15% per year.

Analysis issues

Types of data and distribution considerations

There are two basic types of data–discrete or categorical, and continuous or count data. Two subclasses within the discrete types of data are worth distinguishing–nominally and ordinally scaled data. In the continuous class two types are commonly identified as well–interval and ratio-scaled variables. Count data such as the number of natural teeth or the number of gingival sites with bleeding within a subject can be viewed either as discrete or continuous, but usually are analysed as continuous data.

Nominally scaled data have unrelated discrete classes, which have no natural rank order among them. The location of a cancerous or precancerous lesion within the oral cavity is a nominally scaled variable. Summary measures for this type of data include frequencies, percentages and ratios of frequencies or percentages. In contrast, an ordinally scaled variable possesses a natural ordering. Variables such as size of a cancerous lesion or a staging of an oral cancer would be ordinally scaled variables. Summary measures for such data would include not only frequencies or percentages, but would now include ranks within the sample, medians, percentiles or other statistics based on ranks.

For continuous-type data one usually has a unit of measure. Differences in scores can be computed, and differences of the same size represent similar differences in the variable being assessed. It may be a concentration ($\mu g/l$), measure of heat ($^\circ C$), or the percentage of sites with bleeding. One could even have a unit-free measure, such as the ratio of two scores. The strongest level of measurement is a ratioscaled variable. These variables have a true zero, meaning that a 0 represents the absence of the condition being measured. In clinical research the zero may be a true zero or something which 'behaves like' zero, in the sense of being too small to be detectable. Chemical concentrations below the threshold of detection are examples. For continuous variables one can use the mean or median as a measure of the centre of the data, and the range, standard deviation or coefficient of variation as a measure of variability. Ratios of two means, ratios of two variances, or of a standard deviation to a mean (coefficient of variation) are other possible summary measures.

In dental research multiple measurements for each subject are made at any clinical examination. This introduces a complex dependent data structure into the database due to the correlations of observations made within the same subject. One method of reducing this complexity is to compute subject-based summary measures. For example, in a coronal caries examination 128 measurements are made per subject (excluding third molars). A nominally scaled variable is scored for each site, i.e. the surface is diagnosed as sound, carious, filled or missing (to keep it simple). This scale is partially ordered in the sense that anything but a sound call represents some evidence of disease, and thus could be considered as ordered. However, a 'natural' ordering for the D, F and M categories is probably not that 'natural'. One commonly used subject-based summary measure is the number of carious, filled and missing surfaces for the subject, otherwise known as the DMFS index. This variable is a count variable and behaves more like a continuous variable than discrete. Thus a blurring between the types of measurements can easily occur merely by this common transformation. Another summary measure is the trivariate subject-based summary measure V = (DS, FS, MS), indicating the vector of total carious, filled and missing surfaces, separately. A subject with a V = (3, 8, 4) would have a DMFS score = 15.

A popular index of gingival inflammation is the Löe–Silness index (Löe and Silness, 1963). This index has four values: 0, 1, 2 and 3, representing no inflammation, mild inflammation, bleeding with pressure and spontaneous bleeding. Gingival inflammation is sometimes assessed at two sites per tooth, again producing multiple measurements per subject. This is clearly an ordinally scaled variable measured at each site. The mean gingival inflammation score for all sites and the percentage of sites with bleeding are two commonly reported subject-based summary measures. In each instance one transforms an ordinally scaled variable into a continuous variable.

The converse can also occur. One may measure *Streptococcus mutans* in colony-forming units (CFU) per millilitre, but then collapse the scale by reporting persons having 10^6 or more CFU. Much information is discarded when this is done, but sometimes the percentage of subjects with concentrations of 10^6 or larger is the focus of that specific analysis. In this case a continuous-type measurement is transformed into a dichotomous one. Thus, the scale of measurement can become blurred during different phases of the study. However, the distinction should be understood because it is directly related to the choice of statistical methods appropriate for the data under study.

Analytic considerations may also affect the choice of scale of measurement. One might directly measure the number of CFUs of *S. mutans*. However, analytical comparisons between groups are usually based on the log counts rather than the CFUs themselves. Statistical issues are involved in making a decision as to whether the statistical analyses should be performed on data measured on the original scale or after a logarithmic, square root, logit or rank transformation is made.

A decision must also be made regarding whether treatment group comparisons will be based on differences in means or on the ratio of means. In a caries clinical trial will the focus be on the mean number of DMF surfaces saved $(\bar{x}_C - \bar{x}_T)$ by using test product T compared to a control product C, or on the percentage reduction $(\bar{x}_C - \bar{x}_T)/\bar{x}_C$ in new disease (DMFS) of T relative to C?

Reliability of measurement

An important consideration in all research is to use variables which are valid and reliable. Validity of measurement is difficult to demonstrate. One needs to have a gold standard which can serve as the true value to establish validity. Reliability determinations can sometimes be used to assess validity but more often they are used to assess the reproducibility of the measurement. A reliable measurement may not be valid. For instance, a laboratory measuring device may systematically underestimate a chemical concentration by 10%, but do this consistently. This instrument may be very reliable because it produces virtually identical readings on repeated evaluations of a sample, but they are biased, and therefore are not valid.

Reliability is extremely important when assessing medical or dental conditions or disease, or laboratory assays for concentrations of a substance in specific body fluids or tissues. The investigator has the responsibility of demonstrating that all clinical or laboratory data analysed are reliable. In a dental caries study the ability of the clinical examiners to score the disease should be documented. Procedures for evaluation of the reliability of two examiners for scoring caries in children (continuous response) and gingival inflammation in adolescents (categorical response) will be presented and discussed here.

Continuous responses

The criteria for dental caries that will be employed are studied and discussed among the examiners who will be participating in the study. Experienced examiners may require less time to review the criteria. A sample of children (usually between 20 and 35 subjects will be sufficient) is selected whose ages represent those for the population to be investigated (10–12-year-old group is used here). For simplicity we will assume 10 children are examined by two investigators. Each examiner is scheduled to examine the 10 test subjects for dental caries. This must be done independently so that one examiner is not aware of how the other examiner is scoring or has scored individual subjects. The data for each examiner are recorded and put on a disk or file and checked for obvious coding errors. Next the DS, FS, MS, DFS and DMFS totals are calculated for each subject as scored by each examiner. Ideally each examiner should produce the same set of scores. However, slight variations in the application of the criteria to individual situations will inevitably result in disparate scores, even among experienced examiners.

In Table 9.2 hypothetical caries scores made by two examiners for 10 subjects are presented to illustrate the procedure used to evaluate interexaminer reliability. If the reliability of a single examiner were desired, that examiner would make repeated caries assessments for the test subjects. The resulting reliability would be termed intraexaminer reliability. Only the interexaminer procedure will be presented here. Slight differences in scores between examiners

Table 9.2 Hypothetical data for 10 subjects

Subject	Age (years)	Examiner 1 DS	FS	MS	Examiner 2 DS	FS	MS
1	11	2	8	0	1	8	0
2	10	0	2	0	0	2	0
3	11	0	0	0	0	0	0
4	12	0	0	0	1	0	0
5	10	4	6	0	5	5	0
6	12	2	3	0	0	3	0
7	11	0	0	0	0	0	0
8	12	1	0	0	2	0	0
9	10	2	4	0	1	4	0
10	11	3	5	0	0	4	0
Mean	11	1.4	2.8	0	1.0	2.6	0

DS = Decayed surface; FS = filled surface; MS = missing surface.

for specific subjects are evident from Table 9.2, but on average the DS, FS and MS means are similar. How different can they be and still consider the examiners reliable? One could check for significant differences in mean caries scores for these examiners by using a paired *t*-test. However, examiner differences can often be statistically significant, but clinically trivial. A better measure of the difference is to compute a correlation between these scores, called the intraclass correlation coefficient. The exact form of the intraclass correlation coefficient will depend on the design of the study. This correlation coefficient assesses the relative importance of the variation between examiners as a function of the variation among subjects. Specifically, we define:

$$\rho = \frac{\sigma_s^2}{\sigma_s^2 + \sigma_x^2 + \sigma_e^2}$$

where σ_s^2 represents the variation among subjects, σ_x^2 variation among examiners, and σ_e^2 the random error. This correlation coefficient is different from the usual Pearson correlation coefficient. The Pearson correlation coefficient is not appropriate to use for reliability purposes, although occasionally its value will closely approximate the intraclass correlation. In this example the Pearson correlation coefficients (r_p) are 0.60, 0.99 and 0.94 for the DS, FS and DFS scores, respectively. The intraclass correlations (r) are estimated by using formula (1) or (2) depending on whether one views these two examiners as the only examiners of interest (fixed) or as representative of examiners scoring dental caries (random). The formulas are (Fleiss *et al.*, 1979, Kingman, 1986):

$$r_f = \frac{MSS - MSE}{MSS + (m-1)MSE}$$

Table 9.3 Analysis of variance table for intraclass correlation example. Model is DMFS = subject + examiner + ε

Source	df	SS	MS	F-value	p-value
Model	10	255.60	25.56	22.55	0.0001
Error	9	10.20	1.13		
				$R^2 = 0.9616$	
Summary of results for model components					
Subjects	9	253.8	28.2	24.88	0.0001
Examiners	1	1.80	1.8	1.59	0.2393

df = degrees of freedom; *SS* = sum of squares; *MS* = mean square.
MSS = 28.2, MSX = 1.8, MSE = 1.13.
$r_{fixed} = (28.1 - 1.13)/(28.1 + 1.13) = 0.923$.
$r_{random} = 10(28.2 - 1.13)/[10(28.2) + 2(1.8) + (10(2) - 10 - 2)1.13] = 0.919$.
See text for details.

Table 9.4 Reliability assessed by κ statistic

Examiner 1/2	0	1	2	3	Total
0	40	10	1	0	51
1	15	15	3	0	33
2	0	4	7	2	13
3	0	0	1	2	3
Total (2)	55	29	12	4	100

Observed agreement = 0.64; expected agreement = 0.393; unweighted κ = 0.407.

for examiners considered as a fixed effect, and

$$r_r = \frac{n(MSS - MSE)}{nMSS + mMSX + (nm - n - m)MSE}$$

for examiners considered to be random. Here *n* represents the number of subjects, *m* the number of examiners, MSS, MSX and MSE the mean squares for subjects, examiners and error, respectively. The corresponding analysis of variance is presented in Table 9.3. It is easily shown that the corresponding reliabilities are 0.60, 0.99 and 0.92 for DS, FS and DFS scores, respectively when examiners are random; and 0.59, 0.99 and 0.92 for examiners as fixed (see the section on analysis of variance methods later in this chapter for a more complete discussion).

Categorical responses

For categorical outcomes the κ statistics are often used to evaluate examiner reliability. In Table 9.4 hypothetical gingival inflammation scores for 100 sites examined by two examiners are presented. The frequencies for the diagonal cells represent sites for which the examiners agreed. The total percentage observed agreement was 64%. However, some of this agreement can be attributed to chance agreement, given that the examiners both found that inflammation was present for 45–50% of the sites. The scores for proficient examiners should agree on substantially more of the sites than would be expected by chance. The κ statistics provide one method for adjusting for chance agreement and assessing the reliability of these examiners (Fleiss, 1981; Kingman, 1986; Dunn, 1989). The unweighted κ is

$$\kappa = \frac{p_o - p_e}{1 - p_e}$$

where p_o represents the proportion of observed agreement, and p_e represents the proportion of expected agreement. They are computed by using:

$$p_o = \Sigma p_{ii} = 0.40 + 0.15 + 0.07 + 0.02 = 0.64$$

where p_{ii} are the ith diagonal cell entries, and

$$p_e = \Sigma p_{iT} p_{Ti}/n$$
$$= 0.2805 + 0.0957 + 0.0156 + 0.0012 = 0.393$$

where p_{iT} and p_{Ti} are the totals for the ith row and ith column respectively. Then κ becomes

$$\kappa = \frac{0.64 - 0.393}{1 - 0.393} = \frac{0.247}{0.607} = 0.407$$

This value of κ represents a modest level of agreement. It is clear from the table that the examiners have difficulty in making the distinction between 0 and 1 scores, although here the net effect on the prevalence is minimal. The disagreement here follows a random pattern. One would like to see κ values of 0.70 or higher. Weighted κ can also be calculated to diagnose examiner disagreement, identifying what parts of the scale are the most difficult to distinguish. The weighted κ use weights assigned to each cell frequency. These weights can be viewed as assigning full credit to real agreements and partial credit to examiner disagreements which are relatively minor (Kingman, 1986).

Common statistical models

Continuous responses

Analysis of variance methods

These models generally focus on relationships among categorical explanatory variables and the continuous response variable. The Student t-test is probably the most familiar analysis of variance procedure, with one explanatory variable having two levels. For one explanatory variable having more than two levels, it is known as the one-way analysis of variance model. The multiway analysis of variance models are models having more than one discrete explanatory variable. The general purpose of these models is to examine the joint effect of each explanatory variable on the response variable. For multiway analysis of variance models one can derive adjusted group effects given the presence of other discrete variables in the model. A two-way analysis of variance model for caries scores as a function of examiner and subject could be written as:

$$\text{DMFS} = \mu + \text{Subject} + \text{Examiner} + \varepsilon$$

In Table 9.3 the analytical results for the DMFS scores are presented for the examiner reliability study involving two examiners and 10 subjects, as mentioned previously. The purpose of this study was to evaluate how well these examiners could score caries. The interpretation of the findings given for the model line indicates that the joint effect of subjects and examiners was significant, with 96% of the variance in caries scores explained by differences among subjects and examiners. However, an inspection of the lower portion of the table presents the findings for each effect separately. The small p-value associated with the subjects effect merely indicates that the 10 subjects participating in this study had different caries scores. The mean caries scores for the two examiners are presented in the last line of Table 9.2. The test statistic for examiners can be used to test for examiner bias. The associated p-value = 0.2393 suggests no indication of examiner bias present. The mean squares MSS, MSX and MSE for subjects, examiners and error can be obtained from Table 9.3. They are 28.2, 1.80 and 1.13 and produce the intraclass correlation coefficients 0.918 for examiners considered as a random effect and 0.922 for examiners considered as a fixed effect. The procedure PROC GLM in SAS (Version 6.08) was used to run this analysis.

Linear regression models

Continuous oral health outcomes can often be modelled by regression models, as described in Chapter 5. The standard form for three explanatory variables is given by:

$$Y_i = \beta_0 + \beta_1 X_{1i} + \beta_2 X_{2i} + \beta_3 X_{3i} + \varepsilon_i$$

where Y is the response variable, and X_1 and X_2 are the explanatory variates, and ε_i is the random error associated with Y. We will rewrite this model as

$$E(Y|X\text{'s}) = \beta_0 + \beta_1 X_{1i} + \beta_2 X_{2i} + \beta_3 X_{3i}$$

Almost all statistical software packages have a multiple regression program which can be used to obtain estimates for the unknown parameters, their standard errors, tests for significance of each effect in the model and various options which can be used to assess the fit of the

Table 9.5 Regression analysis table for tooth loss example. Model is TL $= A + E + G + \varepsilon$

Source	df	SS	MS	F-value	p-value
Model	3	4.01	1.34	2.93	0.0375
Error	96	43.81	0.46		
			$R^2 = 0.7300$		

Summary of results for model components

Variable	df	Estimate	std error	t-value	p-value
Intercept	1	-2.00	5.55	-0.36	0.7202
Age	1	0.397	0.05	7.58	0.0001
Education	1	-0.67	0.35	-1.92	0.0625
Gender	1	-0.32	1.03	-0.31	0.7577

model. Confidence intervals for effect estimates can be derived from the output provided. Some packages provide confidence intervals for the model parameters explicitly. One measure of fit of the model routinely provided is the R^2 statistic, which measures what percentage of the total variation in the data can be explained by the explanatory variables collectively. Many other measures of goodness of fit are optional in some packages, and many regression diagnostics are also available (SAS/STAT 1989, BMDP 1990, SPSS, 1990).

Often one of the explanatory variables, say X_1, represents the exposure variable, or the primary variable of interest, and the other variables X_2 and X_3 (and others when appropriate) are covariates or confounders which are to be controlled for, prior to estimating the association between Y and X_1. Legitimate confounders are variables which are associated with the response variable Y and with the exposure variable X_1. The value for the regression coefficient of the exposure variable in the model with the confounding factors included should be substantially different from its value without the confounders included. A more detailed discussion of these methods can be found in almost all statistical texts (see Kleinbaum *et al.*, 1988 for an excellent description of these methods).

In Table 9.5 the output from PROC REG in SAS (version 6.08) is presented for a hypothetical sample of 42 adults, ranging in age from 30 to 65. The response variable is the number of teeth lost to disease, investigated here as a function of age, number of years of formal education and gender. The R^2 value for this model is 0.73,

indicating that 73% of the variation in tooth loss is explained by the three factors in the model. The regression coefficient corresponding to education is marginally significant ($\beta = -0.67$) and that of age ($\beta = 0.397$) significant. The interpretation of the education coefficient is that, on average, for each additional year of formal education, subjects have 0.67 more teeth. The $\beta = 0.397$ value for age is the average additional loss of teeth projected per year increase in age. The coefficient for gender (not significant) indicates that for any specification of level of age and formal education, females have on average 0.32 more teeth than males (a consequence of the coding scheme: males $= 0$, females $= 1$). The decision as to whether to retain gender in the model can be investigated by fitting the model with gender removed. If this were done, one obtains new regression coefficients for age, ($\beta = -0.69$) and education ($\beta = 0.39$). These are essentially the same as those obtained by the model in which gender was included. Thus, gender would not be considered a confounder here. Whether it is retained or dropped from the model may also depend on other considerations.

Categorical responses

Chi-square (χ^2) methods

For studying associations among categorical variables, ordered or unordered, data are often displayed in two-way or higher-way tables. In Table 9.6 the frequencies of subjects in a gingivitis study are presented by presence or absence of gingival bleeding and the average oral hygiene intensity practised by the subject. Inspection of Table 9.6 suggests that the percentage of bleeding versus no bleeding is not constant across levels of oral hygiene. The χ^2 test is routinely used to test whether the percentage of bleeding is constant across levels of oral hygiene. The computed $\chi^2 = 9.55$, with an

Table 9.6 Frequency of gingival bleeding and oral hygiene intensity

Oral hygiene	Bleeding absent	Bleeding present	Total
Rarely	5 (35.7)	9 (64.3)	14
Occasionally	11 (47.8)	12 (52.2)	23
Once a day	20 (64.5)	11 (35.5)	31
Twice a day	25 (78.1)	7 (21.9)	32
Total	61	39	100

associated $p=0.0228$, based on a χ^2 with 3 df. For an $r \times c$ the χ^2 test for testing the independence of two factors has $(r-1) \times (c-1)$ df. However, the oral hygiene variable is an ordinally scaled variable. Given that the proportions of subjects with bleeding gums are different, one could ask whether there is a trend in the prevalence of bleeding gums as a function of the intensity of oral hygiene. The χ^2 test for linear trend can be used to investigate a linear trend in these proportions (Rosner, 1986). The $\chi^2 = 9.42$ for 6 has 1 df, with an associated $p=0.0021$. The evidence of a decreasing trend in the prevalence of bleeding as the intensity of oral hygiene increases is strong.

The odds ratio is a popular statistic to use for assessing association between categorical variables. Suppose one again considers the data presented in Table 9.6. The percentage of subjects with gingival bleeding was 64.3% for the rarely practised category, whereas the percentage was 21.9% for the twice-a-day group. The odds of gingival bleeding for a category is given as the percentage with bleeding divided by the percentage without bleeding. Thus the odds are 64.3/35.7% = 1.80, or 9 to 5 for the rarely category. Similarly the odds are 21.9/70.1% = 0.28, or 7 to 25 for the twice-a-day category. The odds ratio of bleeding in the rarely category compared to the odds for bleeding in the twice-a-day category is defined as the ratio of their respective odds. Thus, the odds ratio (OR) becomes:

$$OR = \frac{9/5}{7/25} = [9(25)]/[7(5)] = 6.43$$

The odds ratios for each category compared with the twice-a-day category are $OR_1 = 6.43$, $OR_2 = 3.90$, and $OR_3 = 1.96$, respectively. The interpretation is that the odds of bleeding are about 6.4, 3.9 and 1.96 times as great for a person who brushes rarely, occasionally or once a day compared with a person who brushes twice a day. The standard error of the log (OR) for the brushes rarely versus twice a day is approximately:

$$\text{s.e.}(\log(OR)) = \sqrt{\frac{1}{a}+\frac{1}{b}+\frac{1}{c}+\frac{1}{d}} = \sqrt{\frac{1}{5}+\frac{1}{9}+\frac{1}{25}+\frac{1}{7}}$$

$$= 0.70$$

A 95% confidence interval for the OR is derived by computing the 95% confidence interval for the log(OR), using $[\log(OR)-1.96$ s.e.$(\log(OR))$, $\log(OR)+1.96$ s.e.$(\log(OR))]$ and then exponentiating these end-points to obtain the 95% confidence interval for the odds ratio. The log(OR) for the brushes rarely versus twice-a-day comparison was 6.43. We obtain

$$CI[\log(OR)] = [1.86 - 1.96(0.70), 1.86 + 1.96(0.70)]$$

$$= [0.49, 3.23]$$

as the confidence interval for the log(OR). After exponentiating these values we obtain [1.63, 25.3] for the confidence interval for the OR.

The Mantel–Haenszel test procedure is another alternative for categorical data. The original Mantel–Haenszel test was derived for the purpose of comparing odds ratios from several 2×2 tables, where the individual tables presented results for different levels of possible confounding variables. Later they extended it to include the $2 \times k$ table, where a mean response for the ordinal variable was derived based on specific weights assigned to the k categories (Selvin, 1991). The analysis of odds ratios for an exposure variable in the presence of several confounders can also be performed by logistic regression models.

Further oral health examples using these methods are described in Chapter 5. Many other procedures are available for analysing ordinal categorical data. These would include ridit analysis, rank sum test (i.e. Wilcoxon–Mann–Whitney), cumulative logit models, and the proportional hazards model (Agresti, 1984).

Logistic regression models

For categorical responses logistic models are frequently used. They are flexible and can accommodate both categorical and continuous explanatory variables. They can be fitted to data derived from case-control, cross-sectional and prospective studies. Estimates of odds ratios are easily derived from these models. Furthermore, if the prevalence of the disease is small, the odds ratio can also be used to estimate the relative risks of developing the disease in a case-control study. The dichotomous response case will be briefly discussed here. Multilevel discrete outcome variables can often be fitted with polychotomous logistic models (Hosmer and Lemeshow, 1989). Many software packages contain a logistic regression procedure. It will be assumed here that the value $Y=1$ represents disease (or the presence of the condition of interest) and the $Y=0$ represents no disease (absence of the condition of interest). Some care must be used since two different coding schemes are used for the design variables. The reference cell method codes the dichotomous X_1 variable using 0 (unexposed) and 1 (exposed). The deviation from means method codes the X_1 variable using the values -1 (unexposed) and 1 (exposed). The logistic model is given by:

$$E(Y|X's) = \frac{e^{\beta_0 + \beta_1 X_1 + \beta_2 X_2 + \beta_3 X_3}}{1 + e^{\beta_0 + \beta_1 X_1 + \beta_2 X_2 + \beta_3 X_3}}$$

Rather than model Y directly, the logit transformation of Y is taken, here given as

$$logit[E(Y|X's)] = \log \frac{E(Y|X's)}{1 - E(Y|X's)}$$
$$= \beta_0 + \beta_1 X_1 + \beta_2 X_2 + \beta_3 X_3$$

and the explanatory part of the model becomes identical to the linear regression model given previously. The maximum likelihood method used to fit the logistic model requires an iterative computational process to obtain estimates of model parameters. The resulting β estimates and their standard errors are computed by the software programs. If reference coding is used for the exposure variable X_1, its β coefficient is easily interpreted. The quantity e^β for the variable X_1 represents the odds ratio of disease for the exposed compared to non-exposed. If one is using the deviation from means coding the odds ratio for X_1 is represented by 2β, not β. In this case the standard error of the odds ratio would be 2 [s.e.(β)], which will also affect the limits of the confidence interval for the odds ratio.

In Tables 9.7 and 9.8 the results are presented for a hypothetical case-control study of the risks of smoking and alcohol consumption on the development of oral cancer. Smoking experience was dichotomized and coded as 0 for non-smoker and 1 for a smoker; alcohol consumption was also coded as 0 for a non-drinker and 1 for a drinker. In Table 9.7(a) the raw data are presented together with the crude odds ratios and the univariate analyses for smokers, alcohol consumers and subjects exposed to both factors separately. The crude odds ratios are derived in Table 9.7(b) as 1.64 for smoking and 1.80 for alcohol consumption. These odds ratios ignore the status of the other risk factor under study. The effect of single or joint exposure to smoking and alcohol consumption was next evaluated. In

Table 9.7(c) the odds ratios for a single exposure and joint exposure compared with neither exposure are derived. These odds ratios were found to be 1.46, 1.49 and 3.11 for smoking only, alcohol only and for both smoking and alcohol, respectively. If they were additive on the logit scale, the separate odds ratio scale would be multiplicative. Thus, the expected odds ratio for joint exposure would be $OR_{SA} = OR_S \times OR_A = 1.46 \times 1.49 = 2.18$. This value is

Table 9.7 Distribution of oral cancer by smoking and alcohol status

(a) Data

	Disease present		Disease absent	
Exposure	Alcohol		Alcohol	
Smoking	Yes	No	Yes	No
Yes	78	124	36	122
No	52	106	50	152
Total	130	230	86	274

(b) Crude odds ratios

Exposure	Smoking		Alcohol	
Disease	Yes	No	Yes	No
Yes	202	158	130	230
No	158	202	86	274
OR	1.64		1.80	

(c) Summary of odds ratios for different exposures compared with neither smoking nor alcohol exposure

Disease	Smoke only		Alcohol only		Both	
	Yes	No	Yes	No	Yes	No
Yes	124	106	52	106	78	106
No	122	152	50	152	36	152
OR	1.46		1.49		3.11	

OR = Odds ratio.

Table 9.8 Logistic regression analysis table for oral cancer example. Model is logit $E(y)$ = Smoker + Alcohol

Source	df	β	s.e.	Wald χ^2	p-value
Summary of results for the multiplicative model					
Intercept	1	-0.4120	0.1175	12.29	0.0005
Smoker	1	0.4805	0.1515	10.06	0.0015
Alcohol	1	0.5774	0.1664	12.04	0.0005
Summary of results for the synergistic model					
Intercept	1	-0.3604	0.1265	8.11	0.0044
Smoker (S)	1	0.3767	0.1797	4.40	0.0360
Alcohol (A)	1	0.3997	0.2350	2.89	0.0891
S × A	1	0.3573	0.3348	1.14	0.2859

somewhat less than the observed value of 3.11. A statistical model having an interaction term included can be used to compute a significance test for a synergistic effect between smoking and alcohol consumption. The results for fitting the synergistic and additive models to the logits are presented in Table 9.8.

These logistic regression models can be used to interpret the associations for each risk factor separately, as well as jointly. The non-significance of the interaction effect in the synergistic model suggests that the difference between the 3.11 observed and 2.18 predicted odds ratio for joint exposure are explained by chance differences. Analytically this can be seen by focusing on the $\beta = 0.3573$ for interaction. If one computes $OR_\alpha/OR_e = 3.11/2.18 = 1.43$, and then takes its log, one obtains the value 0.357, given in Table 9.8. Thus the interaction is a comparison of the observed odds ratio for joint exposure with the expected odds ratio under a multiplicative model. If the test for interaction had been significant then the effect of smoking would have had to be estimated separately for each level of alcohol consumption. Since the effect is not significant we can eliminate that effect and fit the reduced model, labelled the multiplicative model.

The estimates for the odds ratios of smoking and alcohol consumption are now 1.62 and 1.78, respectively. The confidence intervals for these odds ratios can be derived by computing the limits $[\beta - 1.96 \text{ s.e.}(\beta), \beta + 1.96 \text{ s.e.}(\beta)]$ from 8. Then these limits are exponentiated to obtain limits on the odds ratio scale. The confidence interval for the log odds ratio for smoking is given as [0.1836, 0.7774], which becomes [1.20, 2.18] for the odds ratio itself. This odds ratio for smoking represents the effect of smoking given the distribution of alcohol consumption present in this population. Similarly the confidence interval of the log odds ratio for alcohol can be derived as [0.2512, 0.9035], which produces the interval [1.19, 2.45] for alcohol consumption.

The confidence intervals for the odds ratios when interaction is present are more complex (Kleinbaum, 1994) and will be omitted here.

Point and interval estimation and hypothesis testing–interpretations

The practice of reporting *p*-values from statistical tests has proliferated in the literature. Occasionally this can lead to fallacious interpret-

ation by some researchers deducing clinical importance from statistical significance, while others falsely conclude no association exists when non-significant *p*-values are observed. Although *p*-values can be informative when accompanied by appropriate statistical summaries, the potential for overinterpretation of study findings exists and is commonplace in the literature. The ideal study would be designed in such a manner as to equate statistical significance with clinical importance. This is seldom possible because the degree of knowledge about disease patterns and distributions continues to remain incomplete. Therefore statistically significant findings, even though they represent small clinical differences, will continue to be reported. The ultimate importance of such findings will be decided by the experts in that clinical subject matter area.

It is therefore sound practice to report point and interval estimates in published reports of community health studies. An observed per cent reduction in dental caries attributed to a new dentifrice as compared with an active control dentifrice is insufficient. It should be accompanied by its standard error and a confidence interval. A significance test can sometimes adequately summarize the important findings, but a confidence interval quickly conveys the important study findings. Significance tests can certainly be useful, especially when model-fitting and developing strategies for analysing multivariate databases.

References

Agresti, A. (1984) *Analysis of Ordinal Categorical Data,* John Wiley, New York.

BMDP Users Guide vols 1 and 2 (1990) BMDP Statistical Software, University of California Press, Los Angeles.

Division of Epidemiology & Oral Disease Prevention (DEODP) (1989) *Oral Health of US Children.* NIH publication no. 89-2247.

Dunn, G. (1989) *Design and Analysis of Reliability Studies.* Oxford University Press, New York.

Fleiss, J.L. (1981) *Statistical Methods for Rates and Proportions,* 2nd edn. John Wiley, New York.

Fleiss, J.L. (1986) *Design and Analysis of Clinical Experiments.* John Wiley, New York.

Fleiss, J.L., Slakter, M.J., Fischman, S.L., Park, M.H. and Chilton, N.W. (1979) Interexaminer reliability in caries trials. *Journal of Dental Research* **58**: 604–609.

Hosmer, D.W. and Lemeshow, S. (1989) *Applied Logistic Regression.* John Wiley, New York.

Kingman, A. (1978) Adequate cohort sizes for caries

clinical trials. *Community Dental and Oral Epidemiology* **6**: 30–35.

Kingman, A. (1986) A procedure for evaluating the reliability of a gingivitis index. *Journal of Clinical Periodontology* **13**: 385–391.

Kleinbaum, D.G. (1994) *Logistic Regression. A Self-learning Text.* Springer-Verlag, New York.

Kleinbaum, D.G., Kupper, L. and Muller, K.E. (1988) *Applied Regression Analysis and Other Multivariate Methods*, 2nd edn. PWS-Kent, Boston, MA

Löe, H. and Silness, J. (1963) Periodontal disease in pregnancy. I. Prevalence and severity. *Acta Odontologica Scandinavica* **21**: 533–551.

Morton, R.F., Hebel, J.R. and McCarter, R.J. (1989) *A Study Guide topidemiology and Biostatistics.* Aspen Publishers.

National Caries Program, NIDR (1982) *The Prevalence of Dental Caries in US Children, 1979–1980.* NIH publication no. 82-2245, Bethesda, MD.

Rosner, B. (1986) *Fundamentals of Biostatistics*, 2nd edn. Duxbury Press, Boston, MA.

SAS/STAT (1990) Users Guide, vols 1 and 2, 4th edn. SAS Institute, Cary, NC.

Scheaffer, R.L., Mendenhall, W. and Ott, L. (1990) *Elementary Survey Sampling*, 4th edn. PWS-Kent, Boston, MA.

Selvin, S. (1991) *Statistical Analysis of Epidemiologic Data.* Oxford University Press, New York.

SPSS-X (1988) Users Guide, 3rd edn. SPSS, Chicago, ILL.

SYSTAT (1994) Users Guide SPSS, Chicago, ILL.

10

Principles of health economics

B. Alexander White and Alexia Antczak-Bouckoms

Community oral health–an economic perspective

Constrained resources and rising health care costs have heightened awareness of policy-makers, public health officials, employers, insurers, practitioners and consumers regarding the need to ensure that appropriate and cost-effective health care services are available. There is increasing evidence that too many resources are being spent without a commensurate improvement in overall health (Banta and Bekaney, 1981; Fuchs, 1993). Not all programmes provide the same level of health improvement, and there can be substantial variations among these programmes in the economic cost. Quantification and comparison of the costs and health consequences of alternative programmes are critical elements to ensure that individuals and communities are receiving appropriate, effective and cost-effective health services. The purpose of this chapter is to review various methods of assessing these costs and health consequences, including cost minimization, cost–benefit, cost-effectiveness and cost–utility analyses. Steps used in conducting such analyses will be described, and examples of the application of these methods to community oral health programmes will be presented.

Information on economic evaluation of community oral health care programmes should be of interest to individuals, oral health professionals, programme administrators and policy-makers who are faced with decisions regarding allocation of limited health care resources. This chapter is not intended to provide the reader with a detailed discussion of the methods used in such analyses. Rather the potential application of these methods to community health programmes and the strengths and limitations of such information will be described. Readers interested in additional methodological discussion are referred to other texts (Weinstein and Stason, 1977; Drummond, 1980; Weinstein and Fineberg, 1980; Warner and Luce, 1982; Drummond *et al.*, 1987; Sox, 1988; Luce and Elixhauser, 1990; Kamlet, 1992; Petitti, 1994).

Types of economic evaluations

Underlying economic evaluations of health care programmes is the premise that for any given level of resources available, decision-makers seek to maximize the total aggregate health benefits conferred to an individual or a population (Weinstein and Stason, 1977). Alternatively, decision-makers attempt to achieve a specified level of health at the minimum cost. Implicit in this formulation are two points central to economic evaluations. First, both the costs and consequences of the programmes under consideration are quantified and used in the analysis. Without assessing the costs associated with a programme, one cannot determine whether the additional health benefits of one programme relative to another are worth the additional costs. Second, comparisons are made

Are both costs and consequences of the alternatives examined

		NO		YES
		Examines only consequences	Examines only costs	
Is there comparison of two or more alternatives?	NO	**1A PARTIAL EVALUATION 1B** Outcome description	Cost description	**2 PARTIAL EVALUATION** Cost-outcome description
	YES	**3A PARTIAL EVALUATION 3B** Efficacy or effectiverness evaluation	Cost analysis	**4 FULL ECONOMIC EVALUATION** Cost-minimization analysis Cost-effectiveness analysis Cost–utility analysis Cost–benefit analysis

Fig. 10.1 Distinguishing characteristics of economic evaluations of community health care programmes. From Drummond *et al.* (1987), with permission.

between two or more alternative programmes. It is impossible to ascertain whether use of a given level of health resources provides the maximum health benefits to an individual or population without comparisons between and among competing health programmes.

Based on these characteristics, Drummond and colleagues (1987) proposed a scheme for characterizing economic evaluations of health care programmes (Fig. 10.1). When only one programme is being considered, an evaluation is more appropriately referred to as a description of the programme (cells 1A, 1B, and 2) rather than an analysis (cells 3A, 3B and 4). Some evaluations examine only the consequences of alternative programmes (cells 1A and 3A) while others examine only costs (cells 1B and 3B). Evaluations of the type found in cell 1A describe the consequences of a single programme without regard to cost. Cell 3A represents the most common type of studies reported in the literature, namely randomized clinical trials and observational studies of two or more interventions. Cell 1B describes the costs associated with a single programme, while cell 3B describes the costs of two or more alternative programmes. Neither assesses the consequences. Cell 2 describes both the costs and consequences of a single programme. Full economic evaluations are found in cell 4 and are the focus of this chapter.

Cost-minimization analysis

One type of economic evaluation is cost-minimization analysis (Drummond *et al.*, 1987; Eisenberg, 1989). Such analyses identify and compare the costs of alternative health programmes, without explicitly estimating concomitant health consequences. Implicit in this type of analysis is that the health consequences associated with each programme are equivalent. Results of cost-minimization analyses are reported usually as cost per service provided (e.g. cost per sealant placed or cost per fluoride application). For example, such analyses assume that sealants placed by dental auxiliaries and by dentists are equally effective. The goal then is to identify the least expensive strategy to attain the desired outcome. When alternative programmes that yield varying levels of health benefits are being compared, cost-minimization analysis is not a useful methodology. However, other economic assessment approaches, such as cost–benefit analysis, cost-effectiveness analysis and cost–utility analysis, extend the analysis to compare explicitly the costs and health consequences of a health programme.

Cost–benefit analysis

Cost–benefit analysis, and related cost-effectiveness and cost–utility analysis, quantify the costs and health consequences associated with a health care programme. The distinguishing feature of cost–benefit analyses is that monetary values are assigned to both the costs and health consequences. Cost–benefit analysis provides a way to assess whether the benefits are worth the costs since both outcomes are measured in the same units.

Comparisons of the costs and health benefits in a cost–benefit analysis may be accomplished in one of two ways. One may calculate the net health benefit of a particular programme by subtracting the cost from the benefit. If the difference is positive, then the benefits outweigh the costs. If negative, the costs outweigh the benefits. Alternatively, one may determine the ratio of the benefits to the cost. If the ratio is greater than one, the benefits exceed the costs, while if the ratio is less than one, the costs exceed the benefits.

The economic value of health consequences has been assessed in a number of ways, including the economic market value of an item or commodity; a person's willingness to pay for a particular health consequence; policy-makers' views about the value of a particular service; or practitioners' views or professionals' opinions, such as court awards for the value of particular adverse health states (Drummond *et al.*, 1987).

A significant limitation to cost–benefit analysis is that the health consequences must be measured in economic terms (Weinstein and Stason, 1977). Patients, clinicians, policy makers, payers and society often have a difficult time in placing a monetary value on health. Consequently, cost-effectiveness analysis and cost–utility analysis are more commonly used methodologies to assess health care programmes.

Cost-effectiveness analysis

Cost-effectiveness analysis differs from cost–benefit analysis in the valuation of health consequences. Unlike cost–benefit analysis, cost-effectiveness analysis allows the use of a variety of measures of health effects. For many preventive and treatment interventions targeted toward general health, health effects are measured as reduced incidence rates of diseases or events, changes in clinical findings or laboratory tests, years of life, or quality-adjusted life years (QALYs; Weinstein and Stason, 1977). Measures of the health consequences of oral health programmes have included tooth surfaces saved from decay,

decay-free years (DFYs), days of standard discomfort, tooth years and quality-adjusted tooth years (Antczak-Bouckoms and Weinstein, 1987; Tulloch and Antczak-Bouckoms, 1987; White *et al.*, 1989). The ratio of marginal costs to marginal health outcomes of one programme relative to another yields a cost-effectiveness measure. In general, programmes associated with lower marginal cost-effectiveness ratios are preferable to those with higher marginal cost-effectiveness ratios. Comparisons between different types of programmes are limited by the extent to which health consequences of alternative programmes can be measured in the same unit. For example, it would be impossible to compare two programmes if one were measured as cases of oral cancer detected and the other as changes in caries incidence rates.

Cost–utility analysis

The final methodology to be discussed here is cost–utility analysis. Cost–utility analysis differs from cost-effectiveness analysis only in the assessment of the health consequences. In cost–utility analyses, health consequences are measured in units that estimate the quality of the health outcome associated with a particular intervention (Weinstein and Stason, 1977; Drummond *et al.*, 1987; Kamlet, 1992). Most often, health outcomes are reported as QALYs, and the results of cost–utility analyses are reported as cost per QALY.

Cost–utility analysis requires that the health consequences of a programme be measured as final rather than intermediate effects. For example, intermediate measures, such as changes in caries incidence rates or cases of oral cancer identified through a screening programme, cannot be converted into QALYs. However, number of years with a caries-free dentition or number of years of life gained because of early detection of oral cancer can be used in cost–utility analyses. In such cases, both changes in morbidity and/or mortality resulting from a health care programme and the quality of life associated with that health state can be reflected in a single measure.

Cost–utility analysis may be useful when quality of life is *the* important outcome (Drummond *et al.*, 1987). For example, when comparing alternative programmes for the prevention of dental caries, mortality is not usually one of the expected outcomes. Rather, changes in the patient's physical function, freedom from pain, improved social function and psychological well-being are more relevant health consequences. Cost–utility analysis would be beneficial in such situations. In addition, cost–utility analysis can be helpful when a wide range of health care programmes are being assessed, each having a different measure of effectiveness. For example, when used as measures of the consequences of health care programmes, QALYs or quality-adjusted tooth years provide a way to compare preventive strategies targeted toward dental caries, therapy for moderate to severe periodontal diseases and restorative dental care.

Just as there are situations in which cost–utility analysis is advantageous, there are also instances where cost–utility analysis should not be used (Drummond *et al.*, 1987). When only intermediate effectiveness data are available, such as the number of carious lesions averted secondary to a prevention programme or number of cases of oral cancer identified through a screening programme, it is difficult to assess the impact on quality of life or to convert these measures into QALYs. In addition, when the data show that the alternatives are equally effective, identification of the least expensive option through cost-minimization analysis is sufficient. When quality of life is important and can be captured by only a single variable measured in easily understood natural units, cost-effectiveness analysis may be sufficient. For example, one may compare several alternative programmes that affect quality of life through measures such as days of standard discomfort (Tulloch and Antczak-Bouckoms, 1987). Finally, cost–utility analysis should be avoided when the time, effort and resources associated with obtaining and using quality of life measures are judged to be too costly relative to the additional information provided.

A number of methods have been proposed to assess quality of life associated with various health states (Torrance *et al.*, 1972; Weinstein and Fineberg, 1980; Llewellyn-Thomas *et al.*, 1984; Drummond *et al.*, 1987; Froberg and Kane, 1989a, 1989b; Petitti, 1994). These approaches include the standard gamble, time trade-off, and direct rating scales. A detailed discussion of the advantages and disadvantages associated with these methods is beyond the scope of this chapter.

Stages of economic analysis

The stages one uses to conduct an economic analysis of alternative health care programmes are shown in Table 10.1. This is a synopsis of steps that have been reported elsewhere (Weinstein and Stason, 1977; Office of Technology Assessment, 1980; Weinstein and Fineberg, 1980; Drummond *et al.*, 1987; Sox, 1988; Warner, 1989; Petitti, 1994). Each of these will be discussed and illustrated using as an example a comparison between a programme that applies dental sealants and a programme that encourages regular recall examinations and placement of conservative amalgam restoration in the prevention and treatment of caries. It is assumed that these programmes cannot be conducted simultaneously.

1 Define the health intervention under consideration and specify the perspective(s) of the analysis

Economic assessment of community oral health programmes can be used to evaluate a variety of programmes. These may include screening programmes to detect dental caries, periodontal diseases or oral cancer; preventive programmes such as community water fluoridation, fluoride mouthrinse or dental sealant programmes; diagnostic tests to detect risk for and presence of disease; and therapeutic interventions aimed at reducing or eliminating pathology.

Evaluation of the programmes under consideration requires that a well-specified question be posed (Drummond *et al.*, 1987). A question such as: Are dental sealants worth the cost? is not sufficiently specific to address cost-

Table 10.1 Stages of economic evaluation

1 Define the health intervention under consideration and specify the perspective(s) of the analysis

2 Identify and describe alternatives

3 Identify, measure and value costs

4 Identify and measure health consequences and other impacts of the health intervention

5 Discount future costs and effectiveness

6 Account for the uncertainties that may exist in the analysis

7 Address ethical issues

8 Present and interpret results

effectiveness issues. An example of a suitable question may be: From the perspective of (a) patients and (b) the community oral health director, is a programme that applies dental sealants in a school-based setting to prevent pit-and-fissure caries preferable to a programme of regular recall examinations, health education and treating caries lesions in private dental offices with conservative amalgam restorations as the lesions develop? An important part of this question is the identification of the viewpoint for the analysis (Weinstein and Fineberg, 1980; Drummond *et al.*, 1987; Sox, 1988; Eisenberg, 1989; Petitti, 1994). A variety of viewpoints may be taken, including that of the patient, the clinician, the third-party payer (public or private) or society (the broadest, most inclusive perspective). The viewpoint of the analysis dictates which costs and consequences are relevant.

2 Identify alternatives

Cost-effectiveness analysis compares the costs and consequences of two or more alternative programmes. To compare programmes and to determine the applicability of the analysis to other programmes, a detailed description of the competing programmes must be provided. Appropriate assessment of the costs and consequences depends on the identification of who does what to whom, when, where, how often and what the results of the programme are (Drummond *et al.*, 1987). To ensure a complete comparison of alternative strategies, one should also consider a 'do nothing' or status quo strategy. In comparing a dental sealant programme with an existing programme that restores carious lesions as they develop, as specified above, answers to the examples of questions shown in Table 10.2 should be

Table 10.2 Examples of the types of questions that must be addressed to identify fully alternative community oral health programmes

Question	Alternative 1: Sealant programme	Alternative 2: Regular recall, health education and conservative amalgam restorations
Who?	Who conducts the clinical examination? Who determines whether sealants are indicated? Who applies the sealants? Who evaluates the sealants after placement? Who conducts the recall examinations? Who determines if caries are present? Who places the amalgam restoration if caries develop?	Who conducts the clinical examination? Who provides the health education? Who ensures that patients come in for regular examinations? Who determines if caries are present? Who places the amalgam restoration if caries develop?
Does what?	What kind of dental examination is provided? Are radiographs taken? What teeth will be sealed? What kind of sealant material will be used? What kind of amalgam material will be used?	What kind of dental examination is provided? Are radiographs taken? What kind of amalgam material will be used? What kinds of education materials are required?
To whom?	What age groups will have their teeth sealed? Will all children in a specific age group receive sealants or will only high-risk children be treated?	What age groups will receive health education and treatment if caries develop? Will all children in a specific age group receive care or will only high-risk children be treated?
When?	When will the examinations occur? When will the sealants be placed? When will the sealants be evaluated?	When will the examinations occur? When will the education take place? When will amalgam restorations be placed? replaced?
Where?	Where will the examinations occur and where will the sealants be placed (e.g. school clinic, mobile van, community health centre, private dental offices)? Where will the carious lesions be treated?	Where will the examinations occur? Where will the health education take place? Where will carious lesions be treated?
How often?	How often will recall examinations occur to examine individuals for dental caries? How often will failed sealant application be redone?	How often will recall examinations occur to individuals for dental caries? How often will health education occur? How often will amalgam restorations be replaced?
What are the results?	How many teeth/individuals were at risk for caries? How many teeth were sealed? How many dental sealants had to be replaced? How many carious lesions developed? How many amalgam restorations were placed or replaced?	How many teeth/individuals were at risk for caries? How many carious lesions developed? How many amalgam restorations were placed or replaced?

provided to identify fully the alternatives. For any analysis, the relevant questions will be determined by the perspective of the evaluation.

3 Identify, measure and value costs

Once the question being addressed is specified, the costs and consequences can be considered. The relevant costs that should be included in the analysis are dictated by the perspective of the analysis. From a patient's perspective, costs may be limited to out-of-pocket expenses for provision of services, insurance premiums for coverage of dental services or taxes used to support public programmes. In addition, averted costs are also important from a patient's perspective. These include, for example, any savings that may be attributable to prevented disease. From a clinician's perspective, applicable costs may be those associated with the purchase of equipment, rent for clinic space, supplies or additional personnel required to implement a programme. Costs for a third-party payer may include the amount of reimbursement for covered services. Societal costs generally include all costs associated with a programme, without regard to the person or organization that incurs the costs. Averted costs would be included as well.

Methods for assessing costs associated with a health care programme have been developed and applied more commonly to medical services, technologies and procedures than to dental services. Application of these methods directly to dental care should be done with caution (Antczak-Bouckoms *et al.*, 1989). Standards have been less well-developed for the assessment of dental costs. For example, there are no institutional structures, such as hospitals, that can serve readily as a basis for cost comparisons. This is an area in need of further development.

Costs can be categorized in a variety of ways, and the same descriptive term may refer to different components (Petitti, 1994). One way of categorizing costs in community oral health programmes is shown in Table 10.3 (Antczak-Bouckoms *et al.*, 1989). In most analyses, all components of cost cannot be identified and are not included; however, each analysis should state explicitly which costs are included and which are not.

An important caveat in estimating health care costs is the distinction between costs and charges (Finkler, 1982). Charges are the amount that health care practitioners and institutions attempt to recover for the provision of a treatment or service. Payment for that service (reimbursement) is the amount that the

Table 10.3 Definitions and examples of dental costs

Type of cost	Definition	Example
Direct	Costs wholly attributable to the service in question	Equipment acquisition, improvement, labour, materials
Indirect (overhead)	Costs shared by many services concurrently and not directly traceable to a particular service	Rent/building depreciation; upkeep; support services; maintenance, utilities, administration
Fixed	Costs that remain at the same level regardless of the number of services delivered; can be direct or indirect	Rent, supervisor salary; dental chair
Variable	Costs that may vary in direct proportion to the volume of services rendered	Disposable materials, dental chart, dental radiographs
Semivariable	Fixed and variable costs that vary with volume, but not proportionally	Phone service with monthly cost for basic service plus additional costs for long-distance calls
Average	Cost per service or per patient (i.e. total costs divided by number of services delivered or patients treated)	Cost per patient screened in a disease detection programme
Incremental (marginal)	Costs of providing one additional service, or treating one additional patient	Costs of treating an additional patient; costs of sealing the fourth tooth in a patient having already three sealed teeth; cost of detecting an additional case of disease
Opportunity	Costs incurred when a particular strategy is chosen over another	Cost of lost productivity in place of employment while medical care is delivered to an employee
Induced costs (and savings)	Costs and savings of resources; expenditures that are added or averted because of an initial service or procedure	Tests added or averted or treatment added or averted secondary to adoption of a particular strategy

From Antczak-Bouckoms *et al.* (1989), with permission.

practitioner or institution actually receives from a patient or third-party payer. The cost of a treatment or service is the economic measure of the resources required to provide that treatment or service. Costs include the direct costs (e.g. equipment, labour and materials), overhead costs (e.g. fraction of other costs allocated to the programme) and other indirect costs. Use of charges rather than costs may lead researchers to draw unwarranted conclusions about the economic efficiency of one programme relative to another (Finkler, 1982).

Cost-effectiveness analysis compares the costs and consequences of two or more programmes. It is always comparative. Determination of the comparative costs between programmes requires use of the incremental or marginal cost associated with a programme rather than the average cost of the programme. The incremental cost is the extra cost of providing one additional service or treating one additional patient. In contrast, the average cost is the mean cost per service or per patient. Average costs are not comparative and are not useful or appropriate costs for economic evaluation (Finkler, 1982; Detsky and Naglie, 1990).

Sources of cost data

A variety of ways have been suggested to estimate the costs associated with a health care programme. Weinstein and Fineberg (1980) proposed the methods shown in Table 10.4. This approach could be applied to estimating the costs associated with the sealant programme and the recall, education and conservative treatment

Table 10.4 Components of cost and basis for estimating production costs for a community-based oral health care programme

Component	Basis for estimating cost of component
Direct	Total of equipment, labour and materials
Equipment	Depreciated cost divided by frequency of use
Labour	
Dentist's time	Professional fee
Other personnel's time	Hours worked times wages per hour
Materials	Cost per procedure
Indirect (overhead)	Fraction of other facility costs allocated to this procedure

alternative. Sources of cost data are variable depending on the type of programme being evaluated and the perspective of the analysis. Cost estimates for medical services often come from third-party databases (public and private). As noted earlier, however, the organization of the dental care delivery system is different from that of the medical care system. In many countries, public or private insurance coverage for dental services is limited. Consequently, data sources that may be available for estimating the costs of certain medical procedures or services provided in institutions such as hospitals may not be available for estimating the cost of dental services. Sample surveys of the market value of goods and services may be used to estimate cost when other data sources are not available.

4 Identify and measure health consequences and other impacts of the health intervention

Prior to conducting any economic evaluation, scientific evidence must be available that clearly documents the effectiveness of the programmes under consideration. A programme or intervention is effective if it can be shown to be beneficial as the programme or intervention normally would be used in everyday practice with the majority of patients and clinicians. If effectiveness data are not available, then one should not conduct an economic assessment.

As with estimating the costs of a community-based programme, assessment of the health consequences of alternative programmes is dependent on the perspective of the analysis. Health consequences may include the community; subpopulations within a community that may be designated by age, gender, race, race-ethnicity, income level or other sociodemographic and economic variables; or individuals within a community. The health effects of community-based programmes are measured generally at the population or subpopulation level. Evaluations of these programmes generally assume a societal perspective.

A variety of measures may be used for assessing the health consequences of community-based oral health programmes. To date, most community-based programmes have focused on the prevention of dental caries, and effectiveness measures have reflected this emphasis. For example, surfaces saved or caries prevented have been reported, as have changes in the incidence rate of dental caries (White *et al.*, 1989). As noted earlier, these measures are intermediate measures of the outcomes associated with community-based oral health programmes. As such, these measures cannot be used to assess the impact of dental caries on quality of life. Other measures that have been used less frequently, such as number of DFYs secondary to a preventive programme or the number of quality-adjusted tooth years (Antczak-Bouckoms and Weinstein, 1987; Weintraub *et al.*, 1993), provide an estimate of the ultimate effectiveness of these programmes. The health consequences of the sealant programme and the regular recall, health education and conservative amalgam alternative might be measured as changes in the incidence rates of new carious lesions between the two programmes, number of DFYs or quality-adjusted tooth years. The two programmes could not be compared if the health consequences were specified in different units (e.g. number of sealed teeth and number of filled teeth), unless one considers these two outcomes equivalent.

As comparative costs (as opposed to average costs) of alternative programmes are the appropriate economic measure, so too are comparative or marginal measures of effectiveness. Marginal effectiveness provides an estimate of the additional health benefits that may be achieved by implementing one programme instead of another.

Table 10.5 Hierarchy of types of evidence used in practice guideline development

Strength of evidence	Source
Ia	Evidence obtained from meta-analysis of randomized controlled trials
Ib	Evidence obtained from at least one randomized controlled trial
IIa	Evidence obtained from at least one well-designed controlled study without randomization
IIb	Evidence obtained from at least one other type of well-designed quasi-experimental study
III	Evidence obtained from well-designed non-experimental studies, such as comparative studies, correlational studies and case studies
IV	Evidence obtained from expert committee reports or opinions and/or clinial experience of respected authorities

From Agency for Health Care Policy and Research (1992), with permission.

Sources of effectiveness data

Data on the effectiveness of community-based oral health programmes may be obtained in a variety of ways. Ideally, data would be available from an experimental study design, such as a randomized clinical trial, that evaluates the effectiveness of two or more alternative strategies. However, randomized clinical trials are often not available and data must be obtained from other sources. Table 10.5 illustrates a hierarchy of types of evidence used in the development of clinical practice guidelines (Agency for Health Care Policy and Research, 1992). Discussion of methods for meta-analysis and conduct and evaluation of clinical research is beyond the scope of this chapter and is available in other texts (Petitti, 1994; White and Antczak-Bouckoms, 1995).

5 Discount future costs and effectiveness

Assessments of alternative community-based programmes are done at some point in time, usually the present. However, the costs and consequences associated with these programmes do not necessarily occur at the same time. For example, consider the two alternative programmes that seek to prevent dental caries over a 10-year period. One programme places dental sealants on the occlusal surfaces of permanent teeth for all children in a community. Sealants that are lost are replaced if no caries are present. Another programme does not place sealants but institutes a regular recall and health education programme. If caries develop, conservative amalgams are placed.

Over a 10-year period, costs would occur or recur over time. The sealant programme would require significant resources in the early years while the recall, education and treatment programme might require approximately equal levels of resources over the 10-year period. Likewise, the benefits attributable to the two programmes, as measured by caries incidence rates, DFYs or quality-adjusted tooth years, may occur differentially during the time period. Some individuals may not develop caries during the entire period. Others may develop caries in each year of the 10-year period. Still others may develop caries in each of 2 years in the 10-year period. If a policy-maker had to determine which of these two programmes was more cost-effective, then the differential timing of the costs and benefits would have to be considered.

To account for these differences, the value of the future costs is reduced or discounted. 'Discounting is a process for computing how much a dollar, payable one or more years from now, is worth today' (Weinstein and Fineberg, 1980). The basis for discounting is individuals' time preference for money. Money that is not spent today can be invested to yield a larger amount of real money in the future. Consequently, one should determine the present value of future money when assessing the costs of alternative programmes.

Although more controversial, one should also discount future health benefits (Weinstein and Fineberg, 1980). Years of life in the future are valued less than present years of life. While health benefits cannot be invested as can money to yield larger benefits, health benefits are being valued relative to discounted money and therefore should be discounted. In addition, as Keeler and Cretin (1983) pointed out, inconsistencies in the results of economic evaluations are noted when one fails to discount health benefits but discounts costs. For example, for any programme worth implementing this year, there is an alternative programme whose costs relative to health consequences are less if implementation is delayed a year. The future value of money is less than the present value of money. Without discounting health consequences, this year's health effects are equal to next year's health effects, and next year's discounted costs are less than this year's costs. Consequently, failure to discount health consequences leads one to delay starting a health programme, since the cost-effectiveness ratio will be more favourable next year.

6 Account for the uncertainties that may exist in the analysis

Estimates of the costs and health consequences of community-based oral health programmes come from a variety of sources. Each source has associated with it some level of uncertainty and imprecision. Assessing the extent to which the results of the analysis change based on variation in the inputs is known as a sensitivity analysis and is an important part of any economic evaluation (Weinstein and Fineberg, 1980; Drummond *et al.*, 1987; Sox, 1988; Petitti, 1994). Sensitivity analysis can be done on estimates of cost, effectiveness, probabilities of various events, discount rates or the structure of the programme itself. The impact of these variables may be considered singly (one-way sensitivity analysis) or two or three variables may be considered together (two-way or three-way sensitivity analysis). If small variations in any input to the analysis change the relative cost-effectiveness of one programme to another, then additional data may be necessary to estimate the input more precisely. Alternatively, if the conclusions vary little while the inputs are varied over a wide range, then one can have increased confidence in the results.

7 Address ethical issues

Economic evaluations are intended to assist decision-makers in allocating limited health care resources. Results of these analyses are not intended to be used without appropriate consideration of the ethical issues associated with the decision. Economic evaluations do not address issues of equity and distribution (e.g. who benefits and who pays). Health care programmes that benefit the poor, the elderly, individuals living in rural areas or other groups who may be at increased risk for disease may not be cost-effective relative to other programmes that benefit different groups. That one programme is more cost-effective relative to another is an important consideration in the decision-making process; however, it is not the only consideration.

8 Present and interpret results

Results of an economic evaluation may be presented in a variety of ways. One way to present such information is shown in Table 10.6. In this case, three programmes were evaluated, including the two programmes described earlier in the chapter and a 'do nothing' or status quo option. In this example, costs are measured in US dollars and the expected effectiveness is measured in DFYs. The programmes are listed in order of increasing expected effectiveness. The marginal cost and effectiveness are determined by obtaining the difference between two programmes. For example, the marginal cost and effectiveness of the recall, education and amalgam restoration programme is the difference between the recall programme ($100 000; 25 000 DFY) and the next least expensive programme. In this example, the next least expensive programme is the status quo ($75 000; 17 000

Table 10.6 Example presentation of hypothetical results from an economic evaluation of two community-based oral health programmes

Programme	Expected cost	Expected effectiveness (DFYs)	Marginal cost	Marginal effectiveness	Marginal cost-effectiveness ratio
Status quo	$75 000	17 000			
Recall, education, amalgam restorations	$100 000	25 000	$25 000	8000	$3.13 per DFY
Sealant programme	$150 000	40 000	$25 000	15 000	$3.33 per DFY
			$50 000		

DFY = Decay-free year.

DFY), resulting in a marginal cost of $25,000 and a marginal effectiveness of 8000 DFY. The marginal cost and effectiveness of the sealant programme are determined in a similar manner. The ratio of the marginal cost to the marginal effectiveness yields a marginal cost-effectiveness ratio.

Generally the marginal cost-effectiveness ratios will identify one of four relationships between alternative programmes: one programme will cost more and be more effective; one programme will cost more and be less effective; one programme will cost less and be more effective; and one programme will cost less and be less effective. In the first case, if a programme costs more but is more effective, the decision-maker must determine whether, relative to other potential uses for limited resources, the additional health benefit is worth the added cost. In the second case, if a programme costs more and is less effective, the programme should never be adopted, whether resources are limited or not. In the third case, programmes that cost less and are more effective should always be adopted. Finally, programmes that cost less but are less effective provide options to decision-makers in times of retrenchment and budget cutbacks.

The results of the hypothetical analysis suggest that each of the two options in this example costs more and is more effective than the next best alternative. Interpretation of these findings might be as follows: if one is not willing to spend $3.13 per DFY, then resources should be allocated toward the status quo programme. However, if one were willing to spend at least $3.13 and not more than $3.33 per DFY, then one should implement the recall, education, and amalgam restoration programme. Likewise, if one were willing to spend at least $3.33 per DFY, then one should allocate resources toward the sealant programme.

Presentation of the results of an economic evaluation requires more information than just a display of the marginal costs and consequences of competing programmes (Drummond *et al.*, 1987; Petitti, 1994). Such factors as the perspective of the analysis, the time horizon used, sources of costs and effectiveness data and the discount rate used should be stated explicitly. Assumptions and judgements used in the analysis should be pointed out to the reader. As noted earlier, sensitivity analyses should be done to assess the effect of changes in the inputs on the results. Presentation of the results in such a manner allows the reader to assess the applicability of the results to his or her own programme.

Assessing the quality of economic evaluations

Evidence suggests that the quality of economic evaluations is quite variable. For example, in a review of general medical, general surgical and medical subspecialty journals, Udvarhelyi and others (1992) identified 77 cost–benefit and cost-effectiveness analyses published between 1978 and 1980 and between 1985 and 1987. These articles were reviewed and scored based on the degree to which each of six principles identified by the authors were identified. These principles represented a synthesis of the literature describing appropriate methods for cost-effective analysis and economic evaluation of health care practices. The authors stated that failure to address these principles would compromise an appropriate minimum standard for conducting and reporting cost–benefit and cost-effectiveness analyses. Of the 77 articles reviewed, only three adhered to all six principles. The median number of principles to which the articles adhered was three. Based on these findings, the authors concluded that greater attention should be devoted to ensuring that appropriate methods were used in conducting economic evaluations, and users of such information were cautioned to consider the methods of the analysis when interpreting the results. Unfortunately, there is no evidence to suggest that economic analyses conducted on oral health programmes do not suffer from the same limitations.

Indeed, a recent critical review of methods for the economic evaluation of fissure sealants concluded that 'in order for dental public health planners to make informed decisions regarding the use of fissure sealants, more appropriate and properly executed economic evaluation is required' (Lewis and Morgan, 1994). Specifically, one of the problems identified in the review was the quality of outcome measurement. When comparing these types of problems, the choice may be between a sealed sound tooth versus a filled (with associated pain and discomfort) sound tooth. Some authors have equated success (health) with an adequately restored tooth or perhaps a minimum of three restored surfaces (Smales, 1982; Lennon *et al.*, 1984). A more acceptable measurement of dental health equates with sound, completely unfilled teeth (Stamm, 1983). This approach has been used in the example given earlier where the effectiveness of the programmes was measured in DFYs.

Decision-makers, faced with allocating resources among competing oral health programmes, must identify relevant studies that have been published and determine which studies are useful to help inform the decision. For example, decision-makers should determine whether published studies used reliable methods. To assist readers in critiquing the published literature, Drummond *et al.* (1987) have suggested a checklist of questions that may be useful in assessing an economic evaluation (Table 10.7).

A second important aspect of assessing the usefulness of economic evaluations is the extent to which study results can be applied to another setting (Drummond *et al.*, 1993). Differences in the perspective of the analysis, specification of alternative programmes, sources of cost and effectiveness data, discount rates, time horizon and other factors may render two studies incomparable. In addition, differences in the organization of health care systems, the types of personnel employed and the sites of care delivery may make it difficult for the analyst to compare studies conducted in different countries. Consumers of such information must assess the appropriateness of study results in the context of these concerns.

Limitations of economic evaluations

Despite the many advantages of economic evaluations in assisting decision-makers, there are significant limitations that must be considered when using these approaches. These include: determination of the effectiveness of a programme; equity and distribution of costs and health consequences; use of saved resources; and resources required to conduct economic evaluations. Each of these is discussed below.

First, effectiveness must be established prior to conducting an economic evaluation. If the effectiveness of an intervention has not been established, an economic evaluation should not be considered, since there is no basis on which to estimate the health consequences. Data may be available for many community-based oral health programmes, but its quality and usefulness must be assessed.

Second, ethical issues are not addressed generally in these types of evaluations. The

Table 10.7 A proposed checklist for assessing economic evaluations in health care

1 Was a well-defined question posed in an answerable form?
2 Was a comprehensive description of the competing alternatives given? (i.e. can you tell who? did what? to whom? when? where? and how often?)
3 Was there evidence that the programme's effectiveness has been established?
4 Were all the important and relevant costs and consequences for each alternative identified?
5 Were costs and consequences measured accurately in appropriate physical units (e.g. hours of nursing time, number of dentist visits, lost workdays, gained life-years)?
6 Were costs and consequences valued credibly?
7 Were costs and consequences adjusted for differential timing?
8 Was an incremental analysis of costs and consequences of alternative performed?
9 Was a sensitivity analysis performed?
10 Did the presentation and discussion of study results include all issues of concern to users?

From Drummond *et al.* (1987), with permission.

equity and distribution of the costs and health consequences must be considered. Health programmes for certain high-risk groups may never be shown to be cost-effective relative to other health programmes; however, these high-risk groups may be the most vulnerable individuals in a population, and programmes aimed at improving their health status may be of highest priority. As a matter of public policy, decision-makers may allocate resources toward programmes aimed at improving the health of high-risk groups, regardless of the results of an economic evaluation. Further background to such considerations can be found in Chapters 3 and 16 of this book.

Third, economic evaluations assume that resources freed or saved by adopting more cost-effective programmes will be used in alternative ways that are also cost-effective. For example, suppose two programmes, A and B, were evaluated, and programme A was found to be less costly and more effective than programme B. However, programme B was currently in place. If the decision-maker reallocated resources from programme B to programme A, thereby improving health benefits at a lower cost, then the marginal savings attributable to this change should be allocated to another programme that is also cost-effective relative to its alternatives.

Finally, economic evaluations themselves require resources. Conducting a cost-effectiveness analysis to determine how best to allocate $1000 may require that a sizeable portion of the sum be spent in conducting the evaluation itself. In this case, economic evaluation may not be justified. There is no minimum level of expenditure or health impact above which an economic evaluation should always be done and below which should never be done. The needs of the decision-maker, the level of available resources, the ease of obtaining cost and effectiveness data and the importance of the decision should all be weighed carefully in deciding to undertake an economic evaluation.

Use and misuse of the term 'cost-effective'

Given the pressures on health care budgets and the ongoing efforts to allocate limited resources between and among competing priorities, the term cost-effective increasingly has been used to describe the advantages of particular programmes even in the absence of research data. Screening, diagnostic and treatment programmes have been portrayed as cost-effective without any analysis or formal comparison. Doubilet and colleagues (1986) have noted that cost-effectiveness is often misused in the literature when describing medical applications. Ways in which cost-effectiveness is used incorrectly include claiming an intervention is cost-effective when cost data are provided but effectiveness data are not available, when effectiveness has been established but no cost data are reported, or when neither cost nor effectiveness data are reported. Cost-effective does not mean cost saving (i.e. that a strategy is cost-effective only if it saves money in the absence of effectiveness data) or that the most effective programme is the programme associated with the least cost. Nor does cost-effective refer to the most effective programme without information on the costs associated with that programme. The term cost-effective should be restricted to instances in which the following criteria apply. A programme is cost-effective relative to alternative strategies if it is:

1. less costly and at least as effective;
2. more effective and more costly, its additional benefit being worth the added cost;
3. less effective and less costly, the added benefit of the alternative programme not worth the added cost.

Conclusions

Allocating limited resources among a variety of health care programmes poses many challenges for policy-makers. Decisions are made routinely regarding trade-offs between different types of programmes (e.g. preventive, screening or treatment) using different types of health care personnel (e.g. physicians, dentists, dental auxiliaries or community health workers) in different settings (e.g. the community, the hospital, the physician's office, the dentist's office, the school or work site), each associated with different costs and health consequences. Yet it is difficult, if not impossible, for the costs and health consequences of these alternative programmes to be considered explicitly and objectively without quantitative methods. Economic evaluations, such as cost-minimization, cost–benefit, cost-effectiveness and cost–utility analyses, help guide the decision-maker through this process. When used appropriately, these techniques can be powerful aides, helping to quantify the costs and consequences of health programmes for individual patients, for a population or in the formulation of policies regarding utilization and reimbursement. Used improperly, these techniques may only add to the confusion that already exists. Limited resources may be squandered, and health consequences may be minimized rather than maximized.

References

Agency for Health Care Policy and Research (1992) *Acute Pain Management: Operative or Medical Procedures and Trauma.* AHCPR publication no. 92-0032. Rockville, Maryland.

Antczak-Bouckoms, A.A. and Weinstein, M.C. (1987) Cost-effectiveness analysis of periodontal disease control. *Journal of Dental Research* **66**:1630–1635.

Antczak-Bouckoms, A.A., Tulloch, J.F., White, B.A. and Capilouto, E.I. (1989) Methodological considerations in the analysis of cost effectiveness in dentistry. *Journal of Public Health Dentistry* **49**:215–222.

Banta, H.D. and Bekaney, C.J. (1981) Policy formulation and technology assessment. *Milbank Memorial Fund Quarterly* **59**:445–79.

Detsky, A.S. and Naglie, I.G. (1990) A clinician's guide to cost-effectiveness analysis. *Annals of Internal Medicine* **113**: 147–154.

Doubilet, P., Weinstein, M.C. and McNeil, B.J. (1986) Use and misuse of the term "cost effective" in medicine. *New England Journal of Medicine* **314**:253–256.

Drummond, M.F. (1980) *Principles of Economic Evaluation in Health Care.* Oxford University Press, Oxford.

Drummond, M.F., Stoddart, G.L. and Torrance, G.W. (1987) *Methods for the Economic Evaluation of Health Care Programmes.* Oxford University Press, Oxford.

Drummond, M., Brandt, A., Luce, B. and Rovira, J. (1993) Standardizing methodologies for economic evaluation in health care. *International Journal of Technical Assessment and Health Care* **9**:26–36.

Eisenberg, J.M. (1989) Clinical economics: a guide to the economic analysis of clinical practices. *Journal of the American Medical Association* **262**:2879–2886.

Finkler, S.A. (1982) The distinction between cost and charges. *Annals of Internal Medicine* **96**:102–109.

Froberg, D.G. and Kane, R.L. (1989a) Methodology for measuring health-state preferences: I. Measurement strategies. *Journal of Clinical Epidemiology* **44**:127–139.

Froberg, D.G. and Kane, R.L. (1989b) Methodology for measuring health-state preferences: II. Scaling methods. *Journal of Clinical Epidemiology* **44**:345–354.

Fuchs, V.R. (1993) No pain, no gain: perspectives on cost containment. *Journal of the American Medical Association* **269**: 31–633.

Kamlet, M.S. (1992) *The Comparative Benefits Modeling Project: A Framework for Cost–Utility Analysis of Government Health Care Programs.* Report to the Office of Disease Prevention and Health Promotion. Public Health Service, US Department of Health and Human Services, Washington, DC.

Keeler, E.B. and Cretin, S. (1983) Discounting of life-saving and other non-monetary benefits. *Management Science* **29**:300–306.

Lennon, M.A., O'Mullane, D.M. and Taylor, G.O. (1984) A pragmatic clinical trial of fissure sealants in a community dental service programme for 6–10 year old children. *Community Dental Health* **1**:101–109.

Lewis, J.M. and Morgan, M.V. (1994) A critical review of methods for the economic evaluation of fissure sealants. *Community Dental Health* **11**:79–82.

Llewellyn-Thomas, H., Sutherland, H.J., Tibshirani, R. *et al.* (1984) Describing health states: methodologic issues in obtaining values for health states. *Medical Care* **22**:543–552.

Luce, B.R. and Elixhauser, A. (1990) *Standards for Socio-economic Evaluation of Health Care Products and Services.* Springer-Verlag, Berlin.

Office of Technology Assessment (1980) *The Implications of Cost-effectiveness Analysis of Medical Technology. Introduction and Background.* Washington, DC.

Petitti, D.B. (1994) *Meta-analysis, Decision Analysis, and Cost-effectiveness Analysis.* Oxford University Press, New York.

Torrance, G.W., Thomas, W.H. and Sackett D.L. (1972) A utility maximization model for evaluation of health care programs. *Health Services Research* **7**:118–133.

Smales, R.J. (1982) Fissure sealants versus amalgams: clinical results over 5 years. *Journal of Dentistry* **10**:95–102.

Sox, H.C. (1988) *Medical Decision Making.* Butterworths, Boston.

Stamm, J.W. (1983) The use of fissure sealants in public health programmes: a reactor's comments. *Journal of Public Health Dentistry* **43**:243–246.

Tulloch, J.F. and Antczak-Bouckoms, A.A. (1987) Decision analysis in the evaluation of clinical strategies for the management of mandibular third molars. *Journal of Dental Education* **51**:652–660.

Udvarhelyi, I.S., Colditz, G.A., Rai, A. and Epstein, A.M. (1992) Cost-effectiveness and cost–benefit analyses in the medical literature: are the methods being used correctly? *Annals of Internal Medicine* **116**:238–244.

Warner, K.E. (1989) Issues in cost effectiveness in health care. *Journal of Public Health Dentistry* **49**:272–278.

Warner, K.E. and Luce, B.R. (1982) *Cost-benefit and Cost-effectiveness Analysis in Health Care.* Health Administration Press, Ann Arbor, MI.

Weinstein, M.C. and Fineberg, H.V. (1980) *Clinical Decision Analysis.* W.B. Saunders Company, Philadelphia.

Weinstein, M.C. and Stason, W.B. (1977) Foundations of cost-effectiveness analysis for health and medical practices.

New England Journal of Medicine **296**:716–721.

Weintraub, J.A., Stearns, S.C., Burt, B.A. *et al.* (1993) A retrospective analysis of the cost-effectiveness of dental sealants in a children's health center. *Social Science Medicine* **36**:1483–1493.

White, B.A. and Antczak-Bouckoms, A.A. (1995) Improving oral health through systematic reviews and meta-analysis.

In: *Disease Prevention and Oral Health Promotion: Socio-dental Sciences in Action* (Cohen, L.K. and Gift, H.C., eds), pp. 455–479. Munksgaard, Copenhagen.

White, B.A., Antczak-Bouckoms, A.A. and Weinstein, M.C. (1989) Issues in the economic evaluation of community water fluoridation. *Journal of Dental Education* **53**:646–657.

11

Principles of oral health promotion

Lone Schou and David Locker

Introduction

This chapter provides an introduction to health promotion, its origins, principles and concepts. It also demonstrates how these principles and concepts may be applied to oral health. Health promotion is distinct from disease prevention and health education in both its aims and its strategies. It is a comprehensive approach to enhancing the health of families, communities and populations which both complements and challenges the approach on which formal health care systems are based. From its perspective, health is both an individual and a social responsibility that is best secured by collaborative actions at all levels of society. As such it represents a major shift in emphasis involving a new vision of health and how it is to be achieved.

The origins of health promotion

After the Second World War, the governments of most industrial nations began to invest heavily in health. Government policy at this time was largely concerned with developing health services, such as hospitals and primary care facilities, and ensuring that those in need had access to them. In the UK, for example, 1948 saw the founding of the National Health Service, while in Canada during the 1960s and early 1970s, universal publicly managed health insurance schemes were established enabling all Canadians to obtain free medical and hospital care. Even within the more private system of the USA, government legislation encouraged the

development of health-related resources, in the form of biomedical knowledge, health personnel and health care facilities (Green and Kreuter, 1990) and, through Medicaid and Medicare programmes, made health services more readily available to the old and the poor.

Green and Kreuter (1990) have referred to this period as one of resource development and redistribution. The assumption which gave rise to the policy initiatives implemented by governments during this period was that better access to high-quality health services inevitably led to better health. This assumption began to be questioned in the 1970s and it is now increasingly accepted that spending more money on health services will have only a limited impact, if any, on the health of the population. For example, the provision of free health care in the UK did not in and of itself eliminate the health gap between the wealthy and the poor. Even though the investment in health services rose steadily during this period, both in absolute expenditures and relative to gross national product, mortality and morbidity statistics have remained inversely related to socioeconomic status (Marmot *et al.*, 1991).

As the costs of medical services continued to rise, governments began to turn their attention to cost containment (Green and Kreuter, 1990), finding ways of reducing or stabilizing costs while continuing to secure improvements in health. In the USA, for example, emphasis came to be placed on the role of health education in promoting self-care and reducing utilization of services, and upon new forms of medical practice such as Health Maintenance Organizations in which the prevention rather than cure of disease was encouraged through the way in which health professionals were paid.

At the same time it was recognized that the major health problems of modern populations, particularly the poor, were and continue to be chronic degenerative disorders such as cancer, heart disease and cardiovascular disease, which were expensive to manage but could not be cured. However, many of these disorders could be prevented by changes in personal behaviours or the social and physical environments in which people lived (Lalonde, 1974). Consequently, a better understanding of the causes of ill health and mortality reinforced the emerging interest of governments in disease prevention and health education (Green and Kreuter, 1990).

A final factor that encouraged the development of alternative approaches to population health was an increasing scepticism concerning the role of medicine and the formal health care system in bringing about reductions in mortality and morbidity. The historical research of McKeown (1979) demonstrates quite convincingly that improvements in health over the past 200 years were the product of rising standards of living, improvements in diet and improvements in sanitation and water supplies. Since medicine had very few effective remedies prior to 1930 it could not have made a major contribution. For example, 90% of the decline in mortality from tuberculosis had occurred before chemotherapy and BCG vaccination became available. Rather, improvements in the social and physical environment decreased exposure to infectious disease and increased host resistance to microorganisms. Similarly, social, economic and environmental factors have also played an important part in the improvements in oral health occurring over the last 50 years (Murray, 1983).

The work of Cochrane (1972) was also influential in reappraising the contribution of medical practice to health. He suggested that there was no evidence that many of the drugs and procedures routinely used in medicine were effective in terms of securing benefits for the patient, and advocated the widespread use of randomized clinical trials to ensure that all treatments used resulted in health gains.

This kind of thinking began to be reflected in government documents released during the mid to late 1970s (Lalonde, 1974; Department of Health and Social Security, 1976). These provided the first step in the development of a new approach to population health–that of health promotion. As described below, this is a complex and comprehensive approach which rejects much of the philosophy on which health service provision has been based. In certain respects, dentistry has been something of a pioneer in terms of this new way of thinking, with its long-standing focus on environmental change in the form of community water fluoridation and changing personal behaviours such as diet and oral hygiene to decrease the risk of oral disease. Nevertheless, health promotion has come to mean much more than is implied by these concerns. While it involves the prevention of disease and behaviour change through health education, it goes far beyond them.

Before defining health promotion and outlining its principles, it is necessary to consider what is meant by the term health and to review different approaches to improving the health of populations.

The concept of health

Central to the health promotion approach is a conception of health and what it means to be healthy. A useful point of departure for this discussion is the famous and much maligned definition of health offered by the World Health Organization (WHO) in 1948. This defined health as 'a complete state of physical, mental and social well-being and not merely the absence of disease and infirmity'. While the health promotion approach lays great emphasis on this notion of well-being, most health services and health care practice have been more concerned with the eradication of disease. This has in particular been the case in dentistry where the development of oral health care services in most western countries has followed a specific pattern. Early in its history dentistry was predominantly concerned with the treatment of pain and its main orientation was the extraction of teeth. A more restorative orientation followed based on technological advances and this is giving way to a preventive approach also based on the development of technologies such as sealants.

In spite of its obvious limitations, the WHO definition of health was a useful one in that it began to clarify the essential distinction between disease and health. In this context disease is a relatively narrow concept and may be taken to refer to pathological processes which compromise the anatomical or physiological integrity of the body. Health refers to something much broader and is largely concerned with individuals' subjective experience of their body and their selves and its consequences in terms of the conduct of daily life. While disease belongs to the realm of biology, health belongs to the realm of sociology and psychology, encompassing as it does feelings, behaviours and, ultimately, the quality of life.

The breadth of what we mean by health was amply demonstrated by a definition offered by the WHO in 1984 which extended and clarified its 1948 formulation. This definition has been usefully summarized by Epp (1986) in the following way:

> Today we are working with a concept which portrays health as part of everyday living, an essential dimension of the quality of our lives. Quality of life in this context implies the opportunity to make choices and to gain satisfaction from living. Health is thus envisaged as a resource which gives people the ability to manage and even to change their surroundings. This view of health recognizes freedom of choice and emphasises the role of individuals and communities in defining what health means to them.

As Labonte (1993) has argued, these definitions lead us to the conclusion that disease and health are separate and discrete events. Though they may be related in certain circumstances, they often occur and are experienced separately. This is easily demonstrated by reference to the simple model depicted in Figure 11.1.

This model suggests the following, much of it credible in terms of our personal everyday experience. First, it is often–and perhaps usually–the case that we can be diseased without it impinging on our well-being or sense of self. This is represented by sector A. Common dental disorders such as caries and periodontal disease provide an admirable example of this. Sector B represents a situation in which disease becomes so damaging that it compromises our sense of well-being, such as dental diseases which are causing acute or chronic pain. Finally, sector C suggests that just as we may feel healthy in the presence of what may be severe disease, it is also the case that we may experience negative changes to our well-being in the absence of a detectable disease process. Many older people complain of a discomforting feeling of mouth dryness even though salivary flow appears normal. It is also the case that no underlying pathology can be detected in many who experience chronic facial pain. As we explain below, this means that disease is only one of many threats to health. Perhaps this is best clarified further by outlining some of the components of health and well-being (Labonte, 1993):

1 feeling vital, full of energy;
2 having good social relationships;
3 experiencing a sense of control over one's life and living conditions;
4 being able to do things one enjoys;
5 having a sense of purpose in life;
6 experiencing being part of a community.

Note that this is a positive definition of health, but one that is confined to western cultures. What is meant by good health varies considerably across societies and social groups, according to their own values, expectations and philosophies.

How does this apply to oral disorders? It is not an exaggeration to state that the main aim of organized dentistry has been the eradication of disease from the mouth and the replacement of teeth lost to disease or trauma. From the point of view of this contemporary definition of health, the aim should be to obtain and maintain a functional, pain-free, aesthetically and socially acceptable dentition for the lifespan of most people (Sheiham, 1992). Oral disease needs to be treated to the extent that it compromises this aim. A good example of the difference in the two approaches is given by tooth loss. While the traditional view has emphasized the importance

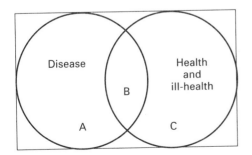

Fig. 11.1

of replacing all missing teeth, recent evidence has shown that two complete dental arches are not necessary for adequate function and aesthetics (Leake *et al.*, 1994). That is, missing teeth may not have a negative impact on health and well-being and treatment is not warranted until they do.

To the extent that diseases of various kinds may impinge on this state of positive health, the prevention of disease and its treatment when it has not been prevented form a part–albeit only a limited part–of health promotion. Seen from this perspective, maintaining or enhancing the health of individuals and communities is a much broader task than providing preventive or treatment services to address disease.

Strategies for improving health

The seminal document in terms of the development of the health promotion approach was a 1974 report issued by the Canadian government written by Lalonde, the then Minister of Health (Lalonde, 1974). The document identified four major determinants of health: human biology, health care organizations, personal behaviours and lifestyles and the environment. The last three identify three distinct but ultimately complementary strategies for addressing health problems. These have been described in detail by Labonte (1993) who labelled them the medical approach, the behavioural approach and the socioenvironmental approach. As mentioned above, the medical approach has dominated thinking on health for much of the past century. It has its origins in the 17th century discoveries concerning anatomy and physiology and was consolidated in the late 19th century with the discovery of microorganisms and the rise of the germ theory of disease. Its philosophical roots, however, lie in the Cartesian revolution which deemed that mind and body were separate, the former merely a machine activated by the latter. The essential features of the medical approach are its focus on disease, an engineering approach which is solely concerned with identifying and repairing disease-induced damage to the body and a narrow conception of the causes of disease and the determinants of health. These are characteristically framed in microbiological or physiological terms so that when this approach concerns itself with prevention it considers risk

factors such as cholesterol levels or high blood pressure and the early detection of disease. From this perspective, the object of medical practice is, then, the body and little attention needs to be paid to the person, the family or the community and their role in health and ill health (Townsend, 1990). The determinants of health are agents, such as microorganisms, which need to be identified and eradicated from the body or malfunctions in body systems which need to be corrected.

During the 1970s thinking about health began to consider the part played by lifestyles and behaviours in the onset of chronic degenerative disorders. Although Lalonde's (1974) seminal document also identified the environment as an important determinant of health, its role was largely ignored or, in some cases, explicitly rejected. As a document on the prevention of disease released by the UK government boldly stated, the diseases of modern populations 'are related less to man's outside environment than to his own personal behaviour, what might be termed our lifestyle' (Department of Health and Social Security, 1976). Consequently, 'much of the responsibility for ensuring his own good health lies with the individual' (Department of Health and Social Security, 1976). From this perspective, healthy behaviours and healthy lifestyles, promoted through health education, are the way to improve health. The responsibility of governments and health professionals is to ensure that individuals have access to the knowledge and information necessary to construct healthy lifestyles.

While this approach does recognize that forces other than the health care system influence our health, it has been subject to severe criticism. First, it focuses solely on the individual and assumes that 'unhealthy' behaviours such as smoking, drinking and consuming diets high in fat or sugar are matters of free choice. This overlooks the fact that there are social and cultural factors which shape our behaviour and set limits on our capacity to change. For example, our diets are influenced by advertising, the decisions taken by food manufacturers and the price and availability of different foods in the neighbourhoods in which we live (Townsend, 1990). Nutrition education, for example, is likely to have little effect on the diet of families living in poverty, whose choices regarding what food and where to purchase it are limited by a lack of money.

A second problem with this approach is that it lends itself to 'victim-blaming' (Labonte and Penfold, 1981). Simply put, if a person is sick it is his or her fault. This is explicit in the UK document on prevention (Department of Health and Social Security, 1976) which ascribed many of the UK health problems to 'over-indulgence and unwise behaviour' and in statements by government ministers which indicate that they prefer to see the problem as one of 'ignorance' (Townsend, 1990).

Critics of the behavioural approach do not claim that lifestyles and individual responsibility play *no* part in maintaining or improving health. The claim is that this approach fails to take account of social and economic conditions over which the individual has little or no control. Enhancing that control lies at the heart of the socioenvironmental approach to health. While treatment is the aim of the medical approach and prevention the aim of the behavioural approach, the socioenvironmental approach has as its goal personal empowerment and political action. In this context, empowerment means 'the capacity to define, analyse and act upon the problems in one's life and living conditions' (Labonte, 1993). From this perspective, powerlessness is a major risk factor for disease and ill health (Wallerstein, 1992). Research evidence for this link is to be found in numerous studies which demonstrate that those in lower socioeconomic groups have higher mortality and morbidity rates than those from higher socioeconomic groups and do worse on a wide range of indicators of health and well-being (MacIntyre, 1986). This relationship also holds for oral disease and disorders (Locker, 1989).

The socioenvironmental model is a broad one (Fig. 11.2) and incorporates elements of the medical and behavioural models. Consequently,

it does not deny that these latter approaches have no merit; both have a valuable but limited contribution to make to health.

The socioenvironmental model has as its basis risk conditions which emanate from the social and physical environments in which we live. Poverty, unemployment, environmental pollution, hazardous or stressful work, poor housing, low education, poor diets and discrimination have a direct effect on health and well-being and also affect health through the numerous psychosocial, behavioural and physiological risk factors which they engender. Psychosocial risk factors are perhaps the least familiar (perhaps because the popular press have not given them the same coverage as risk factors such as cholesterol and smoking) but include such things as a lack of social support, a lack of meaningful and satisfying social relationships and more psychologically oriented problems such as low self-esteem and feelings of hopelessness. Also the family, and in particular the quality of marriage, has been shown to have an influence on physical and psychological health (Hobbs *et al.*, 1985; Schmoldt *et al.*, 1989). A recent study from Brazil showed a highly significant negative association between marital quality and the father's, mother's and child's oral health status (Marcenes and Sheiham, 1995). There is some evidence to suggest that, when under stress, people pay less attention to oral hygiene (Fleck-Kandath *et al.*, 1988) and this may explain the relationship between stress and oral disease.

The main implication of this model is that material deprivation and a lack of control over important dimensions of one's life are the main issues that need to be addressed in promoting the health of the population. It is no accident that those countries where the income gap between the rich and the poor is narrowest have the lowest overall mortality rates. Because income has a major impact on our material well-being and the extent to which we can exert control over many facets of our lives, it is an important determinant of health. There is, then, a connection between the WHO definition of health quoted previously (the capacity to act on and change our environment) and this view of the factors influencing health.

Research evidence in support of the socio-environmental model comes from a study of British civil servants which explored the links between the organization of work and health outcomes (Marmot and Theorell, 1988). It

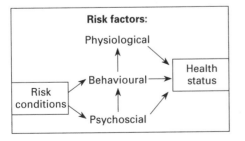

Fig. 11.2 The socioenvironmental approach to health. From Labonte (1993), with permission.

confirmed work conducted in Sweden which showed that cardiovascular disease was more common among those who had a low level of control over their work (Johnson and Hall, 1988). None of the subjects in the British study were living in poverty; nevertheless, there were differences in health status according to occupational grade. Those in the lowest grade had mortality rates three times that of those in the highest grade and higher rates of diseases such as lung cancer and bronchitis. Rates of smoking were twice as high in low- compared to high-grade workers. Another interesting finding was that, while blood pressure levels were similar for low- and high-grade civil servants when at work, they declined much more for the latter than the former when they were at home. This study concluded that the freedom to make decisions at work, particularly when jobs are stressful or psychologically demanding, is linked to at-risk behaviours such as smoking and physiological risk factors such as high blood pressure and health outcomes.

Studies in dentistry have also focused on work and its health effects. Recent evidence has emerged, for example, that stress in the workplace is linked to periodontal disease (Marcenes, 1994). A study of dental assistants found that job stress, job satisfaction and social support at work were associated with mental and emotional well-being (Locker, 1995).

To return to the concept of health outlined above, these studies confirm that the social environments in which we live and work can have a direct impact on our health and an indirect impact by inducing disease.

Defining health promotion

Health promotion is often referred to as a new strategy for improving the health of populations. This is not strictly correct. It is better viewed as the modern equivalent of the public health movement of the 19th century which contributed to the decline of infectious diseases through improvements to the physical environment and the promotion of personal hygiene. It has been defined as 'the process of enabling people to increase control over and to improve their health' (WHO, 1984). To this end, it draws on both behavioural and socioenvironmental perspectives and employs a comprehensive set of strategies:

> Health promotion policy combines diverse but complementary approaches including legislation, fiscal measures, taxation and organizational change. It is coordinated action which leads to health, income and social policies that foster greater equity. Joint action contributes to safer goods and services, healthier public services and cleaner, more enjoyable environments (WHO, 1984).

A major implication of this is that health promotion involves more than the actions of individuals; it involves communities, community groups, formal organizations such as schools or workplaces, pressure groups and political parties and governments at all levels. It recognizes that our health can be influenced in significant ways by the decisions that others take on our behalf and seeks to involve communities in those decisions so that they enhance rather than damage our health. Examples of practical application in oral health promotion involving community-based action are given in Chapter 15.

Health promotion principles

In an early document, the WHO (1984) outlined a set of principles and priorities for health promotion:

1 Health promotion involves the population as a whole in the context of their everyday lives rather than focusing on people who are sick or at risk for specific diseases.
2 It is directed towards action on the determinants of health and requires close cooperation between many different sectors of society.
3 It combines many different approaches and requires organizational change, community development and local activities to identify and remove health hazards.
4 Health promotion aims at effective and concrete public participation and requires that problem-defining and decision-making lifeskills be developed further in individuals and communities.
5 While it is an activity in the health and social fields, it is not a medical service; health professionals have a special contribution to make in the areas of education and advocacy.

The document also indicated that the main aim of health promotion was to increase access to health for all, to reduce inequalities in health and maximize the opportunities people have for improving their health status. Developing an environment conducive to health, strengthening social networks and social supports, promoting healthy behaviours and the capacity to cope and developing and disseminating health knowledge were also identified as important initial goals for health promotion activities.

A later publication, the *Ottawa Charter for Health Promotion* (WHO, 1986) continued the task of identifying activities that were regarded at the heart of the health promotion approach. Five broad actions were specified:

1 *Create supportive environments.* The inextricable links between the environment and health have already been outlined. Creating supportive environments goes somewhat beyond this; it means ensuring that the physical and social environments in which we live maximize the possibility of leading healthy lives. In short, these are environments which 'make healthy choices the easy choices'. A good example is offered by legislation which has banned smoking in the workplace and other public areas. This makes it much easier for non-smokers to escape the effects of second-hand smoke and also acts to support those who aim to reduce or give up smoking altogether. Since smoking is now accepted as a risk factor for periodontal disease, such actions help promote oral as well as general health. An example with respect to dental health would be working with schools to ensure that only sugar-free foods and drinks are available to students.

2 *Build healthy public policy.* Mention has already been made of the fact that decisions taken by organizations at all levels can promote or damage our health. Building healthy public policies means working to ensure that all organizations must take account of the potential health effects of the policies they develop and implement. This is particularly important with respect to central government who control and create policy for diverse sectors such as transportation, agriculture, energy and income, all of which can have important health ramifications. A good example is given by decisions taken by the government of Ontario when faced with the task of reducing public sector spending. Two options were presented: eliminate 40 000 public sector jobs or implement an across-the-board 5% salary cut for all employees. The latter was chosen on the grounds that its negative health impact was likely to be less than the creation of unemployment for substantial numbers of people.

3 *Strengthen community action.* Health promotion involves public participation and works through the actions of communities in identifying priorities, planning strategies and implementing them to enhance health. An important task for health promotion is to increase the ability of communities to recognize and change those aspects of their physical and social environment which are hazardous to health or encourage behaviours likely to damage health. Water fluoridation was implemented in many communities only because dental health professionals were able to work with and obtain the support and involvement of the public in persuading local politicians to implement the measure. Another example is given by Lee (1991) who worked with senior organizations and other interest groups to secure a major reorganization of dental public health service in the city of Toronto. As a result of this, professional and political action services became directed at disadvantaged and high-risk groups such as low-income elderly people and recent immigrants.

4 *Develop personal skills.* Individuals as well as communities can undertake actions to improve their health. However, information and education are necessary to enable them to make choices which promote health and enhance their ability to cope with the stresses and strains of daily life. Such education can be provided in a wide range of settings such as schools and places of work.

5 *Reorient health services.* Health services have traditionally been more concerned with curing disease than promoting health. Consequently, the formal health care system needs to expand its activities beyond the provision of clinical services to address the health needs of individuals and communities and move towards the goal of health gain.

These five strategies have the aim of promoting equity in health by maximizing everyone's opportunities to be healthy, and reducing inequality by ensuring that everyone achieves their health potential.

Promoting oral health

As mentioned previously, dental services have traditionally been concerned with treating and, to a lesser extent, preventing two major diseases–caries and periodontal disease. Other conditions such as mucosal disorders, oral cancer, temporomandibular disorders, salivary problems such as xerostomia and trauma to the teeth and mouth have also been a focus of dental practice. The main factors related to these disorders are dietary sugars, inadequate fluoride intake, poor oral hygiene, smoking, alcohol, stress and accidents. Since most of these factors are implicated in other chronic disorders, promoting oral health and promoting general health are one and the same thing (Sheiham, 1992).

From this point of view, oral disorders are primarily social and political in origin and can only be effectively controlled through appropriate public policies.

Whereas analyses of policies within general health promotion are relatively common, research of policies in oral health have been extremely rare (Schou, 1992). It is perhaps relevant to define briefly the term policy, as it has been classified and categorized in many different ways, and often suffered ambiguity and abuse (Feldman, 1978). Two sharply differing interpretations can be identified. The first and most common usage defines health policies as statements of authority often adopted by governments on behalf of the public in order to improve the health and welfare of the population. Health policy in this sense implies a centrally determined basis for action. A second interpretation suggests that health policy is what health agencies actually do, rather than governmental directives. Defined in this way, policies can be determined only by examining the outcomes of decision-making and, hence, the accommodation of dominance prevailing both within and among organizations. Regarding oral health promotion and oral health policy, three distinctions should be made:

1 policy–authoritative statements of intent;
2 policy output–what, in fact, is done to enforce these intentions;

3 policy impact–the consequences of policy and policy output.

No matter which way we look at policies, it is clear that policy-making is related to the notion of power. In a social context, power may be defined as the capacity of an individual or a group of individuals to modify the conduct of other individuals or groups in the manner desired and to prevent modification of this conduct in a manner that is not desired. Exercise of power in public policy means determining the way decisions are made (Smith, 1976). To illustrate how power is exercised, the model suggested by Smith (1976) may be useful (Fig. 11.3).

Four different types of power involved in policy-making can be distinguished: first, authoritative power. It implies legitimacy–that the person in authority has the right to exercise power and that those over whom the power is exercised recognize this right and therefore their own duty to obey.

The second form of power is that of expertise. To be an authority on a particular subject may give one power. Health professionals in the service of government are said to have power because of authoritative knowledge. The two forms of power, the authority of the office-holder, through legitimacy, and the expert-power can be termed causative–they can produce change in behaviour.

Another form of power is coercive power. When applied to the acts of governments in backing up their decisions with the effective use of sanctions, it is referred to as 'just power'. When applied to groups outside government, it resembles coercion in that threats may be

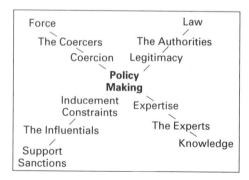

Fig. 11.3 Power in policy-making. From Smith (1976), with permission.

involved. Often the offer of rewards or the use of persuasion are part of the relationship between groups and the government and more appropriately the term 'influence' rather than coercion is used. The concept of 'influence' suggests a relative rather than an absolute power and the interplay of competing influences representing the conflicting interests concerned with practically every policy issue.

Health professionals have the potential of using both coercive or influential powers through support or sanctions and causative power through legitimacy and expertise. Obviously different types of power and different combinations are used relating to particular issues or a particular time in history. In the oral health field, power in the form of expertise may be most effective on issues such as water fluoridation, whereas 'influential power' in the form of support or sanctions may be more useful on issues relating to financing oral health care.

Peter Self (1985) draws a distinction between theories about the use and distribution of power and theories about the influence of personal and social values. He claims that power, on its own, is an inadequate explanatory notion because it leaves out the social meanings which people attach to its use. Authority represents an exercise of power which is supported by social beliefs and norms; and when their supports weaken, the exercise of authority becomes challenged. A 'values' approach is concerned with the procedures and goals which individuals or groups accept as being desirable or necessary, and which they suppose may justify the use of coercive power of government. It appears thus, that based on and supported by social beliefs and norms, oral health promotion needs both expert power and influential power to influence policy, policy output and policy impact.

Sheiham (1995) has identified the following six policy areas as being essential to improving the oral health of the population:

1 a food and health policy to reduce sugar consumption;
2 a community approach to improve body and oral hygiene;
3 a smoking cessation policy;
4 a policy on reducing accidents;
5 policies on water fluoridation;
6 ensuring access to appropriate preventive dental care.

It is hoped that it has become clear from reading this chapter that effective policies for oral health care and the problems posed by oral diseases and disorders are only likely to come about through a health promotion approach.

Key concepts in health promotion

Finally, there are three concepts central to oral health promotion, touched upon in the general description of the approach and its principles, which require further elaboration:

1 *Equity and inequality.* Equity and inequality are linked to social justice and human rights. Equity refers to differences in opportunities to be healthy and inequality to actual and measurable differences in health status. Both terms imply that these differences are unfair and unjust and that society has a moral obligation to minimize them to the extent possible (Whithead, 1991). For example, in Canada, the old and the poor are far less likely than the young and the wealthy to be covered by dental insurance plans even though they have higher dental care needs (Locker and Leake, 1993). Other groups face barriers to adequate dental care because of language and cultural differences. Ensuring that the entire population has access to appropriate and affordable dental care is one step to equity and equality in oral health.
2 *Empowerment.* Empowerment is the most important idea within health promotion. It is often a difficult idea for health professionals to grasp since most have been trained in a model in which the health care provider is an expert and the patient is a recipient of this expertise. It may also be difficult for health professionals to accept, since it requires the transfer of responsibility for and control over health from professionals to people. Nevertheless, the empowerment of others is one of the most important functions of health professionals with respect to health promotion. It involves the provision of health education, teaching people the skills they need in order to use health information effectively and increasing their confidence that they have a choice and can exercise control over the options available to them.
3 *Advocacy.* A second important role for health professionals is that of advocacy for

health. This involves educating politicians, community leaders and other influential individuals such as representatives of the media in order to influence the decisions that have a bearing on the health of the population. In this role, health professionals need to be both technical experts, providing the scientific basis for decision-making, and political activists in mobilizing support for policies which improve health.

Conclusion

Health promotion offers a new and often complex approach to improving both general and oral health. It has sometimes proved to be perplexing to health professionals who have been trained in the biomedical approach and find its concepts and principles unfamiliar. Health promotion shifts the responsibility for health from the formal health care system to individuals, communities and decision-makers at all levels of society. In addition, implementing health promotion requires a different set of skills from those usually learned in schools of dentistry, nursing and medicine. This suggests that the training of health professionals needs to be changed to match the broader role required by the new public health. Training in the behavioural sciences and experience working with communities and interest groups are essential if health promotion is to become a major force in the task of improving the population's health.

References

Cochrane, A. (1972) *Effectiveness and Efficiency: Random Reflections on the Health Service.* The Nuffield Provincial Hospitals Trust, London.

Department of Health and Social Security (1976) *Prevention and Health: Everybody's Business.* HMSO, London.

Epp, J. (1986) *Achieving Health for All: A Framework for Health Promotion.* Minister of Supply and Services Canada, Ottawa.

Feldman, E.J. (1978) Comparative public policy: field or method? *Comparative Politics* 10:288.

Fleck-Kandath, C., Tedesco, L., Keffer, M. *et al.* (1988) Distress and oral health behaviour reports. *Journal of Dental Research* 67(special issue): abstract 1322.

Green, L. and Kreuter, M. (1990) Health promotion as a public health strategy for the 1990s. *Annual Review of Public Health* 11: 319–334.

Hobbs, P.R., Ballinger, C.B., McClure, A. *et al.* (1985) Factors associated with psychiatric morbidity in men: a general practice survey. *Acta Psychiatrica Scandinavica* 71:281–286.

Johnson, J. and Hall, E. (1988) Strain, workplace social support and cardiovascular disease: a cross-sectional study of the Swedish working population. *American Journal of Public Health* 78:1336–1342.

Labonte, R. (1993) *Health Promotion and Empowerment. Issues in Health Promotion Series #3.* Centre for Health Promotion, University of Toronto.

Labonte, R. and Penfold, S. (1981) Canadian perspectives in health promotion: a critique. *Health Education* 4:4–9.

Lalonde, M. (1974) *A New Perspective on the Health of Canadians.* Health and Welfare Canada, Ottawa.

Leake, J., Hawkins, R. and Locker, D. (1994) Social and functional impact of reduced posterior units in older adults. *Journal of Oral Rehabilitation* 21:1–10.

Lee, J. (1991) The reorganization of the city of Toronto dental services: a community development model. *Journal of Public Health Dentistry* 51:99–102.

Locker, D. (1989) *An Introduction to Behavioural Science and Dentistry.* Tavistock/Routledge, London.

Locker, D. (1995) Work stress, job satisfaction and emotional well-being among Canadian dental assistants. *Oral Epidemiology and Community Dentistry* (n press).

Locker, D. and Leake, J. (1993) Inequities in health: dental insurance coverage and use of dental services in older Ontario adults. *Canadian Journal of Public Health* 84:139–140.

MacIntyre, S. (1986) The patterning of health by social position in contemporary Britain: directions for sociological research. *Social Science and Medicine* 23:393–415.

McKeown, T. (1979) *The Role of Medicine: Dream, Mirage or Nemesis?* Blackwell Scientific, Oxford.

Marcenes, M. (1994) Work stress and periodontal disease. *Community Dentistry and Oral Epidemiology*

Marcenes, W. and Sheiham, A. (1996) The relationship between marital quality and oral health status. *Psychology and Health* 11: 357–369.

Marmot, M. and Theorell, T. (1988) Social class and cardiovsacular disease: the contribution of work. *International Journal of Health Services* 18:432–445.

Marmot, M., Kogevinas, M. and Elston, M.A. (1991) Socioeconomic status and disease. In: *Health Promotion Research: Towards a New Social Epidemiology* (Badura, B. and Kickbusch, I., eds). WHO Regional Office for Europe, Copenhagen.

Murray, J. (1983) The changing pattern of dental disease and treatment. In: *The Prevention of Dental Disease* (Murray, J., ed.) Oxford University Press, Oxford.

Schmoldt, R.A., Pope, C.R. and Hibbard, J.H. (1989) Marital interaction and the health and well-being of spouses. *Women Health* 15:35–56.

Schou, L. (1992) *The Role of Oral Health Promotion: An Oral Health Policy. A Comparative Analysis of Two European Countries.* Thesis. University of Edinburgh.

Self, P. (1985) *Political Theories of Modern Government, Its*

Role and Reform. George Allen and Unwin, London.

Sheiham, A. (1992) The role of the dental team in promoting dental health and general health through oral health. *International Dental Journal* **42**223–228.

Sheiham, A. (1995) Development of oral health strategies. In: *Turning Strategy into Action* (Kay, E., ed.) Eden Bianchi Press, Manchester.

Smith, B. (1976) *Policy-making in British Government.* Pittman Press, Bath.

Townsend, P. (1990) Individual or social responsibility for premature death? Current controversies in the British debate about death. *International Journal of Health Services* **20**:373–392.

Wallerstein, N. (1992) Powerlessness, empowerment and health: implications for health promotion programs. *American Journal of Health Promotion* **6**:197–205.

Whitehead, M. (1991) *Swimming Upstream. Trends and Prospects in Education for Health.* King's Fund Institute, London.

World Health Organization (1984) *Health Promotion: A Discussion Document on the Concept and Principles.* WHO Regional Office for Europe, Copenhagen.

World Health Organization (1986) *Ottawa Charter for Health Promotion.* WHO.

12

Principles of health behaviour and health education

Pauline M. McGoldrick

Introduction

This chapter explores an important element in community health research, that of translating the explanations which determine behaviour change into health programmes that are intense and efficacious (Oldenburg, 1994). The chapter also examines the ways in which theories from health and social psychology can come together with the aims of health education to support beneficial changes in health behaviour. The area of health examined is oral health. While the chapter focuses primarily on the psychosocial explanations, it is clear that health involves more than the isolated individual and includes economic, environmental and cultural variables. These factors are considered in Chapters 3, 11 and 15 and complement the approaches in this chapter. The theories chosen in this chapter are those relevant in both dental public health and clinical practice in dentistry. Before embarking on a theoretical pathway it is useful to place oral health in the context of general health.

Oral health in the context of general health

Over the past number of years there has been a dedicated movement towards positive health, healthy lifestyles and increased health choices for everyone. Incorporating and developing measures of quality-adjusted life years (QALY) reflects this trend. Developing appropriate measures for oral health needs is problematic as many oral-health problems are non-life-threatening, and hence efforts to publicize their importance in terms of morbidity are compromised. Furthermore, in terms of quality of well-being, oral health is less weighted when it comes to identifying symptoms which compromise a healthy life (Kaplan, 1994). Nevertheless, the very presence of oral health-related problems in such tabulations indicates its relevance to health and well-being. The development of sociodental indicators to reflect impairment, disability and handicap in oral health is discussed in detail in Chapter 4 of this book. Given the widespread prevalence of dental disease and its painful consequences, poor oral health is without doubt recognized as being relevant to health, well-being, and consequently, quality of life.

The desire to maintain people at an almost perfect state of oral health rather than wait to treat them after they have developed oral or dental diseases has been at the forefront of promoting a healthy lifestyle and modifying habits which prevent optimal oral health status being reached (Taylor, 1990). This is gaining emphasis with the changing dental treatment needs as more teeth are retained through middle age. This will continue as succeeding cohorts of young people have fewer fillings and teeth extracted. Evidence for these developments comes from a number of studies reporting changes in the pattern of dental disease and the delivery of oral health care, all supporting the ensuing emphasis on prevention (Nowak and Anderson, 1990; Mason, 1992; Todd and Lader, 1991). Furthermore, at a contractual level, the role of general dental practitioners strongly incorporates prevention as a core principle, particularly the promotion of self-care behaviours based on a prevention paradigm (Horowitz, 1990).

These factors together with the public's increasing expectation of a natural dentition for life have resulted in an even wider role for the dentist who not only has to continue restorative work but who is now also involved in primary prevention and health education (Levine, 1989). However, despite improvements, resistant groups remain a challenge. Poverty and social stratification continue to be major discriminators of health. Treatment needs differ both locally and nationally. All these factors result in an ever-increasing need for effective prevention at secondary and tertiary levels as well (Craft and Chamberlain, 1992; Brown, 1994). In establishing and promoting oral health goals for the population at large, this heterogeneity makes it difficult to adopt specific models to explain the failure of optimal dental health. A holistic approach to community oral health is thus called for in order to understand the barriers to promoting healthy dental behaviour globally.

Conceptualizing health, health behaviour and health education

Health

To understand the major role that dentistry has been recognized to play in the health of the nation (Harcourt, 1994), an appreciation of what constitutes health and oral health in particular is worthwhile. In earlier days, *health* was a notion based on medical models of disease and thus disease-focused. Today however, the definition of health most employed is the one given by the World Health Organization (WHO, 1964), which states that 'health is a state of complete physical, mental, and social well-being and not merely the absence of disease or infirmity'.

What this definition recognizes relevant to oral health care is, according to Seeman (1989), that the terms 'physical, mental and social ... conceptualise health according to a human-system framework which ... invites a behavioural science-oriented approach to the study of health'. Furthermore, it emphasizes the idea that health goes beyond the realm of the individual to include social, ecological and economic facets of health. In terms of oral health, the focus is no longer just related to treating dental disease *per se*, but to the whole constellation of factors which influence and can prevent it, in particular, psychosocial, economic and cultural.

Health behaviour

The meaning of health behaviour has until recently followed a similar route to health, in that it began its existence as a biological and disease model rather than a psychosocial model (Anderson *et al.*, 1988). Now, however, and in similar fashion to health, emphasis in construing health behaviours has shifted to an understanding of the many social, cultural, economic, long-standing belief and attitudinal factors which affect them. A working definition of health behaviour has been documented by Gochman (1988) and states that health behaviour is:

> those personal attributes such as beliefs, expectations, motives, values, perceptions, and other cognitive elements; personality characteristics, including affective and emotional states and traits; and overt behaviour patterns, actions and habits that relate to health maintenance, to health restoration and to health improvement.

While this definition follows the traditional psychosocial perspective, other definitions are broader in scope, for example, that of Steptoe and colleagues (1994) who define health behaviour as: 'activities undertaken by people in order to protect, promote or maintain health, and to prevent disease'.

There are many realms of behaviours, but in a health context the realms of behaviour which are the most relevant are those that relate to the risk of developing disease or health problems (Baranowski, 1990). Dental health behaviours have been categorized according to 'brushing behaviour', 'complex dental behaviour' and 'sugar behaviour' (Rise and Holund, 1990). Health-related behaviour change would reduce unhealthy behaviours such as sugar in the diet and smoking, as well as increase healthy behaviours such as flossing and dental attendance (Prochaska, 1994). Many general health factors are of direct relevance to oral health, e.g. smoking, diabetes, alcohol, stress, medication (Horowitz, 1990). A distinction is made between health-related behaviours and health-directed behaviours. The latter refer to 'actions which are carried out in the belief that they will benefit health'. The former may have dental health consequences but are undertaken for non-dental health reasons, e.g. reducing sugar in the diet to lose weight rather than for dental health (Freeman and Linden, 1995).

Health education

Oldenburg (1994), reporting on general health promotion, argues that 'with the identification of the importance of behavioural, cultural, social and economic factors as determinants of disease, there is a need for all intervention strategies and approaches, particularly those focusing on lifestyle change, to take account of these'. Health education is one medium generally used to promote health in the population. Health education, thus a functional component of health promotion, is defined in numerous ways and includes:

the process of assisting individuals, acting separately or collectively, to make informed decisions about matters affecting their personal health and that of others (Brown, 1994)

any planned combination of learning experiences designed to predispose, enable, and reinforce voluntary behaviour conducive to health, in individuals, groups, or communities (Frazier, 1992).

Ashley considers the aims of dental health education from three perspectives: adoption of appropriate attitude and lifestyles; making the best of conditions and disorders which cannot be prevented or treated adequately; and encouraging better use of dental services (Ashley, 1989). On the other hand, Croucher (1993) purports health education to be 'a straightforward and unitary activity emphasizing the issue of prevention and changing patient behaviour'.

According to Tones and Tilford (1994), while different definitions will reflect competing ideologies, the mainstay of health education will be based on learning approaches. Furthermore, they argue that given this fact, the definition they offer below will remain unchanged in the face of changing ideologies:

any intentional activity which is designed to achieve health or illness related learning, i.e. some relatively permanent change in an individual's capability of

disposition. Effective health education may, thus, produce changes in knowledge and understanding or ways of thinking; it may influence or clarify values; it may bring about some shift in belief or attitude; it may facilitate the acquisition of skills; it may even affect changes in behaviour or lifestyle' (Tones and Tilford, 1994).

All these definitions highlight the importance of healthy attitudes and lifestyle in much the same vein as health and health behaviour definitions. One presumption which is defined in the statements above is that health education follows a knowledge, attitude and behaviour route, with information being transmitted and attitude and behaviour change taking place. However, there is now much evidence that this is not a linear progression. Knowledge is necessary but not sufficient for behaviour change, as will be demonstrated with reference to the models which help us understand and predict behaviour.

A health psychology perspective

While the definitions of health, health behaviour and health education define outcome, on their own they add little to our understanding of the processes involved or indeed how difficult these can be. What these interpretations presuppose is the link between the basic concept of health, its relation to promoting positive changes in health behaviour and the enhancement of these ideals through health education. In health education the focus is to try to influence behaviour change in individuals by targeting those health-damaging behaviours and replacing them with healthier behaviours.

From this point of view, it seems appropriate that research based on health behaviour be translated into the practices of health education (Anderson *et al.*, 1988). The ideal health message is one that changes a person's health behaviour for the better. However, the step from a health message to a regularly practised health behaviour is big (DiMatteo, 1991). Several factors impinge on an individual's ability to follow healthy practices. How do we explain the process of why one person will adopt a healthy lifestyle while others do not, even if both know that they are at risk of developing dental disease? More specifically, why engage in a particular oral health-related behaviour, such as tooth-brushing twice a day, flossing regularly or attending the dentist every 6 months? We not only have to discover and understand why things exist the way they do, but to learn how things can be made different, i.e. how people can change potentially health-damaging behaviours and adopt health-promoting behaviours.

The traditional focus of health education providing information and determining what changes should be made, in partnership with providing the necessary skills through behavioural strategies, and thus demonstrating how the changes can be made, serves to reduce the interface between health education and the promotion of dental health behaviours (Brownell and Cohen, 1995). In addition, messages need to be tailored to the audience to address social, cultural and environmental barriers to health education. (The effects of social class on dental health and dental attendance have been considered in Chapter 3.)

Determinants of health education

In health education, models are based on two principal approaches: the *applied models* and the *planning models*.

Applied models

The *preventive model* supports a victim-blaming approach through its persuasive and prescriptive stance. The *radical model* has also been criticized for its unethical raising of consciousness without providing the means and resources to change. The *empowerment* model endorses freedom of choice without any guidance over outcome (Tones, 1986; for an excellent review of the three models, see Tones and Tilford, 1994).

Planning models

The planning models can be considered theoretical (Schmidt *et al.*, 1990). They offer guidance, in terms of planning behaviour change programmes in large groups of people, and the evaluation of such programmes. Two of the more common models which will be described here are the *communication–behaviour change* model (McGuire, 1984), and the *precede–proceed* model (Green and Kreuter, 1991). A further model is the *persuasive health message (PHM) framework*

(Witte, 1995). This offers a comprehensive and global guide to developing health education programmes from a psychological perspective.

Communication–behaviour change model

This model, developed by William McGuire, a social psychologist, offers a way of designing public health communication campaigns. However, such strategies which promote the adoption of healthier lifestyles have not been a roaring success (McGuire, 1984). Most of them are based on an information–persuasion model which merely serve to influence knowledge and attitudes without necessarily impacting on behaviour. This is not surprising given the range of outcomes such campaigns are meant to achieve. They are meant to inform people of the health message. They expect listening and understanding, as well as having a positive attitude towards the health message. Implicitly, they expect the acquisition of the skills necessary to modify or change behaviour, or even to learn new skills, and all from a poster or leaflet (McGuire, 1984). McGuire argues that for campaigns to be more successful, they should follow the steps outlined in his communication–behaviour change model. This model provides guidance based on the principles of communication (McGuire, 1984), with the emphasis of the communication being to influence attitude and behaviour change. The model is based on input and output factors. The input factors reflect the health message being sent and the output factors refer to how well the message has been received in relation to any resulting attitude and behaviour change. Hence, for success to occur, the target audience must be exposed to the health message; attend to it; approve of the message and show interest in it; understand it (*knowledge*); acquire the skills to attend to it (*behaviour*); agree to it (*attitude/belief*); incorporate the new attitude and knowledge into memory; undertake information search and retrieval; make decisions from memory recall (*intention/contemplation*); act on this decision (*action*); reinforce behaviour and maintain the new health behaviour over time (*maintenance*).

Persuasive health message framework

The PHM framework identifies two factors in the planning stages of a health campaign which are necessary for success and refers to them as constant and transient factors. The constant factors are those which are applicable to any health message, regardless of the type of message and audience, and should form the basis of all health messages. These are *threat, efficacy, cues* and *audience profile*. Threat relates to the target population's perceptions of *susceptibility* and *severity* of health threat. Efficacy covers both *self-efficacy* and *response-efficacy*, that is, the targeted individuals perceive that they are capable of averting any threat which they may feel. The message contains information about how to cope with and control the threat. This enhances motivation by providing the knowledge and in some cases the means to change. Cues refer to indirect influences on the health message. The *message* itself (pitch, tone, meaning of the language) as well as the *source* (credibility, power, attractiveness) of the message are important variables. Audience profile takes account of the demographic, psychographic and customs or values of the individuals. In this way the health message to be delivered appeals to each of these characteristics of the population.

The transient parts of the health message follow closely the elements of the theory of reasoned action. The framework suggests identification of *salient beliefs*, not just of the targeted audience, but of those in contact with the audience (*salient referents*). Furthermore, the health message must be in keeping with these beliefs (*message goals*). This information provides the basis for determining the threat and efficacy components of the constants part of the framework. Cultural, environmental and mode of message delivery (preferences) feed into the cues and audience profile elements of the framework.

Precede–proceed model

Although similar in its aims to the previous models, the precede–proceed model provides a framework for not only delivering a health education programme but also assessing its ability to meet its aims. The model identifies the necessary steps which must precede a health education programme design and moves on to provide guidance on how to initiate and implement programmes at local, national and international levels. This model identifies nine phases to the design, implementation and evaluation of a health education programme (Fig. 12.1).

In relation to oral health education, the

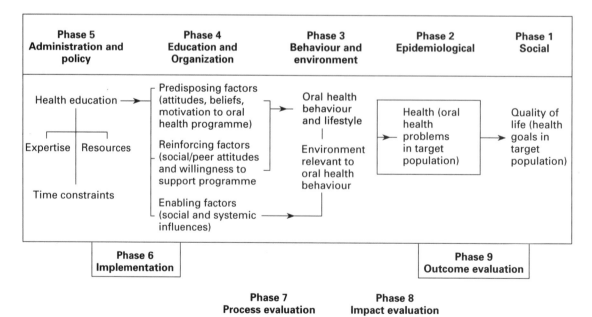

Fig. 12.1 The precede–proceed model for oral health promotion planning and evaluation. Adapted from Green and Kreuter (1991)

planning or precede elements include identifying the health goals of the target population (phase 1), followed by the major oral health-related problems which affect the people (phase 2). The programme is likely to be more successful if the health problems causing the most concern to people are targeted. This has the added effect that people are more likely to want to reduce those problems and therefore, may be more prepared to change their behaviour. In phase 3, the specific influences on the health-related problem need to be identified. The intervention programme will need to address those present behaviours related to oral health, as well as the environmental influences which may impinge on those behaviours (phase 3). Health education plays an important role in this model and a thorough investigation of the factors which influence behaviour change is required (phase 4). These include three variables, first, predisposing factors such as attitudes and beliefs which can increase or decrease the motivation of the individual to change. Second, enabling factors are barriers which originate in society. They include lack of money and lack of control over the promotion of unhealthy behaviours. Third, reinforcing factors relate to positive and negative feedback concerning the behaviours to be changed. Positive reinforcement will increase the likelihood of a behaviour and negative reinforcement will have the same effect.

Once the information concerning the design of a programme has been decided, the next step is to look at the barriers to its implementation, e.g. facilities, expertise, finance. A particular programme design may have to be modified due to administrative constraints. Modifications might include targeting only a small section of those in need or using a less expensive method (phase 5). Implementation of the programme is much more difficult in practice. Unknown difficulties and constraints may come to the surface at this time, leading to a re-evaluation of the original design (phase 6). Evaluation of the programme is comprehensive according to this model and focuses on three directions—process, impact and outcome. Educational and organizational factors which were targeted are examined for success in the process evaluation (phase 7), while the evaluation of the impact of the programme determines whether or not the behavioural and environmental factors were successfully altered (phase 8). Finally, outcome evaluation determines success in terms of improved health and movement towards health goals (phase 9).

Chapter 15 describes a number of evaluations of dental health education programmes as well as some broader programmes in the field of health promotion.

Health education interventions which influence health behaviour change

Health education's sole purpose is to improve health through education (D'Onofrio, 1992). However, health education will only be successful if there is an understanding of the conceptions of health held by the population being targeted for change (Raaheim, 1990).

For the most part dental health education interventions already fall into several categories with much overlap. The first is what Sheiham and Croucher (1994) call 'chairside dental health education' which occurs at the *micro* level. Second, educational interventions can be realized at a community or *meso* level, or can be aimed at the population as a whole, the *macro* level. There is a general belief that most dental health education is carried out in general dental practitioner surgeries at a micro level (Whittle *et al.*, 1994). This area for health education is becoming increasingly important. Yet, prevention both takes place and is most beneficial when it is aimed at all three levels, so optimizing health gain.

A range of health education intervention programmes have been aimed at reducing morbidity from dental disease and promoting the use of dental health behaviours both locally and nationally. Health education interventions vary according to group (small to large) and level of involvement (low to high) and generally range from teaching skills to education or information-giving at an individual, group or community level (Schmidt *et al.*, 1990). Inoculation-based prevention which involves reinforcing already established health-enhancing attitudes, e.g. opposition to smoking which can become challenged in the teenage years (Pfau, 1995), is infrequently used in oral health education. On the whole, persuasive strategies which serve to change already established attitudes and behaviour are the most common.

Oral health education in practice

Mass media campaigns

Mass media campaigns have been employed extensively (Rise and Sogaard, 1988; Towner, 1984; Croucher *et al.*, 1985; Schou, 1987; Croxson, 1993). One campaign developed by the Norwegian Dental Association utilized mass media to increase awareness of periodontal diseases, prevention and behaviour (Rise and Sogaard, 1988). The campaign initially aimed to increase awareness of dental practitioners and then to engage them in promoting the health messages to people visiting dental practices. The methods used in the campaign included written information in the form of a booklet and newspaper articles, together with radio and television broadcasts. Evaluation of this educational campaign revealed an increase in knowledge related specifically to tooth-brushing, but there was no effect on the modification of behaviours related to the development of periodontal diseases.

The authors suggested that, similar to many other mass media campaigns, the current attitudes and beliefs of the audience are reinforced with little effect on changing to alternative behaviours. They highlighted the need for educational programmes which are skill-based in order to influence behaviour change and, in particular, to ensure that the target audience actually understand the information being transmitted. Backer and colleagues (1992) argue that behaviour change can be attained provided the goals are modest and deemed to be achievable. Whilst acknowledging these difficulties with both the present campaign and other similar ventures, the authors offer little in the way of guidance as to how these results could be improved upon and particularly how knowledge can be incorporated into already established value systems. It may be necessary to weave other concepts into intervention strategies designed to change health behaviour, targeting specifically those who perceive themselves to be at risk of developing disease and therefore maximizing health gains for that group. Alternatively, expand the perspective by focusing not just on the individual but adopting a holistic approach considering social, cultural and environmental norms. Clearly, this requires a knowledge of the target group's norms.

Fear communications

Fear-arousing communications have been used with some persuasive effects on behaviour. These communications persuade by highlighting the negative results of not adhering to a health message (Hale and Dillard, 1995). In oral health well-recognized fear appeals include grossly carious teeth, edentulousness and oral cancer. According to some authors, these types of intervention can influence health-related behaviour if the information is perceived as something of importance to the person; if the individual is supplied with alternatives; if he or she feels in control; if he or she has the personal efficacy to change. Barriers may be that the information is too threatening and a dismissal or blocking of the message at a cognitive level leads to a defensive reaction. Often with this type of programme any changes which are made are not maintained. The individual will return to the previous situation when the threat is no longer felt. This method is based on the idea of *cognitive dissonance* which provides a conflict between attitude and behaviour. For example, a picture of grossly carious teeth with information that this can be caused by not brushing regularly may create an uneasy feeling in someone who does not brush his or her teeth regularly, and result in the uptake of this new behaviour.

Evans *et al.* (1970) used a pre-post campaign evaluation including both positive and negative fear appeals. A total of 364 schoolchildren were targeted and subjected randomly to one of five persuasive health messages, thereby creating five experimental groups, in a study into compliance with dental hygiene. Measures of information gained, anxiety, intention to behave, reported behaviour and actual behaviour were gathered before, and on three occasions following, the introduction of the health campaign. When examined in the context of message retention and compliance, the group exposed to the positive appeal gave verbal responses to comply, as well as reporting having complied, at a higher level than those subjected to negative appeals.

Self-directed dental health–skills training and patient information

Promoting self-care behaviours in patients is widespread in general health at a micro/meso level with a high success rate of behaviour change (Watson and Tharp, 1993). Yet, evidence from the dental field suggests that results are not as successful (Horowitz, 1990). In many cases, evidence for the failure of this method of health education in other fields can be applied to the dental area, in particular the claim that 'people do not fail at self-modification because the techniques do not work; they fail because they don't use the techniques' (Watson and Tharp, 1993). Therefore, this type of health education should not only encourage commitment to change and choose a change target, but work out a plan for change, re-evaluating progress and promoting maintenance of successful behaviour change. This process requires a dental health educator to be skilled in teaching the necessary skills to individuals. Skills in this sense extend far beyond the ability to teach, for example, appropriate brushing and flossing techniques. Skills relate to the ability to be able to support the individual to make this behaviour a regular part of life. This type of health education focuses primarily on the individual and his or her particular behaviour. A holistic, individual approach may be particularly appropriate care for patients with more difficult and intractable problems.

A case study published by Horowitz (1990) describes patient education using a self-directed learning programme called the self-care motivation model and demonstrates the use of this programme in the dental field. The aim of this approach is the achievement of health goals through personal growth and awareness. The model emphasizes five key components to influencing dental health-related behaviour change. These include establishing and documenting the dental health outcomes and behaviours for change, patient education to increase awareness and knowledge regarding antecedents and consequences of problem behaviours (thoughts, feelings, actions), increasing patient efficacy and choice, and finally, continuous monitoring and reinforcement. Using a model such as this the author demonstrates how smoking can be extinguished in a patient receiving dental treatment. More importantly however, he suggests that such treatments 'illustrate the potential for dental professionals to facilitate health behaviour change, and promote health enhancement among . . . patients' (Horowitz, 1990).

Alternatively, much of the self-directed health education takes the form of patient information leaflets. While this mode of health education has its merits particularly in relation to increasing knowledge and awareness, its ability to promote health-enhancing behaviours is limited. Nevertheless, unlike the self-directed approach, it is an inexpensive and resourceful way of targeting large sections of the population to consider health changes. Some guidelines are on offer for the production of such patient information in terms of increasing their usefulness to meet the aims of patient education (Newton, 1995). Newton surveyed general dental practice patient information leaflets. He recommends that these leaflets can be more beneficial if attention is paid to the following: appearance in a clear typeface; readability using short sentences, short words, avoidance of technically laden and redundant words, avoidance of unnecessary capitals; being active in language portayal; communication based on a personal or empathic approach.

Health behaviour models

Human behaviour is something with which each of us is familiar, yet when it comes to explaining why we do what we do, our understanding is still very limited (Kaplan *et al.*, 1993). The role which oral health determinants (diet, oral hygiene, smoking behaviours, adherence to dental advice, dentist attendance) play in the development of dental disease has been well-documented. Freeman and Linden (1995) quite rightly suggest that modification of present dental health practices is what is required. However, it is also likely that for some individuals, actually changing unhealthy behaviours and acquiring new skills will be equally important.

To understand the constellation of factors which have been identified as having a role in the execution and maintenance of health behaviours, we must try to explain in a logical way how these come about. Certainly the health education models described offer some insight into the relevant factors. Furthermore, various theoretical models have sprung up in the last 20–30 years which go some way to help us explain what influences health. These add new dimensions to our understanding but a complete integration to health education has yet to be developed. Nevertheless, it is important that health professionals who are involved in health education and the promotion of health-related behaviour understand the theoretical underpinnings of what they strive to achieve on a day-to-day basis.

The theoretical models to be presented can be used to explain many aspects of preventive behaviour at the primary, secondary and tertiary levels. Primary prevention, for example, includes brushing your teeth twice a day (no dental health problems and uses techniques to prevent dental disease). Secondary prevention, on the other hand, may mean attending the dentist for restorative treatment (dental disease treated by routine treatment methods), while tertiary prevention involves care of dentures (measures to replace lost teeth and return function to as normal as possible; Harris and Christen, 1991). Before moving on to a description of the various health-related models available, it is important to note that in their development, numerous concepts have been coined which help us understand the interactions between individuals, behaviour and environment. Each of these concepts will be described in succession.

Health belief model

The health belief model (HBM; Rosenstock *et al.*, 1988) provides us with a specific way of understanding and organizing personal beliefs that are relevant to health behaviour. In this model the authors try to understand the causal processes which underlie human behaviour. *Beliefs* relate to those assertions made by people of the link between an item, behaviour or idea (e.g. tooth-brushing) and some attitude (e.g. is time-consuming). These assertions can be numerous in relation to a specific target; however, only a few of an individual's beliefs will prevail in any one situation, i.e. the salient beliefs (Ajzen, 1991). Beliefs may derive from direct personal experience or vicarious learning and influence both how the person feels and his or her actions (DiMatteo, 1991). Health beliefs are thus those thoughts and feelings that play an important role in the practice or non-practice of health-related behaviours.

According to the HBM, the likelihood that a person will engage in a health behaviour depends directly on the outcome of several factors (Fig. 12.2). *Perceived seriousness* relates to the consequences a person thinks he or she is likely to experience if a health problem develops or the person fails to seek treatment for one. The more serious he or she believes the consequences to be personally, the more likely the individual is to take necessary action to prevent either a health problem developing or progression of an already identified health problem. *Perceived susceptibility* relates to the personal evaluation of the likelihood of developing a particular health problem. The more vulnerable to disease the individual perceives himself or herself to be, the more likely he or she is to take preventive action. A further important variable, *cues to action*, refers to a situation where a person who is made aware of a potential health problem (e.g. by means of a health education programme) is more likely to take preventive action than is someone who is not exposed to such information. The described factors lead the

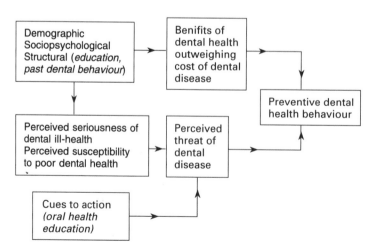

Fig. 12.2 The health belief model: beliefs which affect the uptake of a dental health-related behaviour. Adapted from Rosenstock *et al.* (1988).

individual to make at least two assessments. *Benefits outweighing costs* is the conclusion the individual must come to in order to proceed with a health action. Combined with this is the *perceived threat of the condition* which adds further weight to the likelihood of the person engaging in the appropriate health action. Importantly, the model also considers the demographic, sociopsychological and structural variables which further influence the outcome of following a more adaptive health behaviour.

Although the HBM is one of the most widely cited, it does not explain all of the factors relevant to the adoption of appropriate dental health behaviours. However, it has been applied to the field of dentistry, particularly in the area of dental compliance. In one study looking at the effect of health beliefs on compliance in periodontal patients, Kuhner and Raetzke (1989) assessed the health beliefs of 120 dental patients using a questionnaire based on the HBM. They found that motivation and perceived severity mostly predicted compliance with oral hygiene instruction, with perceived benefits and experience also being important predictors. The authors demonstrated a role for health beliefs in dental compliance with oral hygiene instruction. However, no single variable was able to explain the variance in compliance significantly. The authors conclude that, while the HBM aids us in our understanding of compliance, the process obviously involves more 'complex belief–opinion structures' than those identified in the study.

Protection–motivation theory

Other models have built on the HBM to help us understand further the variables involved in engaging in preventive behaviours. Protection–motivation theory is one such perspective which adds the concept of *efficacy* (belief that a specific preventive measure taken can be effective) to the variables already presented in the HBM. An individual who is self-efficacious believes in his or her capability successfully to carry out the behaviour required to bring about a desired outcome (Bandura, 1986). In other words, self-efficacy explains the role of personal mastery over human behaviour (Taal *et al.*, 1990). Protection–motivation theory, as its name suggests, is the motivation which the individual has, to partake in some kind of health-protecting action.

In this model, the sources of information which can initiate the cognitive mediating processes include both environment (health education) and personal (personality/coping) sources (Fig. 12.3). These sources of information initiate two appraisal processes: threat and coping appraisals. These cognitive processes comprise either the maladaptive or adaptive response(s) and the variables that increase or decrease the probability of the occurrence of the response. The likelihood of an individual being motivated to engage in a health-protective behaviour is dependent on these various cognitive mediating processes. The theory has been used in Figure 12.3 to illustrate the maladaptive response of eating sweets. The factors which increase the probability of continued sweet-eating are the intrinsic rewards such as bodily satisfaction and extrinsic rewards such as peer approval. Factors decreasing the probability of continued sweet-eating are, in a dental health context, beliefs in the severity of dental caries to health caused by eating sweets and in personal vulnerability to the disease. The adaptive response in this case is to stop making the maladaptive response, that is, stop eating sweets. Factors that increase the likelihood of this happening are the belief that it is an effective way to avoid dental caries and the belief that one can successfully stop consuming sweets. Factors decreasing the probability of stopping this behaviour are response costs such as overcoming temptation or the effort required to find alternatives to sweets.

While the merits of both the HBM and protection–motivation theory have been reported in aiding our understanding of the influences on health behaviour change, neither of these specific models, however, has had the success of the more general models of behaviour. In particular, our understanding is increased by those models which focus less on people as rational human beings but on complexities involved in human decision-making regarding health choices, including attitudes as well as beliefs. Two theories in particular are relevant to this general approach–the theory of reasoned action (Ajzen and Fishbein, 1980) and its updated counterpart, the theory of planned behaviour (Ajzen, 1988, 1991).

The theory of reasoned action

In the model of reasoned action, the predictor variable for adoption of health choices is the

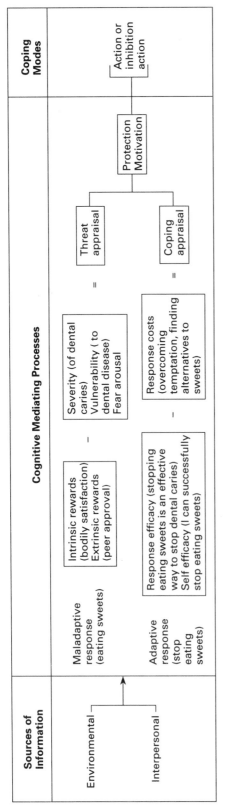

Fig. 12.3 Protection–motivation theory: processes influencing uptake of dental health-enhancing or dental health-damaging behaviours. Adapted from Rogers (1983).

individual's *intention* or commitment to carry out a health-related behaviour. Instead of beliefs being at the forefront, the authors postulate *attitudes* as being more important. An attitude explains the consistent response between an individual's feelings and a particular item or idea. Attitudes are said to stem from beliefs and can range from positive to negative (DiMatteo, 1991). According to this model when demonstrating intention, two considerations are important–the *individual's attitude* and his or her *subjective norms* towards the action. Subjective norms refer to the person's beliefs about what those people he or she considers important want him or her to do.

Hence, individuals' intentions to brush their teeth regularly will be determined by their attitudes towards brushing teeth which in turn will be underpinned by their beliefs in the outcome of competent tooth-brushing. A further factor which influences intention is individuals' representation of local opinions and their motivations relative to these. An example of how this model might work in dentistry is shown in Figure 12.4. An individual believes that tooth-brushing will improve dental health and aesthetics and also believes that others important to them also value this activity. Hence, the person feels motivated to do what is accepted practice in the environment, which leads to the subjective norm that tooth-brushing is an appropriate thing to do. Adding the positive attitude towards tooth-brushing to the above is likely to result in the intention to brush teeth regularly. This would be followed by the behaviour of regular tooth-brushing (this model can also be applied to effective or frequent tooth-brushing).

The theory of reasoned action has been applied to the dental field in a number of studies (Tedesco *et al.*, 1992, 1993; Freeman and Linden, 1995). Tedesco and colleagues have reported on the benefits of this model combined with self-efficacy in predicting oral health behaviour. The investigators enrolled 166 patients who were diagnosed as having mild to moderate gingivitis into the study. Subjects were required to complete a series of seven dental visits spread over 14 months from the date of their first attendance. Both psychosocial (theory of reasoned action questionnaire, self-efficacy assessments, oral health behaviour reports) and clinical (plaque and gingival indices) information were recorded at each visit. Results of the study

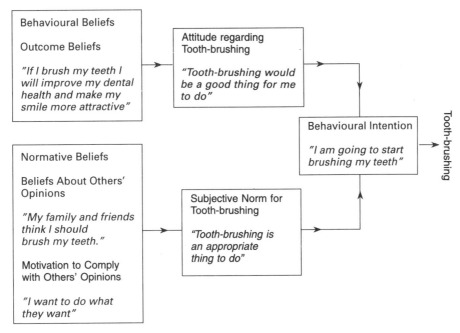

Fig. 12.4 Theory of reasoned action: attitudes influencing adoption of dental health behaviour (tooth-brushing). Adapted from Ajzen and Fishbein (1980).

suggest that on its own the theory of reasoned action could moderately predict brushing and flossing dental behaviours as reported by the participants. However, when self-efficacy was included the variance increased to the high moderate range. When predicting clinical indices, the model of reasoned action and self-efficacy variables did not account for as much variance as expected. The authors acknowledged the need to understand the relevant variables in health-related behaviour uptake and preventive measures and refer to the area of perceived control as one facet which requires further study.

Therefore, the model of reasoned action holds much promise in that behaviours which the individual controls of his or her own volition can be accurately predicted from intentions (Ajzen, 1991). However, certain areas of prediction remain unclear. For example, intending to carry out a health-related behaviour does not automatically predict that the particular behaviour will be carried out, especially if other barriers stand in the way (Baranowski, 1990; Orbell and Sheeran, 1994). Ajzen, however, has drawn on his experience in an attempt to further explain this gap between intention and behaviour by

revising the theory of reasoned action and developing the theory of planned behaviour (Ajzen, 1988, 1991).

The theory of planned behaviour

In this model an additional variable which further helps to predict the uptake of behaviour is *perceived behavioural control*. Perceived behavioural control refers to the individual's felt competency and confidence to perform the behaviour in question and differs considerably from actual control so that it is applicable across a wide range of behaviours and environments. It is a concept similar to Bandura's self-efficacy, mentioned in the protection–motivation model. The theory of planned behaviour continues to recognize the role of intention to perform a behaviour as an essential ingredient in the prediction of behaviour. Here, the central determinant is the motivation of the individual to be prepared to change or modify the behaviour. The three variables involved in this model include attitude and subjective norm as described in the theory of reasoned action, with the addition of perceived behavioural control (Fig. 12.5). According to the model, individuals will have the intention of executing a behaviour

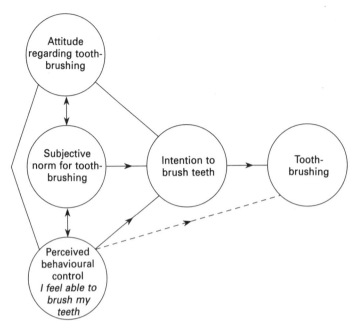

Fig. 12.5 The theory of planned behaviour: attitudes influencing the adoption of tooth-brushing. Adapted from Ajzen (1988).

when they have a positive attitude; they believe that others important to them think it is worthwhile for them to do it; and they believe that they can perform the behaviour with ease, i.e. confidently and competently. Although this model continues to be scrutinized, it has been successful in predicting a variety of health-related behaviours.

One study conducted in the UK examined the utility of the theory of planned behaviour in predicting the ability of mothers with 5–7-month-old babies to restrict the frequency of their children's sugar consumption. Mothers were randomly assigned to attend an education seminar (verbal and written information plus care pack) or enter a no-education control group (Beale and Manstead, 1991). Information for data collection was based on the components of the theory of planned behaviour (behavioural intention, attitude, subjective norm and perceived behavioural control). The results supported the theory of planned behaviour over the theory of reasoned action because the addition of perceived behavioural control increased the prediction of the mothers' intentions to restrict the usual sugar intake of their babies. The authors make the interesting point that, prior to taking part in the study, mothers were not likely to have considered the habitual intake of sugar

for their babies. The authors associate this with the lack of recognition of a link between sugar intake and dental decay, as well as opposing the mothers' already established social patterns or norms and customs.

Two recent studies, part of the Norwegian Longitudinal Health Behaviour Study, applied the models of reasoned action and planned behaviour. These models helped in the construction of persuasive health messages to be used in a dental health education programme (Astrøm and Rise, 1995a, 1995b). The studies were designed to provide a greater understanding of the decision to carry out a particular health behaviour. Increasing our understanding of motivations to change will assist our chances of influencing behaviour. In the latter study (Astrøm and Rise, 1995b), a range of behavioural outcomes were measured prior to a health education programme. These outcomes included behavioural beliefs, evaluation of outcomes, normative beliefs, motivation to comply and perceived barriers. After the health education programme, the results demonstrated that the adolescents who initially had a stronger intention to change behaviour (using dental floss and switching to non-sugared mineral water) were more likely to do so than their peers of the same age exposed to the same messages. These studies support the value of understanding the belief systems of a targeted audience before designing appropriate health education interventions. Studies of this kind can help us avoid ineffective and inappropriate health message campaigns.

The transtheoretical model

Like the theory of planned behaviour, the transtheoretical model helps us to comprehend the role that intention/motivation plays in relation to our understanding of health-related behaviours. This model claims to be much more integrative than those previously outlined (Prochaska *et al.*, 1994). In the transtheoretical model, Prochaska and Di Clemente (1982) propose that we need to consider five processes to understand behaviour change in individuals. These are precontemplation, contemplation, preparation, action and maintenance/relapse prevention. To understand each stage and the processes involved, it is useful to view behaviour from each perspective. Individuals in the *precontemplation* stage are not thinking about changing their behaviour, are not usually aware that they have a problem and often do not present for dental treatment except in an emergency. Those in the *contemplation* stage, however, have an awareness of the problem and are seriously thinking about changing but are not prepared to make any moves in this direction just yet. These people may move on to the *preparation* stage when they are about to take the initial steps to change their behaviour in the near future. In the *action* phase, modifications of behaviour actually begin to happen. Finally, the *maintenance/relapse prevention* stage involves individuals continuing with the change, integrating it into current lifestyles and working to prevent a return to the former behaviour.

Once an individual's stage of change has been assessed relative to the targeted behaviour, the health professional can help the person move in a forwards direction towards a healthier lifestyle (Miller and Rollnick, 1991). These include providing information and feedback in the precontemplation stage so that an awareness of the problem behaviour is increased. Prescriptive advice to someone in this stage can be counterproductive Once the individual is aware of the problem, the person may consider changing, but at the same time, usually sees this as requiring too much effort. Thus, the person

contemplating change may be seen as fluctuating between changing and not changing. The health professional's task is to try to tip the balance in the favour of change. In that way, the person moves into preparation to change and begins to make plans to change his or her behaviour. When the individual has made a decision to change, he or she activates a plan to change or modify the behaviour, i.e. the person engages in particular actions intended to bring about the behaviour, e.g. flossing once a day. However, making a change does not guarantee that the change will be maintained. Barriers or precipitants to relapse need to be identified by the individual. Strategies to overcome these need to be planned in a systematic way if relapses are to be prevented. If the individual does relapse then the process begins again as he or she reverts to one of the previous stages. It has been recognized that people may move several times, including backwards, forwards or sideways across the stages, before change becomes permanent.

Health psychology and community oral health

Dietary and oral hygiene practices are well-recognized as playing a central role in not only the cause of numerous dental diseases but also the uptake of dental health-enhancing behaviours, thus making them appropriate targets for health behaviour change. The models described help us to conceptualize behaviour as a risk factor for dental disease (Schou, 1991). Changing risky behaviours (e.g. infrequent tooth-brushing, poor diet) produces positive changes in dental health; behaviour can be changed and behavioural interventions are the best method to achieve change (Kaplan, 1984). Recently, the importance of cognitive variables (attitudes, beliefs) has been recognized and cognitive-behavioural interventions are becoming the mediation of choice. The models described take account of community-based variables such as attitudes in the theories of reasoned action and planned behaviour; beliefs of the community as in the health belief and protection–motivation models; the presence of environmental constraints and the barriers to volitional control which are often embedded in economic, cultural and broader social norms.

The salience of these models to health

education can be summed up in the words of Hochbaum and colleagues (1992): 'the primary goal of the social and behavioural sciences is to learn to understand the determinants of human behaviour. Working towards this goal, researchers in these sciences have spent years developing and testing theories. It seems foolish for applied fields, such as health education, not to draw on that work'. The combination of these aspects has forced a greater awareness of the need for those involved in dental health prevention to be aware of the interface between theory, intervention and outcome.

From theory to practice

The importance of bridging the gap between psychological theory and health education practice has been much debated. This link generally eludes most health professionals (Witte, 1995) and there appear to be valid reasons for this. Witte outlines several reasons, including the complexity and poor applicability of some theories. However, she does identify the merits of theory as a facilitator to the development of health education interventions. Theories/models can increase understanding of the complex factors associated with prevention by organizing these factors into a coherent and recognizable whole. On the other hand, D'Onofrio (1992) postulates that health educators should not feel constrained and obligated to identify a theory in their health education practices.

For situations where selecting theories to match practice is appropriate, Hochbaum and colleagues make some suggestions which health educators should consider (Hochbaum *et al.*, 1992). These include size of the target audience, whether it be individual, group or community; nature of the target behaviour, e.g. specific, sporadic or invasive behaviour change, or of a personal versus public nature; the match between the target audience beliefs and attitudes and the theoretical perspective underpinning the intervention. Often, health educators will find that no single theory is appropriate to guide their intervention. In this case, it may be more useful to maintain an eclectic perspective based on choosing a range of theoretical models or aspects of those models which might offer help. Anticipating contingencies that may arise when planning a health education programme will facilitate drawing on the theories which best fit

their aims, be they psychological, sociological, educational or a combination of these. Nevertheless, even if the guidelines which are offered by Hochbaum and colleagues are followed, other difficulties will remain. Resources are perhaps the major barrier between theory and practice and, when it comes to interventions, are often in short supply. These resources include time, money and expertise. These factors are not often considered by the theorists whose primary concern is to understand, not intervene.

Given the wide range of knowledge and skills required by health educators to meet the aims of health education, the theories outlined do go some way in helping to identify and understand the factors that are likely to enhance health-promoting behaviours in various situations (Hochbaum *et al.*, 1992). Nevertheless, if theories are to be effective, they need to be carefully chosen, skilfully adapted and applied to the situation. Additionally, a knowledge of the merits and shortcomings of the various models around is required. Choosing which theory to apply requires an experience of the targeted situation/behaviour and the processes in that situation which are facilitated by the theory (Green *et al.*, 1994). Witte (1995) offers similar guidance as to which theory to choose by recommending 'parts of successful and well-tested theories' developed into a framework.

Future considerations–where to from here?

Several developments have led to changes in dentists' practices relating to dental treatment and maintenance of good oral health. Taken together, health professionals work for the common good of the nation, and as such, have an obligation to comply with the recommendations set out by the *Global Strategy for Health for all by the Year 2000* document and the many national targets set subsequently (WHO, 1981). These initiatives clearly implicate a connection between behaviour, lifestyle and health (Diekstra and Jansen, 1990). The need to change unhealthy lifestyle behaviours is supported and accepted. Health behaviour change and health education programmes should support the growth of better health habits using a wide variety of strategies delivered in many different settings (individual/group, clinic/community/work).

There is little doubt that health professionals can influence health behaviour through promoting lifestyle changes, such as dietary, smoking and oral hygiene behaviour change. However, no one claims this to be easy. It is recognized that, so far, much success has been with well-motivated groups, e.g those who actually attend dental practice. Marked socioeconomic differences in health and health-related behaviour have been identified. The difficulties inherent in influencing behaviour change and promoting the adoption of healthy choices across the entire population is evidenced by the ever-continuing level of dental disease and the failure of health education programmes to reach the most health-needy people in the population (Wenzel, 1983). Health education is an important element in helping individuals reach health goals, but much broader perspectives are needed. This involves examining health-related strategies outside of the person–environment and behaviour triangle, to focus on policy, economic and social pathways to promoting the health of the nation.

References

Ajzen, I. (1988) *Attitudes, Personality, and Behaviour.* Dorsey Press, Chicago.

Ajzen, I. (1991) The theory of planned behaviour. *Organizational Behaviour and Human Decision Processes* 50:179–211.

Ajzen I. and Fishbein, M. (1980) *Understanding Attitudes and Predicting Social Behaviour.* Prentice-Hall, Englewood Cliffs, NJ.

Anderson, R., Davies, J.K., Kickbush, I. *et al.* (1988) *Health Behaviour Research and Health Promotion.* Oxford Medical Publications, Oxford.

Ashley, F. P. (1989) Role of dental health education in preventive dentistry. In: *The Prevention of Dental Disease.* (Murray, J.J., ed.), pp. 410–414. Oxford University Press.

Astrøm, A. and Rise, J. (1995a) Drinking of non-sugared mineral water among adolescents: application of an expectancy-value approach. *Community Dental and Oral Epidemiology* (in press).

Astrøm, A. and Rise, J. (1995b) Analysis of adolescents beliefs about the outcomes of using dental floss and drinking non-sugared mineral water. *Community Dental and Oral Epidemiology* (in press).

Backer, T., Rodgers, E. and Sopory, P. (1992) *Designing Health Education Campaigns: What Works.* Sage, Newbury Park, CA.

Bandura, A. (1986) *Social Foundations of Thought and Action: A Cognitive Social Theory.* Prentice Hall, Englewood Cliffs, NJ.

Baranowski, T. (1990) Reciprocal determinism at the stages of behaviour change: an integration of community, personal and behavioural perspectives. *International Quarterly of Community Health Education* 10:297–327.

Beale, D.A. and Manstead, A.S.R. (1991) Predicting mother's intentions to limit frequency of infant's sugar intake: testing the theory of planned behaviour. *Journal of Applied Social Psychology* 21:409–431.

Brown, L.F. (1994) Research in dental health education and health promotion. A review of the literature. *Health Education Quarterly* 21:83–102.

Brownell, K.D. and Cohen, L.R. (1995) Adherence to dietary regimens 1: an overview of research. *Behavioural Medicine* 20:149–154.

Craft, M. and Chamberlain, J. (1992) Generic health promotion and oral health education–why are they separate and what is the interface? *Journal of the Institute of Health Education* 30:50–52.

Croucher, R. (1993) General dental practice, health education, and health promotion: a critical reappraisal. In: *Oral Health Promotion* (Schou, L. and Blinkhorn, A.S., eds), pp. 153–168. Oxford University Press, New York.

Croucher, R.E., Rodgers, A.I., Franklin, A.J. *et al.* (1985) Results and issues arising from an evaluation of community dental health education: the case of the 'Good Teeth programme'. *Community Dental Health* 2: 89–97.

Croxson, L.J. (1993) Periodontal awareness: the key to periodontal health. *International Dental Journal* 43:167–177.

Diekstra, R.F.W. and Jansen, M.A. (1990) The importance of psychosocial interventions in primary health care. In: *Theoretical and Applied Aspects of Health Psychology* (Schmidt, L.R., Schwenhmenger, P., Weinman, J. and Maes, S., eds), pp. 87–101. Howard Academic Publishers, London.

DiMatteo, M.R. (1991) *The Psychology of Health, Illness and Medical Care: An Individual Perspective.* Brooks/Cole, Pacific Grove, CA.

D'Onofrio, C.N. (1992) Theory and empowerment of health education practitioners. *Health Education Quarterly* 19:385–403.

Downer, M.C. (1991) The improving dental health of United Kingdom adults and prospects for the future. *British Dental Journal* 170(4), 154–158.

Evans, R.I., Roselle, R.M., Lesater, T.M. *et al.* (1970) Fear arousal, persuasion and actual versus implied behavioural change. *Journal of Personality and Social Psychology* 16:220–227.

Frazier, P.J. (1992) Research on oral health education and promotion and social epidemiology. *Journal of Public Health Dentistry* 52:18–22.

Freeman, R. and Linden, G. (1995) Health directed and health related dimensions of oral health behaviours of periodontal referrals. *Community Dental Health* 12:48–51.

Gochman, D.S. (1988) *Health Behaviour: Emerging Research Perspectives.* Plenum Press, New York.

Green, L.W. and Kreuter, M.W. (1991) *Health Promotion Planning: An Educational and Environmental Approach.* Mayfield, Palo Alto, CA.

Green, L.W., Glanz, K., Hochbaum, M. *et al.* (1994) Can we build on, or must we replace, the theories and models in health education? *Health Education Research* 9:397–404.

Hale, J.L. and Dillard, J.P. (1995) Fear appeals in health promotion campaigns. In: *Designing Health Messages: Approaches from Communication Theory and Public Health Practice* (Maibach, E. and Parrot, R.L., eds), pp. 65–80. Sage Publications, CA.

Harcourt, J.K. (1994) 1994–The year of oral health. *Australian Dental Journal* **39**:129.

Harris, N.O. and Christen, A.G. (1991) *Primary Preventive Dentistry*. Appleton and Lange, Norwalk, CONN.

Hochbaum, G.M., Sorenson, J.R. and Lorig, K. (1992) Theory in health education practice. *Health Education Quarterly* **19**:295–313.

Horowitz, L.G. (1990) Dental patient education: self-care to healthy human development. *Patient Education and Counselling* **15**:65–71.

Kaplan, R.M. (1984) The connection between clinical health promotion and health status: a critical overview. *American Psychologist* **39**:755–765.

Kaplan, R.M. (1994) The Ziggy theorem: towards an outcomes-focused health psychology. *Health Psychology* **13**:451–460.

Kaplan, R.M., Sallis, J.F. and Patterson, T.L. (1993) *Health and Human Behaviour*. McGraw-Hill, London.

Kuhner, M.K. and Raetzke, P.B. (1989) The effect of health beliefs on the compliance of periodontol patients with oral hygiene instructions. *Journal of Periodontology* **60**:51–56.

Levine, R.S. (1989) *The Scientific Basis of Dental Health Education*. Health Education Authority, London.

McGuire, W.J. (1984) Public communication as a strategy for inducing health-promoting behavioural change. *Preventive Medicine* **13**:299–319.

McGuire, W.J. (1991) Using guiding-idea theories of the person to develop educational campaigns against drug abuse and other health-threatening behaviour. *Health Education Research* **6**:173–184.

Mason, D. (1992) Future relationships of dentistry and medicine in education and practice. *British Dental Journal* **2**:2–4.

Miller, W.R. and Rollnick, S. (1991) *Motivational Interviewing: Preparing People to Change Addictive Behaviour*. The Guildford Press, New York.

Newton, J.T. (1995) The readability and utility of general dental practice patient information leaflets: an evaluation. *British Dental Journal* **178**:329–332.

Nowak, A.J. and Anderson, J.L. (1990) Preventive dentistry for children: a review from 1968–1988. *Journal of Dentistry for Children* **57**(1): 31–37.

Oldenburg, B. (1994) Promotion of health: integrating the clinical and public health approaches. In: *International Review of Health Psychology*, vol. 3 (Maes, S., Leventhal, H. and Johnston, M., eds), pp. 121–143. John Wiley, Chichester.

Orbell, S. and Sheeran, P. (1994) *Protection–Motivation Theory and Intention–Behaviour Consistency*. Poster presented at the European Health Psychology Society, Alicante, Spain. July.

Pfau, M. (1995) Designing messages for behavioural inoculation. In: *Designing Health Messages: Approaches from Communication Theory and Public Health Practice*

(Maibach, E. and Parrot, R.L., eds), pp. 99–113. Sage Publications, CA.

Prochaska, J.O. (1994) Strong and weak principles for progressing from precontemplation to action on the basis of twelve problem behaviours. *Health Psychology* **13**:47–51.

Prochaska, J.O. and Di Clemente, C.C. (1982) Transtheoretical therapy: toward a more integrative model of change. *Psychotherapy, Theory, Research and Practice* **19**:276–288.

Prochaska, J.O., Velicer, W.F., Rossi, J.S. *et al.* (1994) Stages of change and decisional balance for 12 problem behaviours. *Health Psychology* **13**:39–46.

Raaheim, A. (1990) Marketing health and changing behaviour. In: *Theoretical and Applied Aspects of Health Psychology* (Schmidt, L.R., Schwenhmenger, P., Weinman, J. and Maes, S., eds), pp. 141–150, Howard Academic Publishers, London.

Rise, J. and Holund, U. (1990) Prediction of sugar behaviour. *Community Dental Health* **7**:267–272.

Rise, J. and Sogaard, A.J. (1988) Effect of a mass media periodontol campaign upon preventive knowledge and behaviour in Norway. *Community Dentistry and Oral Epidemiology* **16**:1–4.

Rogers, R.W. (1983) Cognitive and physiological processes in fear appeals and attitude change: a revised theory of protection–motivation. In: *Social Psychophysiology: A Sourcebook* (Cacioppo J.T. and Petty, R.E., eds), pp. 153–176, The Guildford Press, New York.

Rosenstock, I.M., Strecher, V.J. and Becker, M.H. (1988) Social learning theory and the health belief model. *Health Education Quarterly* **15**: 175–183.

Schmidt, L.R., Schwenhmezger, J. and Dlugosch, G.E. (1990) The scope of health psychology. In: *Theoretical and Applied Aspects of Health Psychology* (Schmidt, L.R., Schwenhmenger, P., Weinman, J. and Maes, S., eds), pp. 3–28. Howard Academic Publishers, London.

Schou, L. (1987) Use of mass media and active involvement in a national dental health campaign in Scotland. *Community Dentistry and Oral Epidemiology* **15**:14–18.

Schou, L. (1991) Social and behavioural aspects of caries prediction. In: *Dental Caries: markers of High and Low Risk Groups and Individuals* (Johnson, N.W., ed.), pp. 172–197. Cambridge University Press, Cambridge.

Seeman, J. (1989) Toward a model of positive health. *American Psychologist* **44**:1099–1109.

Sheiham, A. and Croucher, R. (1994) Current perspectives on improving chairside dental health education for adults. *International Dental Journal* **44**:202–206.

Steptoe, A., Wardle, J., Vinck, J. *et al.* (1994) Personality and attitudinal correlates of healthy and unhealthy lifestyles in young adults. *Psychology and Health* **9**:331–343.

Taal, E., Seydel, E. and Wiegman, O. (1990) Self-efficacy, protection motivation and health behaviour. In: *Theoretical and Applied Aspects of Health Psychology* (Schmidt, L.R., Schwenhmenger, P., Weinman, J. and Maes, S., eds), pp. 113–120. Howard Academic Publishers, London.

Taylor, S.E. (1990) Health psychology: the science and the field. *American Psychologist* **45**:40–50.

Tedesco, L.A., Keffer, M.A., Davis, E.L. and Christersson, L.A. (1992) Effect of a social cognitive intervention on oral health status, behaviour, reports and cognitions. *Journal of Periodontology* **63**:567–575.

Tedesco, L.A., Keffer, M.A., Davis, E.L. and Christersson, L.A. (1993) Self-efficacy and reasoned action: predicting oral health status and behaviour at one, three and six month intervals. *Psychology and Health* **8**:105–121.

Todd, J.E. and Lader, D. (1991) *Adult Dental Health 1988 United Kingdom.* HMSO, London.

Tones, B.K. (1986) Health education and the ideology of health promotion: a review of alternative approaches. *Health Education Research* **1**:3–12.

Tones, K. and Tilford, S. (1994) *Health Education, Effectiveness, Efficiency and Equity.* Chapman and Hall, London.

Towner, E.M.L. (1984) 'The Gleam team' programme: development and evaluation of a dental health education package for infant schools. *Community Dental Health* **1**: 181–191.

Watson, D.L. and Tharp, R.G. (1993) *Self-Directed Behaviour: Self-Modification for Personal Adjustment.* Brooks/Cole, Pacific Grove, CA.

Wenzel, E. (1983) Lifestyles and living conditions and their impact on health. *European Monographs in Health Education Research* **5**:1–18.

Whittle, J.G., Pitkethly, D. and Wilson, M.C. (1994) A dental health promotion campaign in a shopping centre. *Health Education Research* **9**:261–265.

Witte, K. (1995) Fishing for success. Using the persuasive health message framework to generate effective campaign messages. In: *Designing Health Messages: Approaches from Communication, Theory and Public Health Practice* (Maibach, E. and Parrot, R.L., eds), pp. 145–164. Sage Publications, CA.

World Health Organization (1964) *Basel Documents*, 15th edn, p. 1. WHO, Geneva.

World Health Organization (1981) *Global Strategy for Health for All by the year 2000.* WHO, Geneva.

13

Nutrition, dietary guidelines and food policy in oral health

Andrew Rugg-Gunn

Introduction

All of us eat, but not all of us eat well. In most developed countries, there has never been such a wide choice of foods, often prepared and cooked before purchase, and overnutrition is more of a problem than undernutrition. In contrast, undernutrition is prevalent in developing countries, with starvation common in many areas. Teeth used to be necessary for adequate food preparation, but this role has declined in importance in developed countries and appearance is a much more important reason for keeping teeth than eating. Still, adequacy of a dentition can affect food choice, as we shall see later.

A more relevant line of enquiry is how diet and nutrition affect teeth and their supporting structures. By diet is usually meant the choice of foods and which foods are eaten, while nutrition implies the intake and absorption of nutrients. Diet and nutrition affect the teeth in three ways: the structure of teeth, dental caries and dental erosion. The first is a purely pre-eruptive effect while teeth are forming; erosion is a purely local, intraoral effect on erupted teeth, while caries development is affected by both pre-eruptive and posteruptive influences, although the latter is the more important. Thus diet and nutrition can affect teeth during tooth formation and after eruption in the mouth. The periodontal tissues are also influenced by foods we eat and these will also be considered.

But knowledge of the way in which foods can damage teeth does not necessarily mean that the problem is solved. Alternative behaviours have to be developed and accepted. Advice alone is not enough but has to be supported by actions which make accepting this advice possible–in other words, health promotion. Many of these actions will be required centrally, i.e. on a national basis; others are more appropriate in the community or local setting, while others are best achieved on an individual basis. What is very important is the absence of conflict in the health messages and this has to be worked out at a national and a local level. A discussion on how to achieve uniformity of message will constitute a major part of this chapter.

The effect of nutrition and diet on dental health

Structure of teeth

There are many causes of defects of the structure of teeth (Pindborg, 1982)–nutrition is just one of these. Both the primary and permanent dentition can be affected and the time of the insult can often be identified by the position of the defect in the enamel of the crowns of various teeth, since the chronology of tooth formation is now well-known. A well-recognized defect is linear enamel hypoplasia, which can be seen in the middle third of maxillary central primary incisors and the incisal third of the lateral primary incisors in children in communities in developing countries where malnutrition is prevalent (Sweeney *et al.*, 1971; Enwonwu, 1973;

Infante and Gillespie, 1977). Hypoplasia in primary teeth is more common in low-birth-weight children (Fearne *et al.*, 1990). Childhood and exanthematous fevers have been suggested as a cause of enamel hypoplasia (Jackson, 1961), but other surveys (Wilson and Cleaton-Jones, 1978; Suckling and Pearce, 1984) found no relationship. In a survey of 243 children by Suckling and Pearce (1984), trauma and illness were the only two significant aetiological factors.

Although there is no doubt of the increased prevalence of enamel hypoplasia in children with nutritional deficiencies, the mechanism whereby this occurs was uncertain until Nikiforuk and Fraser (1981) proposed a unifying concept for the aetiology of enamel hypoplasia. Their study involved the thorough examination of 56 patients in Toronto, Canada, over a 25-year period. These patients belonged to three categories of disorders of calcium and phosphate homeostasis. Enamel hypoplasia occurred only in children who had hypocalcaemia, and no relation was observed between enamel hypoplasia and plasma phosphate levels. This theory is compatible with other observations of increased levels of enamel hypoplasia in children with hypoparathyroidism, neonatal tetany and premature birth (Nikiforuk and Fraser, 1981). They note the strong associations between the prevalence of acute diarrhoeal disease and enamel hypoplasia, and hypothesize that chronic diarrhoea causes malnutrition, resulting in hypocalcaemia which leads to linear enamel hypoplasia.

Teeth consist largely of calcium and phosphate and it is not surprising that dietary deficiency of calcium and/or vitamin D has been a prime suspect in the aetiology of enamel hypoplasia. Lady May Mellanby has been by far the most influential worker in this area, particularly between 1920 and 1950. This coincided with the age of discovery of vitamins and Mellanby established, mainly through experiments on dogs, that vitamin D deficiency resulted in a fine type of enamel hypoplasia (Mellanby, 1918, 1923). She also hypothesized that teeth so affected were more prone to dental caries and went on to demonstrate this in two short clinical trials. Mellanby's ideas have not been widely accepted, mainly because the ravages of caries became so severe in the 1950s and 1960s that all attention was given to the posteruption effect of sugars. Her concepts have received some support since Cockburn *et al.* (1980) showed in a

randomized clinical trial that children of mothers in Edinburgh, Scotland, given vitamin D supplement during pregnancy had less hypoplasia in their primary teeth when examined blind at the age of 2–3 years. There is far less controversy, however, in the ability of excessive ingestion of fluoride to cause defects in the structure of dental enamel. This is so well-known that it is unnecessary to report it here and the reader is referred to a standard textbook on fluorides and dental health (Murray *et al.*, 1991) and Chapters 6 and 14 in this book.

In summary, dietary deficiencies and excesses are responsible for defects in the structure of teeth. They are, though, only some of the many causes. The effect of malnutrition is well-recognized in developing countries and it is possible that hypocalcaemia is the uniforming aetiological factor. There is some evidence that correcting deficiency of vitamin D in pregnancy decreases the prevalence of enamel hypoplasia in childhood. Excessive ingestion of fluoride is a very well-recognized cause of defects of the structure of teeth.

Dental caries

The posteruptive effect of diet has much more influence on caries development than any pre-eruptive effect. The pre-eruptive effect should not be dismissed altogether as fluoride can have a significant caries-preventive effect if ingested at optimum levels during tooth formation. Fluoride's very important posteruptive effect often overshadows the still identifiable pre-eruptive effect. Dietary vehicles for fluoride include water (at 1 mg F/l in temperate climates), salt (at 250 mg F/kg), milk (at 5 mg F/l) and fluoride drops and tablets (the dose depending on age). All these fluoride vehicles are discussed in Chapters 7 and 14.

The acidogenic theory of caries aetiology requires that carbohydrates are broken down by bacteria in the dental plaque and the resulting acid causes demineralization at the plaque–enamel interface. Dietary carbohydrates consist very largely of starches and sugars and the evidence linking these with caries development is vast–at least 1500 articles have been reviewed in detail elsewhere (Rugg-Gunn, 1993). From the scientific evidence, it is concluded that:

- sugars are the most cariogenic item in the diet;
- starch can cause caries, especially if finely

ground and heat-treated, but the amount of decay is less than that caused by sugars.

To enlarge on the question of sugars a little, it is useful to examine two issues in a little more detail–first, whether all sugars and sugar-containing foods are equally cariogenic and, second, whether frequency of consumption of sugars is of overriding importance. The common dietary sugars are sucrose, glucose, maltose, fructose and lactose. No other sugar has been shown to be more cariogenic than sucrose. Lactose is the least cariogenic dietary sugar. In comparisons of the cariogenicity of sucrose versus glucose or fructose, it is noteworthy that some American authorities believe that the decline in caries in the USA may be partly due to the change from sucrose to fructose as a major sweetener. Dietary sugars have also been classified according to whether they are milk sugars, intrinsic sugars or non-milk extrinsic (NME) sugars. Cows' (bovine) milk is safe for teeth and indeed has been recommended as a saliva substitute. Human milk has a greater potential to cause caries, due to higher lactose and lower calcium and phosphate levels, but breast-feeding is only associated with caries if prolonged and on demand. Adding sugar to milk makes it cariogenic. Fresh fruit and vegetables are not a threat to dental health. It is the NME sugars in the diet which are clearly linked to caries. The principal sources of NME sugars in the diet which constitute some 70% of all sugars will be discussed in a later section.

There is much evidence that frequency of ingestion of dietary sugars is an important variable in caries aetiology. Since the pH of dental plaque falls each time sugars are ingested, it stands to reason that the more times in a day sugar is consumed, the more times plaque pH will be depressed to a level at which dental enamel may dissolve. Rat experiments have shown clearly that the more frequently they are fed sugar, the more caries develops. However, there is also strong evidence that the amount of sugar consumed, is related to caries development–in some animal experiments, independent of frequency. In most of the epidemiological evidence, sugar intake is quantified in terms of amount rather than frequency. This is not surprising since in human studies, as opposed to animal experiments, there is a very strong correlation between frequency of intake of sugars and weight of sugars consumed. In other words, as one goes up, the other goes up, and vice versa. Both frequency and amount are important and they should not be seen as alternatives.

There are two other aspects of diet and caries which are worth considering. First, whether some foods or components of foods protect against dental caries. The hunt for these so-called protective factors began 60 years ago in South Africa when workers such as Osborn and Noriskin (1937) observed a low prevalence of dental caries in people eating a high-carbohydrate diet. This led to the realization that phosphates, either organic (such as phytate) or inorganic, were capable of reducing the cariogenicity of a carbohydrate diet. A very large number of animal studies were undertaken and some clinical trials. These showed that, while soluble phosphate and organic phosphate, but not calcium, were capable of preventing caries in rats, they were much less successful in preventing caries in human trials. Phytate was the most effective, but it is unlikely to be added to foods since it reduces the absorption of some minerals from the gut. Cheese, as well as protein, fat and casein have been considered as protective factors, with some evidence, but their practical use is at present uncertain.

The last aspect of diet and caries to be considered is the non-cariogenicity of non-sugar sweeteners. The sweet taste is not limited to sugars and an increasing number of compounds have been shown to be possible substitutes for sugar; several of them are approved for use in foods in the UK (Table 13.1). These compounds are usefully considered as either bulk sweeteners or intense sweeteners. Bulk sweeteners are about as sweet as sucrose, gram for gram, and provide nearly as many calories as sugar: they are most often used where bulk is required, such as confectionery. Intense sweeteners are many times sweeter than sucrose and provide very little

Table 13.1 Permitted sweeteners in foods in the UK

Sugars	Bulk sweeteners	Intense sweeteners
Glucose	Sorbitol	Saccharin
Fructose	Mannitol	Acesulfame K*
Sucrose	Hydrogenated glucose syrup*	Aspartame*
Lactose	Isomalt*	Thaumatin*
Maltose	Xylitol*	
	Lactitol†	
	Maltitol‡	

*Permitted 1982; †Permitted 1988; ‡Permitted 1995.

calories: they are used mainly in soft drinks or in combination with bulk sweeteners.

The sweeteners listed in Table 13.1 are non-cariogenic and there is some evidence that some of them may have a minor anticariogenic effect. Xylitol is non-cariogenic. It is not metabolized by the vast majority of plaque organisms and has been shown, in the classical Turku sugar studies (Scheinin and Mähinen, 1975), to result in greatly reduced caries development in subjects whose diet contained xylitol in place of dietary sugars. A number of trials of chewing gum containing either xylitol or sorbitol in place of sugar have been undertaken. These show that sugarless chewing gum not only is non-cariogenic (when compared with sugared gum) but is positively anticariogenic (when compared with no gum). Most people believe this anticariogenic effect is due to the stimulation of fast-flowing saliva which, being alkaline, rapidly raises the pH of dental plaque, encouraging remineralization. The outlook for non-sugar sweeteners is bright and we will return to this subject later when health promotion is considered.

In summary, the most cariogenic item in our diet is sugars: sucrose is the most cariogenic and lactose the least cariogenic. Milk and fresh fruit and vegetables are not seen as cariogenic: milk has been proposed as a saliva substitute, while apples and carrots have been seen as symbols of dental health. NME sugars are the big threat to dental health. Starch can cause caries but much less than that caused by sugars. Staple starchy foods, such as potatoes, pasta, rice and bread, are considered little threat to teeth. If finely ground and heat-treated and especially if mixed with sugars (such as biscuits), starch can cause caries. Some components of foods have been shown to be protective against caries; of these, phosphates have been the most thoroughly studied. Phytate is the most promising but it is unlikely to be used as a caries-protective food additive. Many non-sugar sweeteners have been identified and several are now allowed for general use in foods and drinks in many countries. Bulk sweeteners are mainly used in confectionery and intense sweeteners in soft drinks. They are non-cariogenic or virtually so. In addition, sugarless chewing gum appears to be anticariogenic. For further information on their properties and use in different countries, the reader is referred to Rugg-Gunn (1991, 1993, 1994).

Erosion

Diet is an important and growing cause of dental erosion. There are other causes of erosion of teeth such as regurgitation of gastric fluid and exposure to some industrial acid environments—but dietary acids are the significant factor. Until recently, little was known about the prevalence and severity of erosion in the population. This deficiency was corrected in the UK with the publication of the report on *Children's Dental Health in the United Kingdom 1993* (O'Brien, 1994). One year later a report on the dental health of pre-school children in the UK was published (Hinds and Gregory, 1995). Data from both these studies are given in Table 13.2. The teeth which are most affected are the maxillary incisor teeth, particularly the palatal surfaces, although the labial surface and incisal edge can be affected as well. Erosion is difficult to treat.

Dietary risk factors in dental erosion will vary between populations and between different age groups within populations. In children and adolescents, acid soft drinks are by far the biggest dietary risk factor. Sales of soft drinks have increased rapidly and the prevalence and severity of dental erosion in children seem to have increased in parallel. There has been a large increase in the UK soft drinks market with around 4 000 million litres in 1992 being carbonated. The low-calorie versions have increased their share to around 26%. Overall, food consumption within the European Union (EU) of the original 12 members rose by 9.1% between 1988 and 1993. The most growth was in soft drinks, savoury snacks and frozen fruit

Table 13.2 Prevalence of dental erosion in UK children

	Age (years)		
	$1\frac{1}{2}$–$2\frac{1}{2}$	$2\frac{1}{2}$–$3\frac{1}{2}$	$3\frac{1}{2}$–$4\frac{1}{2}$
Per cent of children with erosion on palatal surfaces of incisors			
Any erosion	9	18	29
Into dentine or pulp	3	6	13

Primary upper incisors (aged 5 years)	
Palatal surfaces	
Any erosion	52%
Dentine/pulp	24%
Permanent upper incisors (aged 14 years)	
Palatal surfaces	
Any erosion	32%
Dentine/pulp	2%

Data from O'Brien (1994); Hinds and Gregory (1995).

and vegetables. The volume of food and drink packaged in cans grew by 18.5%, mostly due to increased soft drinks consumption (Rice, 1995). In older age groups, citrus fruits and vinegar-containing foods may be important dietary risk factors for erosion as well. In a study of adult patients of dentists in Helsinki, Finland, Jarvinen *et al.* (1991) reported that, of the risk factors, the following were ranked in order of occurrence: citrus fruit, other fruit, soft drinks, sports drinks, pickles and apple vinegar.

Nutrition and the periodontium

Periodontal tissues are comprised of epithelium, collagen fibres, blood vessels, other connective tissue elements, cementum and bone. It would be very surprising if nutritional deficiencies did not adversely affect these tissues. There is strong evidence of adverse effects from experiments on rats, guinea-pigs and dogs, but there is much less evidence in humans. Only in the case of scurvy (ascorbic acid deficiency) are the periodontal tissues primarily affected. Overall, periodontal tissues will benefit when nutrition is adequate, but dietary supplementation of nutrients above what are commonly accepted as adequate levels does not seem to improve periodontal health further. Inadequate levels of folate appear to exist in gingival tissues in defined groups of people and delivery of folate to these tissues locally in the mouth (for example in a mouthrinse) can be beneficial. By far the most important way of maintaining periodontal health in humans is regular, thorough physical removal of dental plaque with a satisfactory tooth-brush. For a fuller review of this subject the reader is referred to Rugg-Gunn (1993) and to Chapter 6 of this book in which periodontal conditions are considered in more detail.

The value of teeth in nutrition

Most studies which have investigated the effect of teeth on nutrition have considered two questions: Does a poor dental state affect food choice and, if so, is this potentially damaging to health? and Does a poor dental state affect nutrient intake? The third question: Does a poor dental state affect health? has not been studied, which is a pity as it is the fundamental question. In one of the few good reviews of this subject, Geissler and Bates (1984) are critical of the lack

of good data on this subject. They point out, first, that many of the methods used to assess dietary intake have been poor or, indeed, often unreported; second, that most human studies have not been carefully controlled for social and health factors that affect food choice and nutrition and, third, that extrapolation from animal experiments is not necessarily relevant because of our ability to choose and prepare different foods.

Farrell (1956) investigated the effect of mastication on the digestion of solid foods and concluded that 'The degree of mastication required for maximum absorption of the least digestible foods, was shown to be slight, and to be obtained by persons with dentitions that would normally be termed inadequate'. The number of teeth lost is proportional to the difficulty that people have in eating foods and this, in turn, affects food choice. One aspect of tooth loss which has been addressed by only a small number of people is that tooth loss seems to be a risk factor in death by choking. Anderson (1977) drew attention to statistics which showed that choking on food was more commonly fatal than usually supposed and that poor dental health was often an associated risk factor. Choking on food was estimated by Eller and Haugen (1973) to kill between 2500 and 3900 people per year in the USA and was, therefore, the sixth most common cause of accidental death. Anderson (1977) also drew attention to national statistics from Canada which showed that between 1965 and 1974 there was an average of 372 deaths per year due to inhalation of food. Those under 10 years and over 60 years were at greatest risk. Dentists and dietitians should warn edentulous elderly patients of the need to prepare food adequately for swallowing.

Several researchers have investigated the choice of foods by people with chewing impairments. Heath (1972) identified nuts and tough meat as problem foods in elderly Britons, while Ettinger (1973) identified 27 problem foods, including meat, fruit, salads and some vegetables and crusty bread, in an Australian population. However, there is little evidence that nutrition or health were impaired.

In summary, teeth were essential for the survival of our ancestors, but modern food technology has meant that teeth are much less important for preparing food for swallowing and digestion than previously. Lack of teeth has a marked effect on chewing ability and food choice. In contrast, lack of teeth appears to have little effect on nutritional intake or on serum nutrient levels.

Guidelines for nutrition

Authoritative non-commercial guidelines for healthy eating are extremely useful in helping to inform national policies, community initiatives and individual action. The UK has a history of good authorative reports on various aspects of nutrition, diet and health–most of these are provided by the Department of Health, but also by national bodies responsible for health education, and professional associations. These will be highlighted to appreciate the development of recommendations and the consistency of the advice given before briefly considering their application in health promotion.

The Committee on Medical Aspects of Food Policy (COMA) is a standing committee within the Department of Health in London. It is chaired by the Chief Medical Officer and advises government on food policy as it affects health. Very often the committee establishes panels of experts to look at one particular issue and these temporary panels report to the main COMA committee. One of the first COMA panels to be concerned with dental matters was the Panel on Cariogenic Foods (COMA, 1969). Its terms of reference were to consider the cariogenic action of foods with particular reference in the first place to vitamin supplements as used in babies' comforters, and to make recommendations. The Panel concluded that reservoir feeders, dummies and feeding bottles, when filled with or dipped in sugary and/or acid solutions, including fruit juice preparations, are conducive to rampant caries.

In 1978, a discussion booklet prepared by the Health Departments of Great Britain and Northern Ireland (Department of Health and Social Security, 1978) was published entitled *Eating for Health*. The section on dental caries began:

The United Kingdom has a poor record of dental health. It has never been good, but has become worse over the past century principally through the increasing use of sugar in the diet. Throughout the world the incidence of dental decay in children is related to the consumption of sugar. British people who lived before sugar was in general use had much better teeth than most people have today. During the war, when sugar was restricted, children had less dental decay but, with the advent of peace and the end of sugar rationing, the rate of decay rapidly increased leading to the unnecessary loss of many teeth.

This report also highlighted the concern of the misuse of sugar when a baby is teething. In those days, sugar was used both with dummies and comforters (small bottles or reservoir feeders). The sugar was table sugar, blackcurrant or rosehip syrups, or sweet condensed milk, leading to carious front teeth. In the summary, it was noted that an early introduction to sweet foods may help a child to develop a 'sweet tooth', leading to dental caries and that therefore, the use of sugar and confectionery should be limited.

Infant feeding has been the subject of three COMA reports (Department of Health and Social Security, 1974, 1980, 1988). All three reports strongly reaffirm the desirability of encouraging all healthy mothers to breast-feed their babies. The second and third reports considered dental health, emphasizing the need to restrict sugar consumption in infancy because of the risk of causing dental caries and the development of a sweet tooth, and the need to maximize the use of fluoride, either in water or in drops or tablets. The third report's section on dental health noted that the cariogenic effect of reservoir and dipped dummies was highlighted in the COMA report on cariogenic foods (1969) and that those extreme practices had largely gone. However, sucrose is used to sweeten medicines for children and it urged that alternative non-cariogenic bulk or intense sweeteners should be used instead.

One of the key COMA reports concerning dental health has been the report on *Dietary Sugars and Human Disease* (Department of Health, 1989). Chapters were devoted to sugars and dental caries and to nine conclusions and recommendations which were reproduced in the *British Dental Journal* (Anon., 1990). The principal points are briefly summarized here. Caries risk can be reduced by non-dietary means, particularly the use of fluoride, but these methods offer incomplete protection and some are expensive. The Panel recommended a reduction in the consumption of NME sugars which should be replaced by fresh fruit, vegetables and starchy foods. This recommendation should be brought to the attention of those providing food for families and communities to reduce the frequency with which sugary snacks are consumed. In addition, simple sugars (e.g. sucrose, glucose, fructose) should not be added to bottle feeds; sugared drinks should not be given in feeders where they may be in contact with the teeth for prolonged periods; dummies or comforters should not be dipped in sugars or sugary drinks. The Panel recommended that schools should promote healthy eating patterns both by nutrition education and by providing and encouraging nutritionally sound food choices. The government should seek the means to reduce the use of sugared liquid medicines. In order to facilitate dental practitioners giving dietary advice, on the reduction of NME sugars consumption, it was recommended that teaching of nutrition during dental training should be increased, with professional relations between dietitians and dental practitioners.

This was the first report to divide dietary sugars into intrinsic sugars, milk sugars and NME sugars. This classification has been followed by all subsequent COMA and other authorative reports. It clearly recommended that consumption of NME sugars should be decreased, but did not say by how much. This was left to the COMA report on *Dietary Reference Values for Food Energy and Nutrients for the United Kingdom* (Department of Health, 1991). This Panel agreed with the principal conclusions of the COMA Panel on dietary sugars and proposed that the population's average intake of NME sugars should not exceed about 60 g/day or 10% of total dietary energy. Starches together with intrinsic and milk sugars should provide the main source of carbohydrate food energy (Table 13.3). The subsequent

COMA report *The Nutrition of Elderly People* (Department of Health, 1992a) endorsed the recommendations of the 1991 COMA report on dietary reference values, and proposed that elderly people reduce dietary intakes of fat and simple sugars and increase intakes of starchy foods, non-starch polysaccharides and vitamin D. It was noted that, in some instances, more than the recommended levels of simple sugars may be needed, for example, for very elderly people during episodes of ill health.

In 1994 a report on *Weaning and the Weaning Diet* recommended that mothers should be encouraged and supported in breast-feeding and that milk or water should constitute the majority of the total drinks given (Department of Health, 1994a). Furthermore, other drinks should usually be confined to meal times and not given in a feeding bottle or at bedtime, because of the risk to dental health and that foods and drinks predisposing to caries should be limited to main meal times. Further recommendations were that weaning foods should usually be free of, or low in, NME sugars. The range of such commercial foods should be increased and the sugar content of all weaning foods and drinks should be shown on food labels.

A further COMA report in 1994 examined *Nutritional Aspects of Cardiovascular Disease* (Department of Health, 1994b). This was important since the UK has one of the highest incidences of cardiovascular disease in the world. It is not surprising that the main recommendations were that dietary fat intake should fall (to about 35% of dietary energy). It also recommended that complex carbohydrates, and sugars in fruits and vegetables, should restore the energy deficit following a reduction in the dietary intake of fat and that the proportion of dietary energy derived from carbohydrates should increase to approximately 50% (see Table 13.3).

These Department of Health reports have been supplemented by a variety of other reports. In 1983, the Health Education Council published *A Discussion Paper on Proposals for Nutritional Guidelines for Health Education in Britain*. It is often referred to as the NACNE report as it was prepared by the National Advisory Committee on Nutrition Education (1983). It effectively recommended a halving of sugars consumption from the level of 38 kg/head per year, such that average sucrose intakes be reduced to 20 kg head per year. At the time, the

Table 13.3 Dietary reference values for fat and carbohydrate for adults as a percentage of daily total energy intake (% food energy)

	Individual minimum	Population average
Total fat		33 (35)
Total carbohydrate		47 (50)
Non-milk extrinsic sugars	0	10 (11)
Intrinsic and milk sugars and starch		37 (39)

From Department of Health (1991), with permission.

Table 13.4 World Health Organization nutrient goals—limits for population average intakes

	% of total energy	
	Lower	*Upper*
Fat	15	30
Carbohydrate	55	75
Complex	50	70
Free sugars	0	10
Protein	0	15

From World Health Organization (1990), with permission.

report created much opposition from the food industry for daring to give quantitative targets but, interestingly, NACNE's target of 20 kg sucrose/person per year is equivalent to the recommendations of COMA (Department of Health, 1991) of 60 g person per day. The NACNE targets were expressed in terms of sucrose, while the COMA target was for NME sugars. Furthermore, the recommendations of NACNE (1983) and COMA (Department of Health, 1991) were very similar to the recommendations of the World Health Organization (WHO; 1990), which are given in Table 13.4. The WHO label of free sugars is almost synonymous with NME sugars. The importance of complex carbohydrates in the diet seen in the WHO population nutrient goals recurs in the report from the Royal College of Physicians (1983) on *Obesity*. It recommended reductions in fat and sugar, emphasizing the importance of the fibre-rich starchy components of the diet.

Many professional societies have published policy documents on nutrition, diet and health, for example, that of the British Medical Association (1986) followed the NACNE line closely. The British Dental Association and the British Dietetic Association reiterated and supported the COMA recommendations (Department of Health, 1989, 1991). Not only is there agreement in the published recommendations between professions, but there is also agreement within the dental profession, e.g. the British Association for the Study of Community Dentistry (1985) and the British Society of Paediatric Dentistry (1992) recommended a reduction of intake of NME sugars.

In 1992, a major health initiative was launched in England called *The Health of the Nation*, describing a strategy for health (Department of Health, 1992b). It was especially significant since, for the first time, the document was agreed by *all* the relevant government departments. This was crucial as previously it was very possible for the Department of Health to make recommendations, but the Ministry of Agriculture or Education to take little action to assist in the implementation of these recommendations; occasionally they were antagonistic, as will be described later in this chapter. The *Health of the Nation* initiative was limited to five key areas: coronary heart disease and stroke; cancers; mental illness; human immunodeficiency virus (HIV) and acquired immune deficiency syndrome (AIDS) and sexual health; and accidents. In Scotland (Scottish Office, 1992) a sixth key area (dental caries) was included. One of the products of the *Health of the Nation* initiative was the action plan Eat Well produced by the Nutritional Task Force (Department of Health, 1994c), since diet was recognized as an important risk factor in several of the five key areas. The Eat Well document stated that targets for nutrition and diet were set within the overall context of the COMA dietary reference values (Department of Health, 1991) report.

The current state of dental health and objectives for the year 2003 are given in *An Oral Health Strategy for England* (Department of Health, 1994c). In the section on ways to better oral health, it reiterated the philosophy of the *Health of the Nation* document, listing the Health Education Authority (1989) advice to:

Reduce the consumption and especially the frequency of intake of sugar-containing food and drink, clean the teeth and gums thoroughly every day with a fluoride toothpaste, drink fluoridated water, and attend for regular dental check-ups.

Food and drink manufacturers as well as the pharmaceutical industry can help in this by looking seriously at the composition of their products and replacing cariogenic sugars with less harmful sweeteners, or omitting sweeteners altogether.

School meals have been seen as important, not only because they provide a major proportion of a child's nutrition, but also from the educational viewpoint. The Caroline Walker Trust published *Nutritional Guidelines for School Meals* in 1992. The school meal service is considered in further detail in Chapter 15.

Sugars consumption

Health promotion cannot be targeted successfully without knowledge of eating behaviour. The overriding importance of sugars in caries development has been emphasized, and it is sensible, therefore, to look more closely at the sources of sugars in the diet of those at risk. A fairly full investigation of sugars consumption in young British adolescents was undertaken in 1980 by Rugg-Gunn *et al.* (1986) and repeated in the same location in 1990 (Rugg-Gunn *et al.*, 1993). In the 1990 survey the mean total sugars intake, for both genders, was 118 g/day–equivalent to 43 kg/person per year–in 379 children whose mean age was 11.5 years and mean energy intake 8.42 MJ/day. The mean intake of milk and intrinsic sugars was 28 g/day–11% of total carbohydrate and 5% of total energy intake–while NME sugars consumption was 90g/person per day–35% of carbohydrate and 17% of energy intake. Seventy-six per cent of total sugars consumption was provided by NME sugars; 90 g/day NME sugars equates to 33 kg/person year. It can be seen that these levels are considerably in excess of those consistently and authoritatively recommended in the previous sections of this chapter. When the dietary sources of milk and intrinsic sugars were investigated, milk provided about one-third and fresh fruit and vegetables about two-thirds.

The sources of the NME sugars are given in Table 13.5. Confectionery provided, on average, 30 g of these sugars (and 1 g of milk and intrinsic sugars), soft drinks 24 g of NME sugars, table

Table 13.5 Sources of non-milk extrinsic sugars in 12-year-old Northumbrian children

1980 (n = 405)			1990 (n = 379)	
%	g		%	g
29	24	Confectionery	33	30
19	15	Soft drinks	27	24
23	19	Table sugar	12	11
11	10	Biscuits and cakes	11	10
9	7	Puddings	6	5
2	2	Breakfast cereals	5	5
3	3	Syrups and preserves	2	2
3	3	Other	4	3
100	83	All sources	100	90

From Rugg-Gunn *et al.* (1993), with permission.

Table 13.6 Percentage contribution of food types to average daily intake of non-milk extrinsic sugars for a nationally representative sample of children (n = 1675) aged 1½–4½ in the UK in 1992–93

	%	g
Cereals and cereal products	23	13.2
of which:		
High-fibre and wholegrain breakfast cereals	1	0.8
Other breakfast cereals	3	1.9
Biscuits	7	4.2
Milk products	5	2.9
of which:		
Fromage frais and yogurt	4	2.3
Vegetables, potatoes and savoury snacks	1	0.6
of which:		
Vegetables, excluding potatoes	1	0.6
Fruit and nuts	1	0.6
of which:		
Fruit	1	0.6
Nuts	0	0.0
Sugars, preserves and confectionery	27	15.7
of which:		
Sugar	5	2.7
Preserves	2	1.2
Sugar confectionery	11	6.2
Chocolate confectionery	10	5.6
Beverages	39	22.2
of which:		
Fruit juice	6	3.4
Soft drinks, not low-calorie	32	18.2
Commercial infant food and drinks	1	0.4
Miscellaneous	3	1.5
Total	100	57

Modified from Gregory *et al.* (1995).

sugar 11 g and biscuits and cakes 10 g per person per day. The top two sources–confectionery and soft drinks–provided 60% of NME sugars in these adolescents, and it is not surprising that these two sources are the main target for health education. Total sugars consumption had changed little between 1980 (405 11–12-year-olds) and 1990 (379 11–12-year-olds) at 117 and 118 g, respectively, but over these 10 years, milk and intrinsic sugars intake had decreased from 34 to 28 g/day while NME sugars intake had increased from 83 to 90 g/day. Confectionery is now the second most important source of energy and dietary fat in these children (Adamson *et al.*, 1992).

From the report on the dental health of pre-school children in the UK (Gregory *et al.*, 1995), the average daily intake of total sugars was 87 g with 57 g NME sugars. Confectionery and soft drinks were also the top two sources of NME sugars in the diet, totalling 53% (Table 13.6). As previously described, the current UK recommendation is that the intake of NMEs should contribute no more than 10% of total dietary energy. The Working Group of the Committee on the Medical Aspects of the Weaning Diet considered that this value was also applicable to pre-school children because they are a group at high risk of dental caries (Department of Health, 1994a). The average for all the children was 18.7% with a lower 2.5 percentile of 5.8 and an upper of 35.6, i.e. at worst more than a third of their energy was coming from NME sugars. Overall, beverages contributed one-quarter of the total sugars intake in the children's diet and was typically soft drinks. For these young children, the high percentage of sugar-containing soft drinks was most disturbing and provoked debate in the media on the release of the report. From the dental examination, none of the 105 of 1½–2½-year-olds with the lowest average daily intake of NME sugars had experienced dental caries compared to 8% of those with the highest average daily intakes (Hinds and Gregory, 1995).

International comparisons are difficult, but in one comparison of sugars intake in American and English children (Rugg-Gunn, 1993; Table 13.6), consumption of milk and whole fruit was higher in American children (31% of total sugars

in American children compared with 18% in English children) and consumption of confectionery and table sugar twice as high in English children (36% of total sugars) than in American children (18% of total sugars).

Health promotion perspectives

Dietary recommendations are only of value if they can be implemented. To gain insight into likely change, it is useful to take into account influences on individual dietary intake and known dietary barriers. Figure 13.1 has been constructed reflecting many factors affecting dietary intake. Some of the findings described below are discussed in greater detail in the report of a working party to the Chief Medical Officer for Scotland (*The Scottish Diet*; Scottish Home and Health Department, 1993). These considerations are relevant to a wide range of societies in developed countries.

The traditional pattern of three meals per day appears to be declining, particularly among younger groups in the population. There has been a move to a single cooked evening meal and an increase in snacking. In children from disadvantaged backgrounds, the disadvantage in diet begins from birth with a far lower prevalence of breast-feeding. Children are frequently

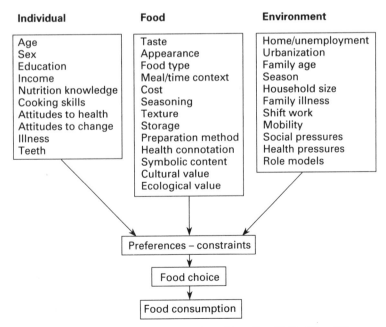

Fig. 13.1 Factors affecting dietary intake. Adapted from Scottish Health and Home Department (1993).

weaned on to an unhealthy diet which is too high in fat, refined extrinsic sugars and in sodium. The diet is typified by daily snacks of crisps, sweets and sugar-containing fizzy drinks.

Higher socioeconomic groups are both more responsive to healthy eating messages and possess the income to make better nutritional choices. In lower socioeconomic groups, responsiveness to healthy eating may be weaker, exacerbated by income constraints. The effort and incentive needed to change established habits, and routines that have led to long-standing dietary inadequacies, are greater in the socially deprived. This is often compounded by a lack of basic food skills and knowledge about how to choose a sensible diet, shop economically, prepare and cook food effectively. Low-income groups spend relatively more of their disposable income on food and replacing dietary items with healthier options can increase the total cost considerably (Cole-Hamilton and Lang, 1986). This is compounded by choice being noticeably limited in shops in socially deprived areas, for example, a marked lack of availability of vegetables and fruit (Mooney, 1990).

Changing consumption of specific food items has been most successfully promoted by the production industry, e.g. the growth in breakfast cereals. However, there is still an enormous imbalance between the amounts spent on advertising healthy and unhealthy foods. For example, in 1991 in the UK, only £4.5 million was spent on advertising fresh fruit and vegetables, compared to £28 million for crisps and snacks and £83 million for chocolate. In the UK, the consumption of fruit and vegetables is relatively low at around 53 kg per capita; it is less than half that of Spain or Greece, with the EU average at almost 81 kg. In the USA, the five-a-day campaign stresses the importance of five servings of fruit and vegetables in the daily diet. This goal is attractive as it is readily understood, based on existing messages, such as 'eat your greens' and 'an apple a day'; it is a simple measure rather than grams or percentages; in addition, the message is positive in being asked to eat more not less.

It is unrealistic to expect rapid societal changes in diet based on mass education alone. A health promotion approach is needed involving cooperation between several government departments. (The theoretical background to this approach is described in detail in Chapter 11 of this book.) However, there are considerable difficulties in overcoming organizational inertia, competing interests and consumer misunderstandings (WHO, 1990).

The interplay between government policy in education compared to health is an interesting one in the UK, where the legislation emanating from one department, Education, has acted to undermine the stated policy of another, Health. This is well-illustrated by the provision of school meals. In the UK, children compulsorily attend school from age 5 to age 16 years. Primary education is from 5 to 11 years and secondary education 12 to 16 years. Typically children attend school from 9.00 a.m. till 4 p.m. and therefore, the midday meal is within school time. Up until 1980, there was a legal responsibility on local education authorities (LEAs) to provide a school meal for all children who wanted one. This meal had to meet prescribed nutritional guidelines. In addition, in primary schools, milk was provided for consumption in the morning break. These two sources of food were particularly important in compensating the diets of children from disadvantaged backgrounds. The 1980 Education Act removed the obligation of school-meal provision and left LEAs free to decide whether or not to provide school meals. They were obliged to provide a meal for children entitled to one free (this could be sandwiches) and adequate facilities for children to eat their own packed lunches. School milk had become discretionary. With the growth in packed lunches brought from home, nutritional inadequacies at home were brought to school, denying the disadvantaged child at least one daily meal that was nutritionally balanced. In 1986, the Social Security Act compounded this further by limiting free school meals to only the very poorest of families. Those families in low-paid work and receiving state augmentation of their income were given extra cash to compensate for the loss. For many senior children, the midday meal has become a plate of chips and a can of fizzy drink. In 1988, the Local Government Act introduced compulsory tendering, further undermining the quality and quantity of school meal provision. The reintroduction of nutritional guidelines for school meals is strongly recommended (Scottish Home and Health Department, 1993) and the Caroline Walker Trust has recently (1992) published *Nutritional Guidelines for School Meals*. This history marks a powerful example of the need for coordinated action between government departments.

Recent successful dietary changes have been seen at the population level in the USA and Norway. Two different approaches have been recognized to bring about their success. In the USA an educational campaign by the American Heart Foundation highlighted the importance of dietary measures and exercise to reduce serum cholesterol levels. The campaign was taken up by other voluntary organizations and led to a widespread change in attitudes. This may have been successful because there is a greater emphasis on personal responsibility for health overlaid with the direct individual financial burden of illness. Incentives for change are greater. In contrast, the Norwegians followed a more classical health promotion route. In developing their nutritional policies, they established a broadly based Nutrition Council involving the agriculture and food industries, public health monitoring, prominent doctors and nutritionists and the public themselves. Both countries have seen a dramatic improvement in health coincident with falls in total fat intake and cigarette smoking.

Tooth-friendly sweets as an example of successful dental health promotion

The tooth-friendly idea is some 25 years old, and began in Switzerland with the development of an intra-oral pH telemetric system which was accepted by the Swiss Health Department as a valid test of non-cariogenicity (Imfeld and Guggenheim, 1990). Progress became more rapid after 1983 when *Aktion Zahnfreundlich* was established in Switzerland, as a partnership between dentists and industry to promote the tooth-friendly idea. A logo (Fig. 13.2) was registered and could be displayed on packets of confectionery which had passed the pH test. A small levy was paid on products carrying the logo, which was used for the generic promotion of the tooth-friendly idea. By 1991, 20% of confectionery carried the tooth-friendly logo, indicating that the product had been shown to be 'safe for teeth'. Over 90% of Swiss children know the meaning of the logo.

Since 1983, seven other countries have followed the Swiss lead (Table 13.7), and there are now four test centres to which confectionery manufacturers can apply to have their products tested. These are Zurich and Berne (Switzerland),

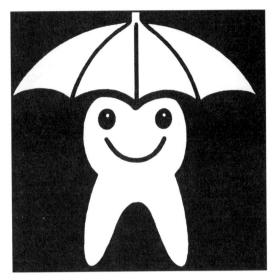

Fig. 13.2 Pictograph of the Mr Happy-tooth. Courtesy of the International Toothfriendly Association.

Table 13.7 The growth of the tooth-friendly concept worldwide: dates of the establishment of national associations

1983	Switzerland
1986	Germany
1991	France
1992	Belgium
1993	UK
	Japan
1994	Italy
1995	Korea

Erfurt (Germany) and Sendai (Japan). In the UK, 1 year after the launch of BATS (the British Association of Toothfriendly Sweets), seven companies have joined and sell tooth-friendly products. As so often happens in other fields, it is the smaller companies who take up the idea first (some changing wholly to sugar-free products) and the larger companies waiting but being forced to join later. The exception to this is presently seen in South America where the tooth-friendly idea is growing fast–here, one big (British-based) manufacturer is showing the way.

These national tooth-friendly associations, such as BATS, are non-profit-making organizations. In the UK, BATS is administered by the British Dental Association and is supported by the Department of Health and the British Society of

Paediatric Dentistry. The levy is currently £0.02/kg confectionery. BATS has now agreed to include infant drinks into the tooth-friendly fold, again, as a way of trying to inform the purchaser.

The tooth-friendly idea is not without its critics. It can be argued that such confectionery is still, largely, empty calories; polyols are known to cause diarrhoea; they may encourage a sweet taste, and they are usually more expensive than their sugar-containing counterparts. On the positive side, the test system is now well-accepted and very unlikely to pass products which cause caries or erosion; confectionery is the target, which is sensible as it is the biggest source of dietary sugars; the purchaser is provided with a choice, and intestinal upsets have not been seen to be a practical problem in Switzerland, nor in the Turku sugar studies where much higher levels of xylitol were consumed. Two further reasons are especially important–first, that tooth-friendly sweets have substituted for sugar-containing sweets rather than added to sales and, second, that there would appear to be a positive benefit to dental health. This is best illustrated in this quote from Marthaler (1990) in his review of changing patterns of caries prevalence in Europe:

In two cases, however, favourable dietary changes are thought to have occurred: the reduction of caries prevalence in Finnish and Swiss children is not likely to be fully explained exclusively in terms of fluorides and improved oral hygiene. In Finland, the widespread use of xylitol as a sweetener may have been a factor in the improvement of dental health; in Switzerland a lowered cariogenic challenge is suggested by the widespread use of nonacidogenic sweets which already in 1985 constituted 10% of the total of sweets sold.

Summary

Nutrition and diet have major influences on dental health. Conversely, dental impairment can adversely affect food choice. Nutrition can affect the structure of teeth, with malnutrition and excessive ingestion of fluoride clearly identified as risk factors. The posteruptive, local intraoral effect of diet is the main cause of dental caries, and dietary sugars are of paramount significance. In order to reduce the risk of caries, both frequency and amount of consumption of NME (free) sugars should be reduced. Dental erosion appears to be a growing problem and this apparent increase in erosion parallels the very great increase in consumption of soft drinks. In the UK, a succession of authoritative, non-commercial reports have urged changes in diet for health–decrease in dietary fats and sugars, and an increase in consumption of starchy foods, fresh fruit and vegetables. This is international advice. Dietary recommendations are only of value if they can be implemented and health promotion is vital to take these measures forward. To reduce risk to teeth in the UK, sugar confectionery and soft drinks are the main targets. Sugar-free confectionery is one option in health promotion and the idea of tooth-friendly sweets is growing internationally.

References

Adamson, A.J., Rugg-Gunn, A.J., Appleton, D.R. *et al.* (1992) Dietary sources of energy, protein, unavailable carbohydrate and fat in 11–12-year-old English children in 1990 compared with results in 1980. *Journal of Human Nutrition and Dietetics* 5:371–385.

Anderson, D.L. (1977) Death from improper mastication. *International Dental Journal* 27:349–54.

Anon. (1990) Dietary sugars and human disease; conclusions and recommendations. *British Dental Journal* **168**:46.

British Association for the Study of Community Dentistry (1985) *Sugar and Dental Caries, A Policy Statement.*

British Dietetic Association (1992) *Position Paper on Sugar.* April 1992.

British Medical Association (1986) *Diet, Nutrition and Health.* British Medical Association, London.

British Society of Paediatric Dentistry (1992) A policy document on sugars and the dental health of children. *International Journal of Paediatric Dentistry* 2:177–180.

Caroline Walker Trust (1992) *Nutritional Guidelines for School Meals.* Caroline Walker Trust, London.

Cockburn, F., Belton, N.R., Purvis, R.J. *et al.* (1980) Maternal vitamin D intake and mineral metabolism in mothers and their newborn infants. *British Medical Journal* ii:11–14.

Cole-Hamilton, I. and Lang, T. (1986) *Tightening Belts: A Report on the Impact of Poverty on Food.* Food Commission, London.

Committee on Medical Aspects of Food Policy (1969) Panel on cariogenic foods; first report. *British Dental Journal* **126**:273–277.

Department of Health (1989) *Dietary Sugars and Human Disease. Report on Health and Social Subjects 37.* HMSO, London.

Department of Health (1991) *Dietary Reference Values for*

Food Energy and Nutrients for the United Kingdom. Report on Health and Social Subjects 41. HMSO, London.

Department of Health (1992a) *The Nutrition of Elderly People. Report on Health and Social Subjects 43.* HMSO, London.

Department of Health (1992b) *The Health of the Nation. A Consultative Document for Health in England.* HMSO, London.

Department of Health (1994a) *Weaning and the Weaning Diet. Report on Health and Social Subjects 45.* HMSO, London.

Department of Health (1994b) *Nutritional Aspects of Cardiovascular Disease. Report on Health and Social Subjects 46.* HMSO, London.

Department of Health (1994c) *An Oral Health Strategy for England.* HMSO, London.

Department of Health and Social Security (1974) *Present Day Practice in Infant Feeding. Report on Health and Social Subjects 9.* HMSO, London.

Department of Health and Social Security (1978) *Eating for Health.* HMSO, London.

Department of Health and Social Security (1980) *Present Day Practice in Infant Feeding 1980. Report on Health and Social Subjects 20.* HMSO, London.

Department of Health and Social Security (1988) *Present Day Practice in Infant Feeding: Third Report. Report on Health and Social Subjects 32.* HMSO, London.

Eller, W.C. and Haugen, R.K. (1973) Food asphyxiation–restaurant rescue. *New England Journal of Medicine* **289**:81–82.

Enwonwu, C.O. (1973) Influence of socio-economic conditions on dental development in Nigerian children. *Archives of Oral Biology* **18**:95–107.

Ettinger, R.L. (1973) Diet, nutrition and masticatory ability in a group of elderly edentulous patients. *Australian Dental Journal* **18**:12–19.

Farrell, J.H. (1956) The effect of mastication on the digestion of food. *British Dental Journal* **100**:149–155.

Fearne, J.M., Bryan, E.M., Elliman, A.M. *et al.* (1990) Enamel defects in the primary dentition of children born weighing less than 2000g. *British Dental Journal* **168**:433–437.

Geissler, C.A. and Bates, J.E. (1984) The nutritional effects of tooth loss. *American Journal of Clinical Nutrition* **39**:478–489.

Gregory, J.R., Collins, D.L., Davies, P.S.W., Hughes, J.M. and Clarke, P.C. (1995) *National Diet and Nutrition Survey: Children Aged 1½ to 4½ Years. Volume 1: Report of the Diet and Nutrition Survey.* HMSO, London.

Hinds, K. and Gregory, J.R. (1995) *National Diet and Nutrition Survey; Children aged 1½ to 4½ Years. Volume 2, Report of the Dental Survey.* HMSO, London.

Health Education Authority (1989) *The Scientific Basis of Dental Health Education. A Policy Document,* 3rd edn. Health Education Authority, London.

Heath, M.R. (1972) Dietary selection by elderly persons, related to dental state. *British Dental Journal* **132**:145–148.

Imfeld, T.N. and Guggenheim, B. (1990) The Swiss association for tooth-friendly sweets (the sympadent association). In: *Sugarless, The Way Forward* (Rugg-Gunn,

A.J., ed.), pp. 197–210. Elsevier Applied Science, London.

Infante, P.F. and Gillespie, G.M. (1977) Enamel hypoplasia in relation to caries in Guatemalan children. *Journal of Dental Research* **56**:493–498.

Jackson, D. (1961) A clinical study of non-endemic mottling of enamel. *Archives of Oral Biology* **5**:212–223.

Jarvinen, V.K., Rytomaa, I.I. and Heinonen, O.P. (1991) Risk factors in dental erosion. *Journal Dental Research* **70**:942–947.

Marthaler, T.M. (1990) Changes in the prevalence of dental caries: how much can be attributed to changes in diet? *Caries Research* **24** (suppl. 1):3–15.

Mooney, C. (1990) Cost and availability of healthy food choices in a London health district. *Journal of Human Nutrition and Diet* **3**:111–120.

Murray, J.J., Rugg-Gunn, A.J. and Jenkins, G.N. (1991) *Fluorides in Caries Prevention,* 3rd edn. Butterworth-Heinemann, Oxford.

National Advisory Committee on Nutrition Education (1983) *A Discussion Paper on Proposals for Nutritional Guidelines for Health Education in Britain.* Health Education Council, London.

Nikiforuk, G. and Fraser, D. (1981) The aetiology of enamel hypoplasia; a unifying concept. *Journal of Pediatrics* **98**:888–893.

O'Brien, M. (1994) *Children's Dental Health in the United Kingdom 1993.* OPCS Social Survey Division. HMSO, London.

Osborn, T.W.B. and Noriskin, J.N. (1937) The relationship between diet and caries in South African Bantu. *Journal of Dental Research* **16**:431–441.

Pindborg, J.J. (1982) Aetiology of developmental enamel defects not related to fluorosis. *International Dental Journal* **32**:123–134.

Rice, S. (1995) West European food and drink packaging. *FT Management Report.*

Royal College of Physicians (1983) Obesity. *Journal of the Royal College of Physicians London* **1**:3–65.

Rugg-Gunn, A.J. (ed.) (1991) *Sugarless, The Way Forward.* Elsevier Applied Science, Essex.

Rugg-Gunn, A.J. (1993) *Nutrition and Dental Health.* Oxford University Press, Oxford.

Rugg-Gunn, A.J. (ed.) (1994) *Sugarless, Towards the Year 2000.* Royal Society of Chemistry, Cambridge.

Rugg-Gunn, A.J., Hackett, A.F., Appleton, D.R. and Moynihan, P.J. (1986) The dietary intake of added and natural sugars in 405 English adolescents. *Human Nutrition: Applied Nutrition* **40A**:115–124.

Rugg-Gunn, A.J., Adamson, A.J., Appleton, D.R. *et al.* (1993) Sugars consumption by 379 11–12-year-old English children in 1990 compared with results in 1980. *Journal of Human Nutrition and Dietetics* **6**:419–431.

Scottish Home and Health Department (1993) *The Scottish Diet. Report on Working Party to the Chief Medical Officer for Scotland.* The Scottish Office, Edinburgh.

Scottish Office (1992) *Scotland's Health–A Challenge To Us All. A Policy Statement.* HMSO, Edinburgh.

Suckling, G.W. and Pearce, E.I.F. (1984) Developmental defects of enamel in a group of New Zealand children, their prevalence and some associated etiological factors. *Community Dental and Oral Epidemiology* **12**:177–184.

Sweeney, E.A., Saffir, A.J. and Leon, R. (1971) Linear hypoplasia of deciduous incisor teeth in malnourished children. *American Journal of Clinical Nutrition* **24**:29–31.

Wilson, R.M.H. and Cleaton-Jones, P. (1978) Enamel mottling and infectious exanthemata in a rural community. *Journal of Dentistry* **6**:161–165.

World Health Organization (1990) *Diet, Nutrition and the Prevention of Chronic Diseases*. Technical report 797. WHO, Geneva.

14

Fluoridation

Sheila Jones and Michael Lennon

Introduction

The main focus of this chapter is water fluoridation. First, the history of the development of water fluoridation as a public health measure to reduce dental caries is outlined. The various legal and decision-making frameworks are then discussed, followed by an overview of the ethical framework within which decisions about fluoridation are taken. A section on the medical safety of fluoridation reviews the relevant reports on the subject. This is followed by case studies of the fluoridation experiences of four countries– the USA, the UK, Ireland and Hong Kong. The topic of water fluoridation is concluded with a brief overview of the extent of water fluoridation worldwide, and discussion of some decisions to cease fluoridation. Finally, other public health approaches to fluoridation, including the fluoridation of salt and milk, are discussed briefly with a particular focus on their comparability to water fluoridation as population approaches to disease prevention.

Historical background

Water fluoride levels and dental fluorosis

The discovery of the dental benefits of fluoride came about almost by accident as a result of the search for the cause of dental mottling (now recognized as dental fluorosis). Endemic 'stained' teeth have been described by observers of various communities in Europe and North

America since the late 19th century (McClure, 1970). Probably the first scientific investigation into the cause of the phenomenon started in 1901 when newly qualified American dentist Frederick McKay decided to investigate a condition which affected most of his patients, and which was known locally as Colorado brown stain. It was believed that the condition, which was characterized by brown or yellow staining of the enamel and often also pitting, was acquired, and that it was associated with geological conditions. Public water supplies were implicated in the aetiology from the late 1920s when two small communities successfully eliminated the condition by changing their water supplies. However, it was not until the early 1930s, when water fluoride analytical methods were refined, that it was possible to suggest that fluoride was the water borne factor causing the problem of dental mottling in many communities in the USA.

The next phase of the investigation was conducted by Dr H. Trendley Dean of the US Public Health Service's National Institute of Dental Research. In 1931 Dean was given the mission 'to resolve the relation of waterborne fluoride to endemic mottled enamel'. This work was to produce the epidemiological studies which established the relationship not only between water fluoride levels and the prevalence of dental fluorosis, but more importantly, between water fluoride levels and the prevalence of dental caries. In order to record quantitatively the various degrees of severity of mottled enamel, Dean developed an index which classified fluoride mottling in six grades: normal, questionable, very mild, mild, moderate and severe (Dean, 1938). The index provided Dean with the necessary tool with which to assess the degree of mottling in the individual, and also to determine 'a numerical weighted index of clinical severity (index of dental fluorosis)' for each group examined (McClure, 1970). This was necessary for the epidemiological surveys and subsequent 'correlation with chemical and other studies'. In 1933 Dean published the first of his systematic surveys of the distribution of mottled enamel in the USA (Dean, 1933).

Water fluoride levels and dental caries

That mottled teeth were no more susceptible to caries than teeth without enamel defects had been recognized by McKay as early as 1929 (McClure, 1970). However, in the early 1940s Dean and colleagues published the now classical '21 cities' studies which clearly demonstrated an

inverse relationship between the fluoride concentration of the public water supplies and the caries prevalence in children aged 12–14 years (Dean *et al.*, 1941, 1942). The most important finding was the 'strikingly low dental caries prevalence ... associated with the continuous use of domestic waters whose fluoride content was as low as about 1 part per million, a concentration which under the conditions prevailing in the localities studied produced only sporadic instances of the mildest forms of dental fluorosis of no practical esthetic significance'. Figure 14.1 shows the prevalence of dental fluorosis (according to Dean's Community Index), the decayed, missing, filled teeth (DMFT) of 12–14-year-olds, and the natural fluoride concentration in water in the 21 cities. From the work of Dean *et al.* it was concluded that a concentration of 1 part of fluoride naturally present per million parts of water was associated with significantly lower levels of dental caries and with an acceptable prevalence of only the

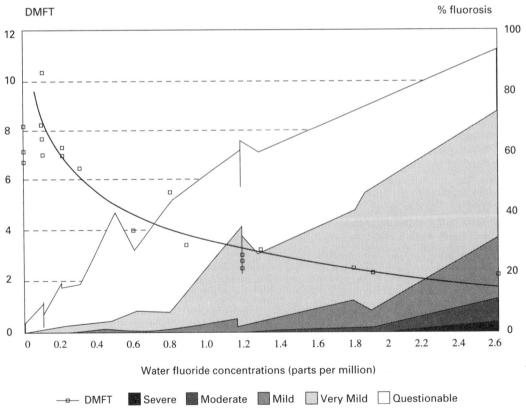

Fig. 14.1 Decayed, missing, filled teeth (DMFT) of 12–14-year-olds, dental fluorosis and water flouride concentrations in 21 US cities 1941–42. Modified from Dean *et al.*, 1941, 1942), with permission.

mildest forms of fluorosis. Thus the 'optimal' level for fluoride naturally present in drinking water was set at 1 part per million (1.0 p.p.m.).

Fluoridation trials in the USA

Dean's work led to the hypothesis that the artificial adjustment of the fluoride level in the public drinking water might also confer the benefits of caries reduction seen in naturally fluoridated regions, whilst minimizing the undesirable effects of fluorosis. Plans for initial fluoridation studies under the auspices of the US Public Health Service were approved by health and local authorities on the basis of there being substantial knowledge of the health of generations of populations drinking water which naturally contained 1.0 p.p.m. fluoride or more.

On 25 January 1945 the first study of controlled community water fluoridation began when Grand Rapids, Michigan became the first community in the world to fluoridate its drinking water artificially. The cities of Muskegon, Michigan (non-fluoridated), and Aurora, Illinois (natural water fluoride level 1.2 p.p.m.) served as controls. Several other studies were soon set up, the objectives being to monitor caries and fluorosis levels in fluoridated and non-fluoridated communities, and to demonstrate the technical and financial feasibility of artificial fluoridation. The first dental data were published in 1950, and the results were so impressive that, in the UK in 1951, the Anglesey County Council agreed to ask the government for a grant to introduce water fluoridation on the island (Griffith, 1956). In 1952 the British government, on the recommendation of the Medical Research Council, sent a delegation to the USA and to Canada (where several studies were also in progress). The task of the British mission included an evaluation of the dental results, consideration of possible effects of fluoridation on general health, and a study of the technical processes involved in artificially fluoridating water supplies (Ministry of Health, 1953).

The UK fluoridation studies

The report of the mission recommended that the British government should consider adopting fluoridation as a public health measure to control dental caries, and recommended the establishment of a series of UK demonstration studies. In 1955 and 1956 UK fluoridation demonstration projects were started in Watford, Andover, Anglesey and Kilmarnock. Due to pressure from antifluoridation activists, Andover and Kilmarnock Councils decided to withdraw from the studies after 2 years and 6 years respectively. Two reports were published after 5 years and after 11 years (Ministry of Health, 1962; Department of Health and Social Security, 1969) confirming the benefits and safety of fluoridation, and by the mid 1960s local authorities throughout the UK, encouraged by the government, were establishing fluoridation schemes. These included schemes in the West Midlands, for approximately 1.2 million people in 1964; the North-east, for approximately half a million people in 1968, and Yorkshire, for approximately 132 000 people in 1968.

The results of the Kilmarnock study were presented as an appendix to the 11-year report (Department of Health and Social Security, 1969). Annual examinations of children aged 3–7 years had continued in both the study and control communities after cessation of fluoridation in 1962. The studies, reported by Professor Mansbridge of the University of Edinburgh, assessed both the effects of $6\frac{1}{2}$ years of fluoridation, and the effects of withdrawal of fluoridation. By 1968, 6 years after the cessation of fluoridation, the prevalence of caries in deciduous dentition in Kilmarnock had deteriorated almost to the level which existed prior to fluoridation, and was again similar to that of the control community which had remained consistently high (Fig. 14.2).

The legal framework and decision-making about fluoridation

Legislation governing fluoridation varies throughout the world. Some countries have no legislation covering fluoridation (e.g. the Netherlands); in others, for example the UK, *enabling* legislation exists; while in some countries, for example Ireland and Singapore, mandatory fluoridation legislation exists. In the USA, no *federal* fluoridation legislation exists; however, states enact their own fluoridation legislation, some of which is enabling, and some mandatory.

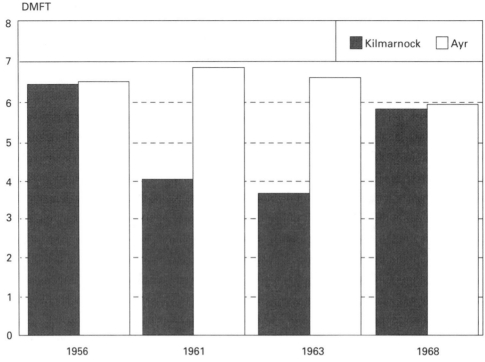

DMFT

Fig. 14.3 Growth of US general population and population served by fluoridated water 1945–1992. Data from USPHS Division of Oral Health (1993).

Absence of fluoridation legislation

As stated, in many countries no fluoridation legislation exists; for example, developing countries where dental caries is not, as yet, a public health problem. Furthermore, in some developed countries water fluoridation has been practised for many years in the absence of specific legislation. In some of these countries challenges to the legality of fluoridation have resulted in the passage of specific legislation, as in the case of the Water (Fluoridation) Act 1985 in the UK. In other countries, for example the Netherlands, such action has resulted in the withdrawal of fluoridation and a continued absence of legislation (König, 1987).

Enabling legislation

Enabling legislation usually takes the form of devolving decisions about the need for fluoridation, and its implementation, down to local level. In the UK the 1985 Water (Fluoridation) Act empowers district health authorities to request water suppliers to adjust

the fluoride content of water supplies to the optimal 1.0 p.p.m.. However, before making such requests health authorities are required to undertake a major public consultation exercise about their fluoridation proposals. Other forms of enabling legislation, e.g. in some American states, require local authorities to ballot their local population before implementing fluoridation proposals.

Mandatory legislation

Mandatory legislation usually allows decisions about fluoridation to be taken centrally. For example in Ireland, as will be described in detail later in this chapter, decisions about whether water supplies for any community shall be fluoridated are taken by the Minister for Health who has the power to require health authorities to arrange for the fluoridation of the piped water supplies within their areas (Irish Government, 1960). Other forms of mandatory legislation exist; in the USA some states require local authorities to ensure that all public water supplies contain optimal levels of fluoride.

Decision-making about fluoridation

The legislative framework surrounding fluoridation directly affects decision-making about fluoridation. Where countries have opted for mandatory legislation it has been suggested that:

> If the issue of fluoridation were left to several health authorities to decide, members of such bodies would be called upon to familiarize themselves with the results of the many dental and medical surveys and researches by which its effectiveness as a safeguard against dental caries has been demonstrated. Members who were unable to do this were likely to be misled and fall victims to the horrific arguments with which propagandists of the 'pure water' school would assail their conscience as well as their ignorance (MacEntee, 1972).

Thus decisions about the need for, and the benefits and risks of, fluoridation are taken centrally. The implementation, and often financing, of such decisions is then for local authorities to oversee. Although such legislation can often be met by opposition (MacEntee, 1972), once enacted, fluoridation should be relatively routine.

In contrast to mandatory legislation, enabling legislation usually means that decisions about fluoridation are taken locally. Such action usually involves public consultation, which unfortunately can sometimes degenerate into an acrimonious exchange of claim and counter-claim as local decision-makers, usually town councillors, and health and water authority members find themselves torn between the scientific and technical advice on the one hand, and the claims of antifluoridationists on the other. The degree of controversy perceived by the decision-maker will critically affect the outcome of such local action, and failure to implement fluoridation is at least as likely an outcome as success (Lennon, 1993).

The ethics of water fluoridation

Consideration of the ethics of water fluoridation does not differ from consideration of ethical issues related to any other aspect of health care. It is generally accepted that the four *prima facie* moral principles–respect for autonomy, beneficence, non-maleficence and justice–plus attention to their scope of application 'encompass most of the moral issues that arise in health care' (Gillon, 1994).

Opponents often claim that water fluoridation is unethical, immoral, or that it is an infringement of the individual's freedom of choice. These claims have been examined by different disciplines over several years, including presiding judges in the high courts in Ireland and Scotland (Mr Justice Kenny, 1963; Lord Jauncey, 1983); the Chairman of the UK Parliamentary Human Rights Committee (Lord Avebury, 1984); and a respected professor of applied philosophy (Harris, 1989). The consensus among these commentators is that there is no moral dilemma about water fluoridation. Indeed, it has been suggested (Harris, 1989), since dental caries is the cause of a great deal of suffering, and fluoridation is a safe and effective measure to reduce the incidence of caries, it could be considered unethical *not* to fluoridate water supplies. Further support is given to the argument that fluoridation is ethical by the fact that the issue has been debated and approved by many bodies of elected representatives in countries throughout the world (see, for example, MacEntee, 1972; House of Commons, 1985; Easley, 1995).

The four principles–respect for autonomy, beneficence, non-maleficence and justice–which generally provide a framework for discussing ethical issues in health care are now discussed briefly. Respect for autonomy is 'the moral obligation to respect the personal freedom of others in so far as such respect is compatible with equal respect for the autonomy of all potentially affected' (Gillon, 1994). In society generally some diminution of individual freedom is accepted for the general good. Most laws and regulations depend on this. In terms of fluoridation, Harris (1989) suggests:

> we should ask not are we entitled to impose fluoridation on unwilling people but are the unwilling people entitled to impose the risks, damage and costs of failure to fluoridate on the community at large? When we compare the freedoms at stake, the most crucial is surely the one which involves liberation from pain and disease.

Beneficence (to help others), and non-maleficence (to do no harm) can be considered together, since when we try to help others we inevitably risk harming them. The aim of health care intervention should be that of producing net benefit over harm. In considering these principles with regard to fluoridation, we must consider not only those who will benefit, but also those in the community who will derive no direct benefit–the edentulous, for example. Clearly the obligation of non-maleficence applies to all affected by fluoridation, whether or not we recognize an obligation of beneficence. In other words, we must be as confident as it is possible to be that fluoridation will do no harm. The question of medical aspects of fluoridation is dealt with in detail below. Suffice to say here, in the words of Sir Richard Doll: 'In so far as I can say anything is safe, I say fluoridation is safe' (Doll, 1989).

Finally we turn to the principle of justice. Equality and fairness are the essence of justice, and water fluoridation, as a public health intervention, epitomizes this principle. Whilst fluoridation benefits everyone with natural teeth, the greatest benefits are obtained by those least able to help themselves: children, and those living in socially deprived communities. Furthermore, those responsible for managing limited health care resources have an ethical duty to use those resources in the most cost-effective way possible. In the words of the UK Minister for Health, 'Fluoridation is simply the most cost-effective public health measure available to reduce unacceptably high levels of dental caries' (Malone, 1995), and as such it represents a public health measure which is entirely in keeping with the principle of justice.

Medical aspects of water fluoridation

The possibility of optimally fluoridated water being harmful to human health has occupied both proponents and opponents of fluoridation from the outset. Of prime concern to proponents of fluoridation has been the need to maintain a watching brief on the health of communities consuming fluoridated water. Indeed, as was described earlier, one of the objectives of the 1950s British mission to the USA and Canada was to consider possible effects of fluoridation on general health. Even earlier than that, Weaver in his 1940's studies of naturally fluoridated communities considered 'the possibility of its [fluoridation] doing any harm' (Weaver, 1948). Since then, and up to the present, the extensive scientific literature on the health benefits and

risks of fluoridation has been the subject of searching reviews by expert committees throughout the world, including the World Health Organization (Expert Committee on Water Fluoridation, 1958; Royal College of Physicians, 1976; National Health and Medical Research Council, 1979, 1985, 1991; Knox, 1985; US Public Health Service, 1991b; US National Academy of Sciences Committee on Toxicology, 1993; Expert Committee on Oral Health Status and Fluoride Use, 1994). None has found evidence that drinking water with a concentration of around 1.0 p.p.m. is harmful to human health. In fact, other than dental fluorosis, only one condition–endemic skeletal fluorosis–is known to result from long-term ingestion of water containing high levels of fluoride. To protect against skeletal fluorosis, the US Environmental Protection Agency has set a maximum contaminant level (MCL) for fluoride in water at 4.0 p.p.m. (Federal Register, 1986). However in Europe the maximum admissible concentration (MAC) for fluoride in water is 1.5 p.p.m. (Commission of the European Communities, 1980) and the World Health Organization's Guideline value for fluoride in water is also 1.5 p.p.m. (World Health Organization, 1993).

In recent years opponents have attempted to link fluoridation with a wide range of diseases and afflictions. Many of these allegations are farcical; for example, that fluoridation makes men 'frisky' (Roberts, 1991). Others are calculated to raise fears in the minds of the public and decision-makers; for example, that fluoridation causes cancer, Alzheimer's disease or that it interferes with the immune function. Such allegations are often couched in pseudoscientific terms and put forward by seemingly well-qualified individuals. Such claims often interest the media, and thus the general public and lay decision-makers are given the impression that there is a scientific controversy about the safety of fluoridation. There is, in fact, overwhelming agreement between the scientific, medical and dental community worldwide that fluoridation of water is a safe and effective public health measure. Nevertheless, research continues, particularly into the effects of fluoride on bone health, and the scientific community will continue to balance the risks and benefits and make policy recommendations accordingly (Medical Research Council, 1993; Hillier *et al.*, 1996).

Fluoridation case studies

Fluoridation in the USA

More people receive fluoridated water in the USA than in any other country in the world–approximately half of all those receiving artificially fluoridated water supplies. The practice of artificial fluoridation of water supplies expanded rapidly in the USA as the results of the controlled fluoridation trials, begun in Grand Rapids in 1945, became widely available. In 1950 the US Chief Dental Officer spoke publicly in favour of water fluoridation for the first time. In 1951 approximately 5 million people were receiving fluoridated drinking water, and by 1952 the number had almost trebled to 14 million.

Figure 14. 3 shows the growth of fluoridation in the USA by population, and demonstrates that steadily increasing numbers of Americans are benefiting from a fluoridated water supply. In 1993 the number of Americans receiving fluoridated water had grown to 145 million.

Forty-two of the 50 largest US cities fluoridate their water supplies. Around 10 million people receive water supplies naturally fluoridated at the optimal level, while a further 135 million receive artificially fluoridated supplies. Thus 56% of the total population (62% of those on public water supplies) benefit. Approximately 10% of the US population does not receive a public water supply.

Small water systems (serving < 500 population) comprise 62.2% of US community water systems, but serve only 2.3% of the population on public water supply systems. Many of these small systems serve American Indian and Alaskan Native reservations. Four hundred and seventy such systems serving 300 000 residents of reservations provide artificially fluoridated water. In addition, school water fluoridation, using schools' own individual wells, is practised in 319 US schools serving a population of approximately 100 000 in communities where a fluoridated public water supply is not available. Schools are fluoridated at 4.5 times the recommended optimal level for communities (USPHS Division of Oral Health, 1993).

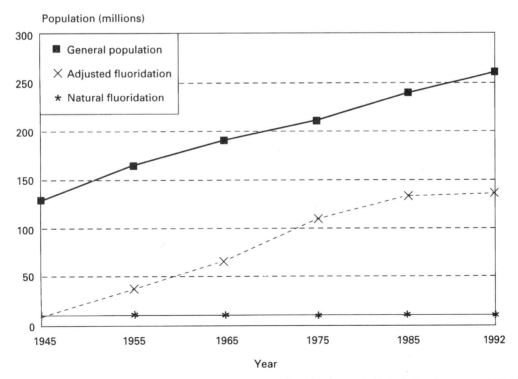

Fig. 14.3 Growth of US general population and population served by fluoridated water 1945–1992. Data from USPHS Division of Oral Health (1993).

Community water fluoridation remains the cornerstone of dental public health policy in the USA (Easley, 1995a). Most of the federal fluoridation promotion and monitoring activity in the USA is undertaken by the Centers for Disease Control and Prevention (CDC)–a branch of the US Public Health Service. Fluoridation engineers and dental professionals provide training and expert advice about fluoridation to state health departments. In addition, federal funding for fluoridation activities is available. Following the early and rapid expansion of water fluoridation in the USA, in 1979 a national target–that 95% of community water systems should be fluoridated by 1990–was set by the US Public Health Service (1979). This target proved too ambitious and was not met, and in 1991 a more realistic target was set. The revised target aims to have at least 75% of community water systems fluoridated by the year 2000 (US Public Health Service, 1991a). This target has already been achieved by 20 states and the District of Columbia; however, to achieve the target nationally, fluoridated water must reach a further 30 million people. In California (the most populous US state) less than 16% of the population receives fluoridated water. Efforts to extend fluoridation in California have met with resistance in the past. However, on 1 June 1995 the California Assembly agreed, by a large majority, the first stage of mandatory fluoridation legislation for the state (Easley, 1995b).

The dental benefits of fluoridation in the USA, and in other countries, are well-documented (Murray *et al.*, 1991). Briefly, early studies of children in newly fluoridated communities demonstrated large reductions in caries prevalence of between 45 and 94% (as described in Chapter 7). Studies conducted between 1973 and 1988 demonstrated that 6–13-year-old children living in fluoridated communities developed fewer new carious lesions than their peers in non-fluoridated communities (on average, 0.8 and 1.5 respectively). Nationwide studies of children's dental health have demonstrated that, in recent years, the differences in caries experience between children living in fluoridated and non-fluoridated communities have reduced. For example, in 1979–80 differences in caries experience of children resident in fluoridated and non-fluoridated communities were demonstrated to be between 30 and 37%, whereas by 1986–87 the differences were 8–18% (Newbrun, 1989).

Opponents of fluoridation have claimed that these recent results show that the claimed benefits of fluoridation have always been exaggerated (Yiamouyiannis, 1990). In fact the reason for this apparent reduction in the effectiveness of water fluoridation in the USA is likely to be a combination of three major factors:

- first, the phenomenon of declining caries prevalence recognized throughout the developed world since the mid 1970s;
- second, the widespread availability of fluorides from sources other than drinking water–for example, fluoridated toothpaste, supplements and professionally applied varnishes and gels;
- finally, the 'halo' effect. This effect, described by Newbrun (1989), occurs when residents of non-fluoridated communities are exposed to the benefits of fluoridation to some degree by consuming foods and beverages manufactured and processed in fluoridated communities. In the USA where 42 of the 50 largest cities are fluoridated this effect is likely to be significant, since it is probable that many large food and beverage manufacturing plants are located in large cities and therefore use fluoridated water during their manufacturing processes.

In 1989 the cost of community water fluoridation in the USA was estimated at between \$0.12 and \$1.31 per person per year depending on the number of people served by the water system. The average cost was \$0.54. In 1992 the benefit-to-cost ratio was 80 : 1–that is, for every dollar spent on fluoridation, \$80 in dental treatment costs was saved (Easley, 1995a).

Water fluoridation in the UK

The progress of fluoridation in the UK following the early demonstration studies is described as this is perhaps an excellent example of the problems of implementing a health promotion initiative. Three phases can be identified as follows.

Period of implementation–1964–74

This period was one of considerable progress. Local government had wide responsibilities including responsibility for public health and for local water supplies, and during this period many local authorities (LAs) throughout the UK introduced water fluoridation schemes on the advice of their medical officers of health. Major schemes were introduced in Birmingham and the West Midlands (1964–68) and Newcastle and parts of the North-east (1968). Many smaller schemes were introduced throughout the UK; for example, in Yorkshire: Grimsby (1971), Scunthorpe (1968), Huddersfield (1970) and Dewsbury (1970); in Cheshire: Chester and Crewe (1975); in Lincolnshire (1970); in Oxfordshire: Oxford (1972) and Wycombe (1973); in Bedfordshire (1972); in Powys (1971); and in Northern Ireland (1973). By 1974 fluoridated water reached approximately 9% of the population (Anon., 1988). Two principal factors brought this period of progress to an end:

- reorganization of local government, including the creation of 10 water authorities for England and Wales, taking the responsibility for water supplies away from LAs;
- reorganization of the National Health Service (NHS), including the creation of area health authorities (HAs), taking the responsibility for public health away from LAs.

Period of stagnation–1975–85

With the exception of the extension of some of the West Midlands schemes, no new major schemes were introduced during this period. Initially, the reasons for this situation are likely to have been related to the changes in responsibilities for water supplies and public health. However, an additional factor–uncertainty about the legality of fluoridation–was introduced in 1978 when a resident of Glasgow applied for an interdict to restrain Strathclyde Regional Council from implementing its decision to fluoridate the water supplies at the request of the local health boards (McKechnie, 1985). (In Scotland regional councils are the water authorities; and the NHS changes had resulted in the creation of health *boards*, not health *authorities*.) This period culminated with the passage of the 1985 Water (Fluoridation) Act which clarified the legal situation, and *apparently* placed responsibility for decisions about water fluoridation in the UK with health authorities (Her Majesty's Government, 1985). At this stage approximately 10% of the population received fluoridated water.

Period of frustration–1986 to present (1996)

By 1986 the general decline in caries prevalence in developed countries was well-established, and in the UK it was recognized that dental caries had become a class-related disease, commoner in poorer communities (Hill, 1989). A clear 'north/south divide' in children's oral health had developed–a trend which was interrupted in the North-east and West Midlands by water fluoridation (Downer, 1989).

Successive British governments since the early 1960s had encouraged water fluoridation, and once the Water (Fluoridation) Act was passed the Department of Health reaffirmed the government's confidence in fluoridation, and issued guidance to HAs on implementation of fluoridation under the new Act. The Act made HAs responsible for the cost of fluoridation, but in its guidance the Department offered HAs financial assistance in meeting some of the costs of fluoridation (Department of Health and Social Security, 1987). In 1986 therefore there was a great deal of optimism in the NHS that the Water (Fluoridation) Act had, at last, opened up the possibility of extending the benefits of fluoridation to communities–mainly in the large urban communities of the North of England, Scotland, Wales and Northern Ireland–where caries rates remained unacceptably high. That optimism was unfortunately misplaced.

With the regional health authority (RHA) adopting a coordinating role, the HAs of the (then) North-western region were the first to attempt to implement the 1985 Fluoridation Act. Their considerable efforts, documented in detail by Taylor (1995), were to prove fruitless, as have the subsequent efforts of HAs in Scotland (Strathclyde Regional Council, 1993), Yorkshire (Yorkshire Water, 1995) and Wessex (Southern Water Services, 1995). The water industry (privatized in England and Wales in 1989) has refused to cooperate with HAs, claiming that the Act gives water suppliers discretion in matters of fluoridation. The government has made it clear that the water industry's interpretation of the law is not what Parliament intended (Malone, 1995). Nevertheless, no new schemes have been implemented under the 1985 Act, and, with some notable exceptions, the industry appears to be resolutely opposed to extending water fluoridation, although remaining willing to continue operating schemes which were established prior to 1985.

Fluoridation remains an important component of the government's strategy for oral health (Department of Health, 1994). Furthermore, the British Dental Association and the British Fluoridation Society (1994) have suggested a target for an increase in coverage from the current 10% to approximately 25% of the UK population to include districts with caries levels above the UK mean (British Dental Association, 1994; Lennon, 1995).

Surveys of children's dental health coordinated by the British Association for the Study of Community Dentistry show that fluoridation in the UK continues to provide considerable dental benefits to children (Pitts and Palmer, 1994). In addition, Thomas and Kassab (1992) have clearly demonstrated that the benefits continue into adulthood. Inequalities in oral health persist in the UK, and the variation in mean disease levels within regions and countries is considerable (Downer, 1994; Pitts and Palmer, 1994). Fluoridation has been shown to reduce social class inequalities in the oral health of children (Carmichael *et al.*, 1980; Ellwood and O'Mullane, 1995); and it is believed that unless fluoridation is extended in areas such as the North-west of England, oral health strategy targets will not be met (Taylor, 1995).

Water fluoridation in the Republic of Ireland

From the mid 1940s in the Republic of Ireland, as in other developed countries, dental caries was recognized as a major public health problem (MacEntee, 1972). Interest in water fluoridation increased following publication in 1955 of the national dental survey (Medical Research Council of Ireland, 1955), and a visit to the Republic by Dr Trendley Dean in 1957 during which he was guest speaker at the Royal College of Surgeons of Ireland. The Minister for Health appointed a Fluorine Consultative Council in May 1956 to examine:

> Whether, with a view to reducing the incidence of dental caries it is desirable to provide for an increased intake of fluorine, and, if the Council considers it so desirable, to advise as to the best method of securing such an increased intake and as to any safeguards and precautions necessary (MacEntee, 1972).

In May 1958 the Consultative Council unanimously agreed 'that an increased intake of fluorine will reduce the incidence of dental caries and that it is desirable to provide for such an increased intake'. The Council further recommended that 'the increased intake of fluorine can best be provided by the fluoridation of public water supplies to the level of 1.0 part per million F'.

In December 1960 the Health (Fluoridation of Water Supplies) Act 1960 became law. However, an unsuccessful legal challenge, the basis of which was the claim by a Dublin resident that the Act was unconstitutional, delayed implementation of the Act for over 3 years. The Act empowers the Minister of Health to require health authorities to arrange for the fluoridation of public water supplies. However, before making such regulations, the Minister is obliged to arrange for a survey of the dental health of schoolchildren within the HA area, and to arrange for an analysis of the public water supplies. The Minister is further obliged to report the results of each, and his subsequent fluoridation regulations to each House of the Oireachtas (Parliament). Thus the Act is mandatory, and only Parliament has the power to question the Minister's decisions about fluoridation.

Between July 1964 and March 1971 water supplies serving 1 386 000 people (47.5% of the total population) living primarily in towns with a population in excess of 5000 were fluoridated (O'Hickey, 1972). By 1995 approximately 67% of the 3.5 million population was served with fluoridated water supplies (O'Mullane, 1996). The requirement of the Health (Fluoridation of Water Supplies) Act 1960 to conduct baseline and ongoing surveys of dental health has ensured that the effectiveness of fluoridation has been monitored since its inception in Ireland. National surveys of children's dental health show that for 5-year-olds and for 12-year-olds between 1961–63 and 1984 there was a major decline in the prevalence of dental caries throughout the Republic of Ireland. However, Table 14.1 shows that this decline, which has been observed throughout the developed world since the mid 1970s, has been much greater in lifetime residents of fluoridated communities than in residents of non-fluoridated communities (O'Mullane, 1996).

A recent survey of the dental health of adults (O'Mullane and Whelton, 1992) found that in adults aged 25 and over the percentage edentulous was considerably lower amongst lifetime residents of fluoridated communities. The mean number of natural teeth present was greater among 45–54-year-old residents of fluoridated communities, while the percentage of exposed root surfaces which were decayed or filled (Root Caries Index) was lower–see Table 14.2 (O'Mullane, 1996). The prevalence of enamel opacities has been monitored in Ireland since 1984. In 1984 the percentage of 8- and 15-year-old children with enamel defects was similar for lifetime residents of both fluoridated and non-fluoridated communities. The only trend to emerge was that diffuse opacities (which are usually associated with fluoride intake) tended to be somewhat higher in the fluoridated group (O'Mullane, 1990). Recent surveys suggest that, over the 10-year period since the 1984 survey, there has been a marginal increase in the prevalence of questionable/very mild opacities (O'Mullane, 1996).

Water fluoridation in Hong Kong

Between 1945 and 1950 the population of Hong Kong increased from less than 750 000 to over 2 million (Hong Kong Government, 1951). The dentist:population ratio was such that it was impossible to cope with the dental needs of the population, and in 1958, with the support of the Hong Kong government and the Hong Kong Dental Society, the World Health Organization's recommendation to implement water fluoridation was agreed (Hong Kong Government, 1958).

During 1961 and 1962, and with the exception of some isolated rural villages, water supplies for the entire population were fluoridated. Initially the fluoride concentration was set at 0.9 p.p.m. during the cooler months, and at 0.7 p.p.m. during summer. In 1967 the level was increased to 1.0 p.p.m. on a year-round basis; then, in 1978 because of concerns about dental fluorosis (discussed below), the level was reduced to 0.7 p.p.m. on a year-round basis. In mid 1988, in response to an observation that very mild fluorosis was still a little higher than expected for areas with optimal water fluoride levels, the level was further reduced to 0.5 p.p.m. (Schwarz and Lo, 1995). The main findings of a 1987 review of surveys of dental health in Hong Kong over the 25-year period since the introduction of water fluoridation (Evans *et al.*, 1987) are summarized below.

Baseline surveys of the dental health of schoolchildren had been conducted prior to the introduction of fluoridation. Further surveys were carried out in 1968 and 1980. The 1968

Table 14.1 Mean number of decayed, missing and filled teeth in 5-year-old (dmft) and 12-year-old (DMFT) residents of each of the eight health boards of the Republic of Ireland in 1961–63, and lifetime residents of the fluoridated (F) and non-fluoridated (NF) sections of those communities in 1984

Health board	5-year-olds			12-year-olds		
	1961–63	1984		1961–63	1984	
		F	NF		F	NF
Eastern	5.6	1.3	2.9	5.2	2.2	3.4
Midland	5.2	1.9	3.0	4.6	2.5	2.5
Mid-western	6.4	2.3	4.0	4.9	3.1	3.7
North-eastern	5.0	1.0	2.1	4.3	2.3	2.8
North-western	5.2	1.7	3.0	4.2	2.4	3.9
South-eastern	6.3	1.9	2.8	5.2	2.2	3.5
Southern	6.4	2.5	4.0	5.4	3.3	4.1
Western	5.0	1.5	2.2	4.2	2.3	3.0
All health boards	5.6	1.8	3.0	4.7	2.6	3.3

From O'Mullane (1995), with permission.

Table 14.2 Percentage edentulous, mean number of teeth present, and Root Caries Index (percentage of root surfaces with recession which have decayed or been filled) in adults resident in fluoridated and non-fluoridated communities in the Republic of Ireland 1989–90

Age (years)	Fluoridated			Non-fluoridated		
	Percentage edentulous	Mean no. of natural teeth present	Root Caries Index	Percentage edentulous	Mean no. of natural teeth present	Root Caries Index
16–24	0.0	27.1	0.0	0.0	27.2	0.0
25–34	0.0	26.1	1.6	3.3	22.9	3.3
35–44	2.4	22.5	2.5	6.1	19.0	8.5
45–54	10.8	16.4	5.4	29.5	10.7	13.4
55–64	33.8	11.6	2.2	47.1	6.8	12.2
65+	42.3	9.2	11.7	54.2	5.9	18.9

From O'Mullane (1995), with permission.

survey included adults, and in 1982 a further survey of Hong Kong adults was conducted. Since almost the entire population of Hong Kong received fluoridated water from 1962, comparisons between fluoridated and non-fluoridated communities were not possible. Thus it was not possible to differentiate reductions in caries prevalence related to fluoridation from those related to a general secular trend. However, it was concluded that: 'The reduction in caries experience was considerable and comparable to that observed elsewhere following the introduction of water fluoridation'.

In the 1960s baseline surveys dental fluorosis prevalence was negligible. By the late 1970s there was an awareness of an increase in the prevalence of dental fluorosis, and in 1978 the water fluoride concentration level was lowered to 0.7 p.p.m.. A 1986 survey of Hong Kong schoolchildren was conducted to determine the effects on dental fluorosis prevalence of reducing the water fluoride level from 1.0 to 0.7 p.p.m. (Evans and Stamm, 1991). The study confirmed that 'the prevalence and severity of dental fluorosis among children in Hong Kong was reduced following the lowering of the fluoride concentration in drinking water'. Evans and Stamm noted that an adjustment of as little as 0.2 p.p.m. had a measurable effect on dental fluorosis with no apparent adverse effect on caries prevention. Several reasons for this were discussed, including the Hong Kong climate and predominant dietary practices.

Extent of fluoridation worldwide

The World Health Organization estimates that approximately 210 million people in 39 countries benefit from artificially fluoridated water. An additional 40 million benefit from a water supply which is naturally fluoridated (Murray *et al.*, 1991; Expert Committee on Oral Health Status and Fluoride Use, 1994). It is difficult to establish precisely the status of water fluoridation worldwide at any given time. However, Table 14.3 presents published data on the subject which gives some indication of its distribution in recent years.

Reasons for cessation of fluoridation

Several communities having initially started fluoridation schemes have since ceased. The reasons for decisions to discontinue fluoridation are usually complex. Opponents of fluoridation often cite examples of such decisions to support their resistance to fluoridation, claiming that governments or community leaders have discontinued fluoridation because of evidence of adverse effects. There is no evidence to support such claims. Decisions to discontinue fluoridation fall into two broad categories: political and economic.

Political reasons for discontinuing fluoridation include:

- decisions by governments not to pursue fluoridation in the face of antifluoridation activity as happened, for example, in the Netherlands (König, 1987), the Czech Republic (Lekesová, 1995); and Finland (Seppa, 1992);
- decisions by water suppliers not to reinstate fluoridation after interruption for technical reasons as happened, for example in Wales (Hulse *et al.*, 1995).

Economic reasons for discontinuing fluoridation include:

- reassessment of the costs and benefits of fluoridation in the light of generalized reductions in caries prevalence. For example, in 1989 the fluoridation plant which had served the community of Watford UK for over 30 years required refurbishment. (Watford was one of the early UK demonstration study communities.) At its January 1991 meeting the local HA approved in principle the fluoridation of Watford's water supply, and referred the matter to the purchasing team for consideration. However, the authority has not allocated resources to reinstate fluoridation since, in light of reductions in caries prevalence particularly in the South-east of England, it now considers the benefit:cost ratio to be unfavourable (Robertson, 1993).

It should be stressed that, so far as we are aware, decisions to discontinue fluoridation have invariably been based on political, technical or economic concerns, and not because of concern about adverse health effects.

Other methods of fluoridation

Salt fluoridation

The World Health Organization recommends that salt fluoridation should be considered as an

Table 14.3 Water fluoridation status worldwide

Country	Artificial: population served	Natural: population served
Anguilla	0	0
Argentina	1 293 685	4 500 000*
Australia	10 666 976	143 443
Austria	0	?
Barbados	0	0
Belgium	0	0
Bermuda	0	0
Bhutan	0	?
Botswana	0	?
Brazil	60 000 000	?
Burkina Faso	0	0
Cameroon	0	0
Canada	9 666 707	210 399
Chile	1 381 948	555 930
China (People's Republic of)	0	?
China, Taipei	0	?
Colombia	29 406 860	600 140
Cook Islands	0	0
Cuba[a]	5 communities: number of people affected unknown	?
Cyprus	0	30 000
Czechoslovakia	1 500 000*	15 000*
Denmark	0	50 000*
Egypt[a]	Pilot study begun in Alexandria: number of people affected unknown	0
Ethiopia	0	?
Fiji	300 000	0
Finland	76 000†	200 000*
France	0	Approximately 3% of population
Gabon	0	1 363 000
Germany[a]	1 500 000	?
Greece	0	0
Grenada	0	0
Guatemala[b]	1 800 000	?
Guyana	45 000	200 000
Haiti	0	11 461
Honduras	0	0
Hong Kong	Total population	0
Hungary	0	30 000*
Iceland	0	0
Iran	0	Several cities: population coverage not known
Ireland (Republic of)[c]	2 345 000	200 300
Israel	1 600 000	75 000
Italy	0	1 community: population coverage not known
Jamaica	0	?
Japan	0	?
Kenya	0	Many water supplies have excessive fluoride levels

Continued

Table 14.3 *(continued)*

Country	Artificial: population served	Natural: population served
Kiribati (Republic of)	0	Estimated 60% of the population
Korea (Republic of)	410 000	0
Lao PDR	0	0
Libya[a]	400 000	1 000 000
Luxembourg	0	0
Malaysia	10 200 000	0
Mali	0	0
Malta	0	?
Mexico	1 000 000	3 000 000
Mongolia	0	?
Myanmar	0	?
Namibia	0	200 000*
Nauru (Republic of)	0	Water supplies imported from Australia and New Zealand, not known if fluoridated
Netherlands	0	0
New Zealand	64% of population	0
Nigeria	0	20 000
Norway	0	10 000
Pakistan	0	0
Panama (1974§)	509 554	0
Papua New Guinea (1975§)	102 000	70 000
Paraguay (1977§)	350 000	3 communities: numbers covered not known
Peru[a]	500 000	80 000
Philippines	5 000 000*	850 000
Poland	80 000	300 000
Portugal	0	0
Puerto Rico (1974)	1 820 000	0
Romania	0	?
Senegal	0	1 000 000
Sierra Leone	0	?
Singapore	100% of population covered	0
South Africa	0	?
Spain	200 000*	0
Sri Lanka	0	15% of the population covered
Sweden	0	750 000
Switzerland	300 000	40 000
Syria	0	0
Taiwan[b]	600 000*	?
Thailand	0	5 000 000
Trinidad and Tobago	0	?
Turkey	0	2–3 areas: numbers covered not known
Tuvalu	0	0
Uganda	0	?
UK[d]	5 400 000	2 359 000
USA[e]	135 000 000	10 000 000
USSR (1977§)	85 communities: number of people affected unknown	15% of the population covered
Uruguay	0	15 000

Continued

Table 14.3 (*Continued*)

Country	Artificial: population served	Natural: population served
Venezuela	0	100 000
Vietnam	4 000 000	0
Zaire	0	600 000
Zambia	0	10% of the population covered
Zimbabwe	0	1 000 000*

Data published by Fédération Dentaire Internationale (FDI) 1990 unless otherwise indicated as follows: [a]DSI (1984); [b]FDI (1981) (data from Fédération Dentaire Internationale, 1984); [c]O'Mullane (1995); [d]British Fluoridation Society (1994); [e]US Public Health Service Division of Oral Health (1993).
*Estimate.
†Discontinued 1992.
‡Former GDR, discontinued since reunification.
§Most recent data.

alternative to community water fluoridation 'where water fluoridation is not feasible for technical, financial or sociocultural reasons' (Expert Committee on Oral Health Status and Fluoride Use, 1994).

Fluoridated salt is currently used in Switzerland–since 1955 (79% of sales), France–since 1985 (40-50% of sales), Costa Rica–since 1987, Jamaica–since 1987 (100% of sales) and Germany–since 1991 (approximately 12% of sales). In addition, fluoridated salt from Jamaica is exported to other West Indian countries (Warpeha, 1994). The introductory stages of salt fluoridation projects have been reached in Mexico and Spain (Expert Committee on Oral Health Status and Fluoride Use, 1994), and several South American countries (Argentina, Chile, Uruguay and Venezuela) are reported to be actively pursuing salt fluoridation (Kermode, 1995). Further details on salt fluoridation from the public health perspective can be found in Chapter 7.

Milk fluoridation

Milk was suggested as a vehicle for fluoride as a possible alternative to water fluoridation in the USA in the early 1960s, and in the UK from the late 1960s (Anon., 1969). Some clinical trials of fluoridated milk have been conducted, and caries levels were lower in groups consuming fluoridated milk (Expert Committee on Oral Health Status and Fluoride Use, 1994). School milk fluoridation schemes, in which children consume 200 ml of milk fluoridated at a level of 5 mg/l (5.0 p.p.m.) daily, have been introduced in Bulgaria, Chile, China and the Russian Federation (Expert Committee on Oral Health Status and Fluoride Use, 1994); whilst in the UK an investigation into the epidemiological, organizational and legal feasibility of school milk as a vehicle for fluoride has been conducted (Jones *et al.*, 1992). A 5-year study is now being conducted by the World Health Organization Collaborating Centre for Oral Health Services Research, University of Liverpool into the benefits and feasibility of integrating the distribution of fluoridated milk (0.5 mg F per 200 ml milk per child per day) into a dental health promotion programme for children aged 3–7 years attending nursery and primary schools in Merseyside.

Meanwhile, the World Health Organization's Expert Committee on Oral Health Status and Fluoride Use recently concluded:

● Fluoridated milk programmes have a limited effect as a public health measure.
● The production of fluoridated milk requires a high level of technical expertise.
● While encouraging results have been achieved, further studies are required before the method can be recommended for widescale use (Expert Committee on Oral Health Status and Fluoride Use, 1994).

The authors have relied extensively on papers presented at the International Symposium on Water Fluoridation held in Birmingham, UK on 1 and 2 June 1995. The proceedings of the symposium will be published as a special issue of the journal *Community Dental Health* in 1996. We acknowledge our debt to all the contributors to that symposium. We are also indebted to the Fédération Dentaire Internationale whose data we have used extensively in compiling Table 14.3.

References

Anon. (1969) Fluoridation of milk (editorial). *British Dental Journal* **127**:441–442.

Anon. (1988) Progress for fluoridation. *British Dental Journal* **164**:337.

British Dental Association (1994) *The Oral Health Strategy: Next Steps.* British Dental Association, London.

British Fluoridation Society (1994) *One in a Million: Water Fluoridation and Dental Public Health.* British Fluoridation Society and Public Health Alliance, Liverpool.

Carmichael, C.L., Rugg-Gunn, A.J., French, A.D. and Cranage, J.D. (1980) The effect of fluoridation upon the relationship between caries experience and social class in 5-year-old children in Newcastle and Northumberland. *British Dental Journal* **149**:163–167.

Commission of the European Communities (1980) Council directive relating to the quality of water intended for human consumption (80/778/EEC). *Official Journal of the European Communities* L **229**:11.

Dean, H.T. (1933) Distribution of mottled enamel in the United States. *Public Health Reports* **48**:703–734.

Dean, H.T. (1938) Chronic endemic dental fluorosis (mottled enamel). In: *Dental Science and Dental Art* (Gordon, S.M., ed.) Lea & Fabiger, Philadelphia.

Dean, H.T., Jay, P., Arnold, F.A. and Elvove, E. (1941) Domestic water and dental caries II. A study of 2832 white children aged 12–14 years, of 8 suburban Chicago communities, including *Lactobacillus Acidophilus* studies of 1761 children. *Public Health Reports* **56**:761–792.

Dean, H.T., Arnold, F.A. and Elvove, E. (1942) Domestic water and dental caries V. Additional studies of the relation of fluoride domestic waters to dental caries experience in 4425 white children aged 12 to 14 years, of 13 cities in 4 states. *Public Health Reports* **57**:1155–1179.

Department of Health (1994) *An Oral Health Strategy for England.* Department of Health, London.

Department of Health and Social Security (1969) *Reports on Public Health and Medical Subjects No. 122. The Fluoridation Studies in the United Kingdom and the Results Achieved after Eleven Years.* HMSO, London.

Department of Health and Social Security (1987) *Health Service Development: Fluoridation of Water Supplies HC(87)18.* DHSS, Heywood.

Doll, R. (1989) *Fluoridation–Safety First.* Interview on British Fluoridation Society Video. British Fluoridation Society, Liverpool.

Downer, M.C. (1989) Time trends in dental decay in young children. *Health Trends* **21**:7–9.

Downer, M.C. (1994) The 1993 national survey of children's dental health: a commentary on the preliminary report. *British Dental Journal* **176**:209–214.

Easley, M.W. (1995a) Celebrating 50 years of fluoridation: a public health success story. *British Dental Journal* **178**:72–75.

Easley, M.W. (1995b) Personal communication.

Ellwood, R.P. and O'Mullane, D.M. (1995) The association between area deprivation and dental caries in groups with and without fluoride in their drinking water. *Community Dental Health* **12**:18–22.

Evans, R.W. and Stamm, J.W. (1991) Dental fluorosis following downward adjustment of fluoride in drinking water. *Journal of Public Health Dentistry* **51**:91–98.

Evans, R.W., Lo, E.C. and Lind, O.P. (1987) Changes in dental health in Hong Kong after 25 years of water fluoridation. *Community Dental Health* **4**:383–394.

Expert Committee on Oral Health Status and Fluoride Use. (1994) *Fluorides and Oral Health. WHO technical report series no. 846.* World Health Organization, Geneva.

Expert Committee on Water Fluoridation (1958) *First Report. WHO technical report series no. 146.* World Health Organisation, Geneva.

Fédération Dentaire Internationale (1984) *World Fluoridation Status: As at 31 December 1984.* FDI, London.

Fédération Dentaire International (1990) *Dentistry Around the World. Basic Facts 1990.* FDI, London.

Federal Register (1986) Vol 51, No 63, 2 April 1986, National Archive and Record Administration, Washington DC.

Gillon, R. (1994) Medical ethics: four principles plus attention to scope. *British Medical Journal* **309**:184–188.

Griffith, G.W. (1956) The introduction of fluoridation in Anglesey. *Health Education Journal* **14**:223–231.

Harris, J. (1989) *The Ethics of Fluoridation.* British Fluoridation Society, Liverpool.

Her Majesty's Government. (1985) *Water (Fluoridation) Act 1985.* HMSO, London.

Hill, F. (1989) Our children's teeth (editorial). *British Medical Journal* **298**:272–273.

Hillier, S., Inskip, H., Coggon, D. and Cooper, C. (1996) Water fluoridation and osteoporotic fracture. *Community Dental Health* (in press)

Hong Kong Government (1951) *Hong Kong Annual Report 1950.* Hong Kong Government Printer, Hong Kong.

Hong Kong Government (1958) *Estimates of Revenue and Expenditure and Explanatory Memoranda 1 April 1957 to 31 March 1958.* Hong Kong Government Printer, Hong Kong.

House of Commons (1985) Water fluoridation bill, House of Commons debate 5 March 1985. *Parliamentary debates (Hansard). House of Commons: official report* **71**:c1091–c1138.

Hulse, G., Kenrick, A., Thomas, H. *et al.* (1995) Welsh water should reinstate fluoridation on Anglesey. *British Dental Journal* **178**:46–47.

Irish Government. (1960) *Health (Fluoridation of Water Supplies) Act 1960.* Stationery Office, Dublin.

Jones, S., Crawford, A.C., Jenner, A.M. *et al.* (1992) The possibility of school milk as a vehicle for fluoride: epidemiological, organisational and legal considerations. *Community Dental Health* **9**:335–342.

Kermode, J. (1995) Personal communication.

Knox, E.G. (1985) *Fluoridation of Water and Cancer: A Review of the Epidemiological Evidence.* HMSO, London.

König, K.G. (1987) Legal aspects related to caries prevention in the Netherlands. In: *Strategy for Dental Caries Prevention in European Countries According to their Laws and Regulations* (Frank, R.M. and O'Hickey, S., eds) IRL Press, Oxford.

Lekesová, I. (1995) Personal communication.

Lennon, M.A. (1993) Promoting water fluoridation. *Community Dental Health* 10:57–63.

Lennon, M.A. (1995) *Handbook of International Symposium on Water Fluoridation, Birmingham UK.* British Fluoridation Society, Liverpool.

Lord Avebury (1984) Fluoridation and individual freedom. *British Dental Journal* 156:277.

Lord Jauncey (1983) *Opinion of Lord Jauncey in causa Mrs Catherine McColl (A.P.) against Strathclyde Regional Council.* The Court of Session, Edinburgh.

McClure, F.J. (1970) *Water Fluoridation–The Search and the Victory.* US Department of Health Education and Welfare, NIH, NIDR, Bethesda, MD.

MacEntee, S. (1972) Fluoridation in Ireland: the spadework. *Journal of the Irish Dental Association* 18:48–52.

McKechnie, R. (1985) The Strathclyde fluoridation case. *Community Dental Health* 2:63–68.

Malone, G. (1995) *UK Minister for Health: Speech to International Symposium on Water Fluoridation Birmingham UK.* British Fluoridation Society, Liverpool.

Medical Research Council. (1993) *Report of the Working Group on Fluoridation of Drinking Water–Link with Osteoporosis.* Report of meeting held 17 December 1993. MRC, London.

Medical Research Council of Ireland. (1955) *Dental Caries in Ireland.* Medical Research Council of Ireland, Dublin.

Ministry of Health (1953) *The Fluoridation of Domestic Water Supplies in North America as a Means of Controlling Dental Caries. Report of the United Kingdom Mission, February–April 1952.* HMSO, London.

Ministry of Health (1962) *Reports on Public Health and Medical Subjects No. 105. The Conduct of the Fluoridation Studies in the United Kingdom and the Results Achieved after five Years.* HMSO, London.

Mr Justice Kenny (1963) *Fluoridation. Judgement delivered by Mr Justice Kenny in the High Court, Dublin, 1963.* Department of Health, Dublin.

Murray, J.J., Rugg-Gunn, A.J. and Jenkins, G.N. (1991) *Fluorides in Caries Prevention,* 3rd edn. Wright, Cambridge.

National Health and Medical Research Council (1979) *Submission to the Committee of Enquiry into Fluoridation of Victorian Water Supplies.* Commonwealth of Australia, Canberra.

National Health and Medical Research Council (1985) *Report of the Working Party on Fluorides in the Control of Dental Caries.* Commonwealth of Australia, Canberra.

National Health and Medical Research Council (1991) *The Effectiveness of Water Fluoridation.* Commonwealth of Australia, Canberra.

Newbrun, E. (1989) Effectiveness of water fluoridation. *Journal of Public Health Dentistry* 49:279–289.

O'Hickey, S. (1972) The progress of fluoridation in Ireland. *Journal of the Irish Dental Association* 18:68–72.

O'Mullane, D.M. (1990) The future of water fluoridation. *Journal of Dental Research* 69:756–759.

O'Mullane, D.M. (1996) Water fluoridation in Ireland. *Community Dental Health* (in press).

O'Mullane, D.M., and Whelton, H. (1992) *Oral Health of Irish Adults 1989–1990.* Stationery Office, Dublin.

Pitts, N.B. and Palmer, J.D. (1994) The dental caries experience of 5-, 12-, and 14-year-old children in Great Britain. Surveys coordinated by the British Association for the Study of Community Dentistry in 1991/92, 1992/93 and 1990/91. *Community Dental Health* 11:42–52.

Roberts, E. (1991) Interview. *Manchester Metro News* 20 September.

Robertson, S. (1993) Personal communication.

Royal College of Physicians (1976) *Fluoride, Teeth and Health.* Pitman Medical, Bath.

Schwarz, E. and Lo, E.C.M. (1995) Oral health and dental care in Hong Kong. *International Dental Journal* 45 (in press).

Seppa, L. (1992) Personal communication.

Southern Water Services (1995) *Southern Says no to Fluoride.* News Release 30. Southern Water Services 20 July 1995, Worthing.

Strathclyde Regional Council. (1993) *Council Minutes.* 30 June 1993.

Taylor, G.O. (1995) North west water and water fluoridation. *British Dental Journal* 178:47–48.

Thomas, F.D. and Kassab, J.Y. (1992) Fluoridation in Anglesey: a clinical study of dental caries in mothers at term. *British Dental Journal* 173:136–140.

US National Academy of Sciences Committee on Toxicology (1993) *Health Effects of Ingested Fluoride.* National Academy Press, Washington DC.

USPHS Division of Oral Health (1993) *Fluoridation Census 1992.* US Department of Health and Human Services Centers for Disease and Prevention, Atlanta, GA.

US Public Health Service (1979) *Promoting Health, Preventing Disease: Objectives for the Nation.* US Department of Health and Human Services, Washington, DC.

US Public Health Service (1991a) *Healthy People 2000: National Health Promotion and Disease Prevention Objectives.* US Department of Health and Human Services, Washington, DC.

US Public Health Service (1991b) *Review of Fluoride Benefits and Risks.* Department of Health and Human Services USPHS, Washington DC.

Warpeha, R. (1994) Salt fluoridation in Jamaica. *West Indian Dental Journal* 1:8–11.

Weaver, R. (1948) The inhibition of dental caries by fluorine. *Proceedings of the Royal Society of Medicine* 41:284–290.

World Health Organisation (1993) *Guidelines for Drinking-Water Quality. Vol 1 Recommendations,* 2nd edn. World Health Organization, Geneva.

Yiamouyiannis, J.A. (1990) Water fluoridation and tooth decay: results from the 1986–1987 national survey of US schoolchildren. *Fluoride* 23:55–67.

Yorkshire Water (1995) *Yorkshire Water not to Fluoridate Region's Water.* News release 107. 12 April 1995.

15

Approaches in oral health promotion

Richard Watt and Sabrina Fuller

Introduction

The central focus of this chapter is to build upon the theoretical principles of oral health promotion presented in Chapter 11 and to present, using a series of practical examples, the process of development, implementation and evaluation of a variety of oral health promotion initiatives based in a range of settings. Particular emphasis will be placed on developing opportunities for those working in oral health promotion to extend their activities out of the traditional health education model to a truly health promotion perspective. Although this chapter will focus on examples of oral health promotion within the UK, the principles developed will have general application in both the developing and developed world.

Initially we will present an overview of key theoretical concerns of oral health promotion which have a direct impact on practical implementation. The planning and implementation process will then be explored in greater depth with the variety of key stages in the process highlighted. The final section of the chapter will present examples of oral health promotion action within a diverse range of settings. These will be used to illustrate the various levels at which oral health promotion can operate and that successful oral health promotion is essentially a multidisciplinary activity.

Translating theory into practice

The World Health Organization (WHO) defines health promotion as:

> The process of enabling individuals and communities to increase control over the determinants of health and thereby improve their health, representing a mediating strategy between people and their environment, combining personal choice and social responsibility for health to create a healthier future (WHO, 1984).

This provides a very useful starting point for an exploration of the practical implementation of health promotion. Of fundamental importance to this definition is the clear recognition for the need to focus action on the prerequisites for health within society. Rather than adopting a 'victim-blaming' approach commonly practised by many health professionals, which focuses attention and preventive action at an individual level, based on the false assumption that individuals have complete control over their lifestyle, health promotion in contrast recognizes the need to change both the conditions in which people live as well as the ways in which they live, to make the healthier choices the easier choices (Milio, 1986). Recognition of the importance to health of the social environment and contexts in which individuals operate has direct and significant implications for those involved in planning and practising oral health promotion. The determinants of oral health are fundamentally linked to the consumption of non-milk extrinsic sugars, control of plaque levels, smoking behaviour, exposure to optimal levels of fluoride and the appropriate use of dental services. Although all these factors are under limited individual control, complex socioenvironmental and political factors are more influential. Nadanovsky and Sheiham (1994) have highlighted the significant contribution of social factors in explaining the improvements in children's oral health that have occurred in the UK during the 1980s. Indeed, Blane (1985) has presented a convincing case that social environments have a greater impact on health than individual behaviours.

It is therefore of critical importance that oral health promoters, in their efforts to improve and maintain oral health, direct attention at improving the environments or settings in which target groups are placed. Such an approach recognizes the impact and influence of a wide variety of institutions and organizations such as schools, hospitals, colleges, leisure centres and the workplace on the lives of most modern citizens and attempts to modify how these organizations cater for their students, staff and clients to ensure that the range of activities and the total environments are conducive and supportive to health (Grossman and Scala, 1994). Hospitals can be modified through the process of organizational development in many ways to make them a more health-promoting place for their clients, workers and visitors in terms of the quality and choices available in the services offered and the overall environment and ethos of the hospital (Baric, 1992). The concept of the health-promoting school will be explored in greater depth later in this chapter.

Recognition and understanding of the social and political determinants of oral health necessitates the adoption of a multisectoral approach and the development of healthy public policies (Milio, 1986). Policies within education authorities, the food manufacturing industry, social service departments, planning departments, water companies and the retailing sector may all have an effect on oral health. Therefore an essential role for oral health promoters is to raise oral health matters on to the policy agendas of these agencies.

Within health services isolation and poor communication between departments who are often striving to achieve similar results often result in duplication of effort, wasted resources and ultimately ineffective interventions. Unhealthy eating practices, poor body hygiene and smoking are all major concerns to a collection of health and other workers. The adoption of a common risk factor approach in which collective action is directed at risk factors which are linked to the development of many diseases, rather than particular diseases, not only reduces duplication, saves resources and improves effectiveness but also reduces the burden on an increasingly cynical public (Grabauskas, 1987).

A central principle of health promotion is the need to involve and respect the contribution of lay people, understand their needs and views and not to impose professional values. Unlike traditional health care practice, which is dominated by professional values, health promotion adopts a participatory approach which aims to involve the customer actively in the entire process of planning, implementing and evaluating interventions. Such an approach requires health professionals to be flexible in their work, to be able to negotiate and communicate shared goals. Indeed, if such an approach is not adopted, interventions designed to produce meaningful change are unlikely to be effective in the long term without public support and understanding.

A wide range of complementary measures are available in health promotion which extend action far beyond the field of health education, the traditional focus for prevention. Although the importance of educational initiatives is clear, it is also very apparent that to enable people to make healthy choices they often need far more than sound knowledge and 'appropriate' attitudes. Actions such as regulatory and legislative change can have a major influence over the environments in which people live to support their health. For example, at a national level supportive and permissive legislation on fluoridation of public water supplies could have major benefits for oral health. Regulatory changes can also be adopted at a more local level in the development of healthy eating and smoking policies within the workplace and in recreational facilities. The impact of fiscal policy on the use and uptake of services and products has been clearly demonstrated. Again, this type of health promotion action can be adopted at many levels within society which all have an influence on health, from the European Union common agricultural pricing policy to the cost of fruit sold within school canteens.

In line with the principle of public participation, self-care and joint ownership for action, community development is another option within a health promotion policy where the needs and values of local communities are central. Indeed, such an approach depends upon members of a particular community identifying causes of ill health and organizing in response to these. Within this model health professionals have a key role to act as resource and facilitator for change but the agenda is decided by the community themselves rather than health workers. Community development is a widely accepted option within a public policy framework. It has been adopted to a very limited extent in oral health promotion, although opportunities do exist in projects such as local food cooperatives.

Traditionally the dominant preventive philosophy within dentistry has followed what could be termed a high-risk approach. This approach recognizes that ill health is not evenly distributed throughout populations and therefore aims to improve the health of the diseased minority by identifying 'high-risk' individuals through screening tests and then to apply preventive or curative measures as required. Although such an approach has been widely adopted by the dental and medical professions, it is seriously flawed and ineffective in producing desired change (Sheiham and Joffe, 1991). Rose (1992) in his classic appraisal of preventive strategies has demonstrated the limitations of this approach and instead has proposed the adoption of a combined whole-population and targeted high-risk approach. The whole-population approach recognizes the importance and influence of social norms within society and therefore attempts to modify these within the whole population as opposed to focusing only on the diseased. For example, within a health promotion policy social environments can be modified by focusing action on the key purveyors of health-related norms within society such as health and education professionals and the media. In conjunction with this population approach, a targeted high-risk approach can be utilized when tackling inequalities is a priority. Such an approach does not attempt to identify high-risk individuals, with all the difficulties that poses, but instead focuses action on high-risk groups and directs action on the determinants of their poor health.

Planning oral health promotion interventions

As in many other services, individuals working in health promotion are under considerable pressure to respond to an array of demands. Working in a pressurized environment often means that services develop reactively. Although common, such an approach can seriously limit their productivity and effectiveness. There is a need to stand back and assess in a more proactive fashion what exactly is the nature and purpose of the service and to plan out a clear and shared direction for future action where it is most needed and most likely to produce beneficial results. However, a rational planning approach in which a whole series of options are identified and assessed before a comprehensive programme is developed is most often not a realistic and practical means of planning. Instead, more of an incremental approach can be adopted where planning is based on developing small-scale change rather than grand plans. This approach recognizes the limited information often available to planners and the uncertain and constantly changing context in which services operate (McCarthy, 1982).

Several theoretical health promotion planning models have been devised which provide some useful insights into the planning processes involved in health promotion (Tones, 1974; Green *et al.*, 1980; Ewles and Simnett, 1992). However, all can be criticized for their rather narrow health education approach which focuses on the educational and behaviour change aspects of health but largely excludes consideration of the social, political and environmental context of health. Indeed, these models propose a planning process which is dominated by health professionals and provides very little opportunity for community involvement. On the more positive side the models do provide a useful guide and framework to follow in terms of the different stages that can be considered when planning a health promotion intervention.

Developing an oral health promotion strategy

In many countries the importance of developing strategic plans for oral health promotion has been recognized. National strategic plans have been published providing guidance and direction to the development of oral health promotion. For example, oral health promotion strategies have been published in both Wales and England (Welsh Health Planning Forum, 1992; Department of Health, 1994a).

Experience from the commercial sector suggests that organizations without a strategic plan shared by all levels within the organization have a limited ability to adapt to changing circumstances and therefore to survive in the long term (Hamel and Prahalad, 1989). In these times of intense competition for resources, successful organizations need a strategy to provide vision, purpose and direction, clarify values, establish priorities and provide a framework for future action (Catford, 1983).

The process of developing these plans is critically important to ensure successful implementation. To produce practical, realistic and relevant oral health promotion strategies an active consultation process needs to be undertaken to enlist support from all relevant sectors. The importance of building effective partnerships in this process should not be underestimated.

Building on the Ewles and Simnett's (1992)

planning model, the development, implementation and evaluation of oral health promotion strategies can be divided into a series of stages which form a circular linking model (Fig. 15.1). The practical issues relevant to each stage will now be described.

Formation of planning and implementation group

The first step is the formation of a strategic planning and implementation group. Members of such a group should have both theoretical and practical experience relevant to the task of developing, planning and implementing oral health promotion strategies. It is essential that a balance is struck between members involved in the implementation and those with a more theoretical interest. The core membership of the group will include oral health personnel but as the strategy develops many other agencies would have a critical role to play.

Identification of resources

The next stage in the process is for the group to identify the range of resources that can be utilized in the development and implementation of a strategy. The most important resource is the availability of appropriate personnel who are experienced and skilled to undertake the range of tasks that are identified. Other key resources which need to be identified include funding to support the strategic planning process and

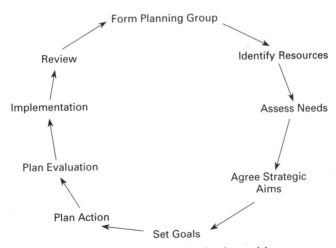

Fig. 15.1 Oral health promotion strategic planning model.

information sources from which key data can be accessed. It would also be very valuable to consult other strategic oral health plans and those produced by some other related field to assess not only their contents but also their approach and the developmental processes adopted.

Needs assessment and priority setting

Before any strategy can be devised the oral health needs of the community being served have to be assessed to enable priorities to be set. Detailed consideration of oral health needs assessment has been covered in Chapter 4 but it is important to stress here that an oral health promotion strategy has to be developed from both normative and lay measures of need. Currently in many health care systems there are major gaps in what is known about the oral health needs of different population groups. Lack of a good information base can often dent enthusiasm and halt progress until it is recognized that in planning all the information that ideally should be available very rarely is. However it is important to consult widely and where possible access information collected by other departments and agencies. For example, public health departments may have information relevant and useful to an oral health promotion strategy such as data on deprivation measures of local communities, dietary patterns of population groups and health services utilization statistics. Once the available oral health needs data have been assessed and initial priorities identified, representatives of local communities should be included in the consultation process.

Agreeing strategic aims

Based on the assessment of oral health needs a strategic direction can then be devised in which a clear set of long-term aims are proposed. These aims provide a overall vision for desired change. For example, in some communities oral health inequalities may have been identified as an area where change is desired and therefore aims are set to reduce unacceptable oral health inequalities between community groups. For example, in the Welsh strategy the following aims were set:

- a significant reduction in the difference

between the levels of tooth decay in Wales and those in the best regions in the UK;
- measurable reductions in the level of periodontal diseases in the Welsh population;
- a reduction in oral pain and discomfort;
- an improvement in people's chances of retaining their own teeth into old age;
- a reduction in years of life lost from oral cancer (Welsh Health Planning Forum, 1992).

Goal setting

Once the strategic aims have been agreed the next step in the process is setting goals that will provide a clear pathway to achieving the aims. Depending on the nature of the strategic aims, a range of different types of goals can be set. Goals can be set in terms of desired changes in oral health status, changes in oral health behaviours or environmental changes relevant to oral health. When goals are set it is essential that consideration is given to how the desired changes can be measured and evaluated. There is little point in setting a goal whose attainment cannot be demonstrated during evaluation. Goals need to be challenging in nature but also realistic and achievable and set in a time scale which is appropriate to the challenge. Initially short time scales are preferable as future circumstances are always uncertain.

Examples of different types of goals set within the Welsh strategy include the following:

Health gain goals

- Increase to 50% the proportion of children aged 5 with no experience of tooth decay, by 2002 (baseline 1991:40%).
- Reduce by 10% the proportion of children aged 11–16 who eat sweets, biscuits, cake or confectionery most days, by 2002 (baseline 1990: boys 74%, girls 65%).

Health education goals

Family Health Service Authorities and district health authorities will by 1997 be able to report that at least 50% of children by age 5 have an understanding of basic oral health principles, and at least 75% by 2002 (baseline not available).

Health promotion goals

- By 1995 district health authorities in collaboration with Health Promotion Authority of Wales and local education authorities and social services should have urged upon all schools the benefits of a healthy eating policy, moving towards the non-availability on their premises of confectionery and fizzy drinks.
- Family Health Service Authorities and district health authorities should by 1997 through coordinated action across Wales encourage fluoridation of water sources covering 60% of the Welsh population and take action to improve uptake of fluoride by those lacking access to fluoridated water (Welsh Health Planning Forum, 1992).

Action planning

The next stage in the process is planning the action required to meet the goals and aims set. The interventions planned need to be linked to the oral health needs and resources identified. Interventions which produce sustained change and result in a modification of the social environments are more important than short-term measures such as tooth-brushing programmes in schools, which are often not sustained in the long term. A range of complementary interventions can be devised which focus on the causes of oral disease. At a local level, as well as providing a range of health education initiatives, a variety of other supporting actions can be planned which focus on changing the environments in which people operate to create a more health-promoting setting. For example, working in a variety of settings such as schools and in primary health care to alter these environments can have a major influence on oral health.

Evaluation planning

Following the development of the action plan careful evaluation of all stages in the process needs to be planned to ensure that a monitoring mechanism is established which can feed back information on progress made at each level. Process and outcome measures can be considered in any evaluation. Process evaluation is essential in any health promotion plan as it assesses the process of implementation, including factors which support or impede progress as well as the reaction of those receiving the programme. The effects of any health promotion intervention can be measured by outcome assessments. Increasing emphasis is being placed on producing outcome measures for both clinical and health promotion interventions, although progress with this task has been limited due to the complexity and costs involved.

Implementation

On completion of all these stages the implementation and evaluation of the strategy can then finally be undertaken. Depending on the nature of the aims and targets set, a phased implementation process is often a preferred means of implementation, small steps building together to achieve significant progress.

Review process

Following the implementation and evaluation stages it is important to review and update the whole planning process. For example, in the light of experience gained, are the goals set achievable or overambitious? Is there a need to access increased funding for training and staff development? Information fed back into the process can help to develop and extend successful practice.

Skills required in oral health promotion

One of the major challenges facing oral health promoters is the acquisition and development of the range of skills required if they are to become involved in the stages outlined above. Traditionally most oral health promoters are trained to perform health education tasks which mostly involve teaching and training individuals and small groups. Although these skills are important, to be involved in a health promotion strategy requires skills in planning and evaluating strategies, in identifying and networking with significant agencies and individuals and in working with groups to maximize their effectiveness. To effect social change requires skills in political lobbying, the ability to influence people with power and to negotiate compromises and agreements. A range of effective communication skills will be required in all of these activities.

Oral health promotion opportunities

This section illustrates the principles already described by identifying a range of settings which can be used to promote oral health. As well as identifying the opportunities and limitations of each, there are examples of process and outcome objectives set for particular interventions and of how their achievement was evaluated.

The primary health care team

Primary health care is the first level of contact individuals, families and communities have with health services. In the UK, the members of the primary health care team include doctors, receptionists, practice nurses, health visitors, district nurses, midwives and social workers. These community-based professionals have a key role to play in the promotion of health. A high proportion of the population has contact with the primary care sector, often over many years, enabling good communication and trust to be developed between users and service providers. Primary health care teams are ideally placed to promote oral health within the context of general health.

One way in which family doctors can successfully be encouraged to promote oral health is through prescribing sugar-free liquid medicines rather than sugar-containing syrups. Prescribing a sugar-free alternative is a relatively small behaviour change on the part of the family doctor, while restricting sweets can represent a major shift in behaviour for a mother (Blinkhorn, 1989). Doctors require evidence of the benefits of sugar-free medicines and advice about how to prescribe them through input at postgraduate meetings, supporting materials and reinforcement of this message at regular intervals (Bentley and Mackie, 1993). Dental health education can tackle this problem. As well as medical practitioners, pharmacists, health visitors and dentists can be included to ensure that parents receive the same message from many sources. One objective of such a campaign could be to increase the proportion of sugar-free compared with sugar-containing medicines prescribed for children by medical practitioners. One way such a campaign can be evaluated is through comparison of the proportions of prescriptions of each type of medicine before and after the campaign (Bentley *et al.*, 1993).

In the UK the member of the primary health care team most closely associated with health education and promotion is the health visitor who acts as an important source of advice, particularly for mothers of young children. They advise mothers throughout the period of primary socialization when parents transmit and children internalize routines of health-related behaviours. Norms, actual or perceived, can be used to encourage the acquisition and maintenance of a routine of behaviour such as dietary preferences by an individual within a group. Patterns of behaviour learnt in early childhood and established as routines eliminate the need to make conscious decisions to choose health-related behaviours in later life. For example, tooth-brushing is carried out more dependably as a habit than as the result of a succession of health-related decisions, and patterns of behaviour learnt at a young age are deeply ingrained and difficult to change (Blinkhorn, 1978). Furthermore, high rates of preference for sweet tastes among 2-year-olds have been related to regular consumption of sugar water (Department of Health, 1994b). Health visitors are therefore a most important ally in the primary prevention of dental disease as they can offer social support for the establishment of healthy dietary patterns as the child is weaned. This is particularly important in deprived communities where existing norms support frequent sugar consumption (Blinkhorn, 1982).

As well as advising on restriction of sugars in the diet, health visitors can advise on dental visiting and brushing with a fluoride toothpaste when the teeth erupt. Other advantages of recruiting health visitors as dental health promoters include their ability to integrate dental health within general health advice and to reinforce this advice at developmentally significant stages. Priority is given to families who need support in the development of parenting skills; these are often the same families whose children are most at risk from dental disease. Health visitors are readily accessible, available and acceptable to mothers. They have access both to clients in their own homes and to community networks, so that they can be involved with prevention at an individual counselling level as well as influencing oral health as part of an overall health promotion strategy. However, often there is a need to increase health visitors' knowledge about oral health messages and the priority they place on oral health advice (Quinn and Freeman, 1991).

One possible solution is to arrange a series of workshops for health visitors. Appropriate objectives might include providing health visitors with an update on the aetiology and prevention of dental disease, particularly in young children, as well as an opportunity to discuss how they might promote oral health in small children as part of their existing role as health educators. Questionnaires before and after the seminars can demonstrate improvements in understanding of the principles of oral health (North West Region Dental Public Health Resource Centre, 1994). The next stage of such a campaign could be to increase the number of children aged 0–2 registered with general dental practitioners. Outcome measures are the number of pre-schoolchildren registered with a general dental practitioner as a result of the campaign; and process measures are to evaluate the role of health visitors in increasing dental attendance of pre-schoolchildren, and to determine the attitudes of health visitors to the campaign (Bentley and Holloway, 1993).

Family doctors and health visitors clearly have a major role to play in promoting oral health. Through the adoption of a team development approach all primary care team members can be encouraged to integrate aspects of oral health promotion into their daily work. For example, district nurses may have a role in identifying oral health needs of their elderly clients and making the appropriate referrals. Other team members involved in child health may consider the practice policy with regards to the distribution of sweets or samples of high-sugar baby foods and drinks and the impact this will have on norms relating to oral health.

Pharmacists and dentists

Although not normally integrated within the primary health care team, other primary health workers are pharmacists, general dental practitioners and community dentists. Pharmacists are in an ideal position to undertake health education in conjunction with other health care professionals. About 6 million visits are made daily to some 12 000 pharmacies in the UK, providing the opportunity for both passive and active health care advice and information to many people. Possible benefits include increased awareness by the public of oral health care messages, increased demand for sugar-free medicines, better selection of suitable oral health aids, regular use of fluoride toothpaste and appropriate use of dental services (Morrow and Maguire, 1989). Pharmacists are seen by the general public, in descending order of importance, as advisers on over-the-counter medicines, symptoms of minor ailments, prescribed medicines and finally general health (Shafford and Sharpe, 1988). There is a need for continuing education for pharmacists if they are to equip themselves for a role in giving advice on oral health, for the provision of suitable health education materials and for interprofessional liaison.

Morrow and McGuire (1989) set two levels of objectives in their project with pharmacists in Northern Ireland. Those relating to process were to provide an appropriate knowledge base for pharmacists whereby they could respond effectively to issues relating to dental care; to design a model dental health promotional initiative for community pharmacy practice; to implement this model initiative in the practice situation, and to conduct a quantitative analysis of the promotion. Outcome objectives were to increase public awareness of the need for proper dental care; to educate the public in the methods of preventing dental disease; to encourage the public to practise effective dental care and to prevent the development of dental caries in children. They fulfilled the process objectives but point to a number of problems in the evaluation of the achievement of outcome objectives, the difficulty of locating the pharmacists' client population, the very high cost of measuring heath gain and the lack of rigorous evaluation techniques which can isolate the effects of a particular campaign.

Primary dental care

General dental practice offers important opportunities for dental health education (Croucher, 1993). The dentist is where people would go first if they wanted information or help about dental health for themselves or their families. Requirements can be included in dentists' contract to secure and maintain the oral health of the patient. The recognition of the value of the multiple-risk-factor approach will encourage dentists to take a larger role in prevention generally, including smoking cessation. Current dental practice tends to adopt a simplistic belief in the effectiveness of giving information in bringing about behaviour change. This approach is centred on the expectations of the professional rather than the needs of the individual. There should be a review of organizational arrangements within dental practice to identify factors which limit the opportunities for health promotion and development of a partnership between patient and dentist to bring about improvements in health (Croucher, 1993). Nettleton (1986) interviewed community dentists and identified a perceived conflict between their role as clinician and that of health educator. Although they saw it as important to communicate with their patients, they were not confident in their own skills in this area. Furthermore they were discouraged by their perception of the patients' lack of receptiveness. She advocates training dentists to improve the knowledge and skills they need to meet the increasing demands for dental health education in this setting.

While the dentist can give advice opportunistically, monitor improvements in health and give appropriate reinforcement, it may be more cost-effective to involve other members of the dental team in teaching the skills of toothbrushing, in dietary counselling or in group health education sessions. Team work is an essential part of an effective practice strategy for prevention. Each team member must know what advice they should be giving and what their role is.

Various initiatives have been undertaken to support the general dental practice team in their role as dental health promoters (North West Region Dental Public Health Resource Centre, 1994). Facilitators were appointed to distribute health education materials to general practice, and arrange training for members of the team. It was found that few practices were aware of the existence of health promotion units in their districts from which they could obtain good health education materials and consequently they were dependent on commercial materials designed primarily to promote a particular product. Seminars for auxiliaries were held on the content and techniques of dental health education. Objectives included increasing knowledge of the scientific basis of health education, improving communication skills and stimulating uptake of formal qualifications in dental health promotion. Participants had a high

degree of satisfaction with the courses, had improved their knowledge, and claimed to be more likely to carry out dental health education as part of their job and to pursue further qualifications in the subject.

Schools

Schools have been the traditional focus for community-based oral health education. They provide a setting for the efficient delivery of health education programmes, giving access to large numbers of children. School is the major agency of secondary socialization, a more formal and detached process than primary socialization which influences decision-based rather than inculcated behaviours. This is when the necessary knowledge for a rational explanation of behaviour is acquired and serves as a reinforcement for its maintenance. One limitation of school health education is that it often takes place too late to initiate habits and routines, as dietary preferences are established before the child starts school (Blinkhorn, 1989). Peer groups' influence increases as the child becomes an adolescent. On the one hand this supports oral health through reinforcing the importance of oral hygiene in the context of grooming and cleanliness (Hodge et al., 1982). On the other hand sweet consumption is encouraged through its symbolic function in demonstrating identification with peer group norms (Rise and Holund, 1990).

Oral health promotion fits comfortably within the overall concept of the health-promoting school. This has three main elements. First, health education is taught through the formal curriculum, integrated into other key areas such as science or personal and social education; second, the nature and quality of relationship between the home and school and the surrounding community, its environment and services is emphasized, and third, considerations of health permeate what is known as the hidden curriculum or school ethos (Scottish Health Education Group, 1989). The hidden curriculum incorporates the example set by teachers, caring relationships within the school and the physical environment including school meals and snacks. Policies on snacks and drinks may form a relatively minor part of a health-promoting school initiative but one that is straightforward to achieve. Such policies limit the frequency of sugar intakes and establish healthy snacks and drinks as a norm. They can also benefit other aspects of the child's education, for example familiarizing the children with foods they may not have access to at home, practising the social skills associated with mealtimes or teaching them the organizational and business skills required to run a tuck shop. Careful planning and cooperation are needed at all levels since, for example, the principle of teachers as role models can be undermined by the teachers themselves. In a study with teenagers in deprived areas of Edinburgh (McKinlay, 1994), pupils often reported teachers being seen smoking from the staffroom window. Some children regularly acted as runners to the chip shop and bakery for teachers.

Health-promoting school initiatives require a multisectoral approach. To develop and implement such a policy successfully will involve collaboration with the local education authority, with headteachers, school governors, teachers and parents, and with dietitians, health promotion officers and school nurses. One objective could be the adoption of a policy promoting healthy eating by the local education authority. As it is difficult to demonstrate immediate health gain associated with such an initiative a system of audit of defined process objectives is advocated (Baric, 1991). These could include the number of schools implementing policy on healthy snacks in relation to what is sold, provided or brought in to school, or in relation to the use of sweets as rewards or birthday treats.

The formal curriculum provides another aspect of the health-promoting school. Children's perceptions change as they age, as do the influences upon them, so that health education should take place as part of a progressive programme which builds on previous learning and allows children to extend their knowledge and skills appropriate to their stage of development. Oral health promotion programmes have been developed for use in nursery, primary and secondary schools (Craft and Holloway, 1983; Towner, 1984; Croucher *et al.*, 1985; Hodge *et al.*, 1987). These tend to be based on experiential learning relevant to pupils' needs and everyday lives.

Health education can be integrated into the regular curriculum, especially if material is adapted to cater for the needs of the students. The role of the dental profession has shifted from that of provider and presenter of dental health

lectures to that of initiator, encourager and supporter of programmes that can be used by teachers in schools (Towner, 1984). Toothpaste companies, national health education authorities and community dental services all produce evaluated dental health education materials for use by teachers in schools. Increasingly it has become necessary to tailor these to the demands of the UK National Curriculum as little time is left for use at the teacher's discretion.

A strategy for schools requires an assessment of the materials and staff time available. On the basis of this, decisions can be made concerning priority groups. Local epidemiological data may be used to identify schools with the greatest dental health need and approach them offering resources and support to address inequalities in dental health within a district. Training workshops for teachers participating in oral health programmes are beneficial in order to update their oral health knowledge and to familiarize them with resources provided. This workshop can also provide an opportunity to discuss the school environment, particularly in relation to snacks and drinks.

A number of evaluations have been carried out of dental health education programmes. The Gleam Team is a flexible teacher-selected dental health education programme for infant schools. The aim of the programme is to promote in infant schoolchildren an awareness about the value of their teeth and the choices involved in achieving good dental health (Towner, 1984). The objectives of the evaluation were to find out whether the programme was generally acceptable to teachers and children and whether it could be used in a variety of different classrooms, that is, its acceptability; to investigate the effects the programme had on children's knowledge on dental health matters, their attitudes and their behaviour in respect to dental health, that is, its effectiveness, and to ascertain the views of teachers on the individual components of the programme, so that materials could be revised before publication. The programme was evaluated by means of questionnaires and interviews with teachers, interviews with children, teachers' records of use, classroom observation and a pilot clinical trial.

Natural Nashers is a British health education programme for early secondary school years which can be generally applied. Changes in pupil knowledge and beliefs were measured using self-complete questionnaires, changes in oral hygiene by assessments of the children's gingival condition, opinions of teachers by questionnaire. Some improvements in knowledge, attitudes and beliefs were demonstrated, the greatest improvements in knowledge occurring where knowledge and attitudes were poor at the outset (Craft and Holloway, 1983).

Community-wide approaches–promoting structural change

A major challenge facing oral health promoters is developing working practices that are placed within a broader community setting which seek to influence the social environments relevant to oral health. Two examples of this type of approach will now be explored–a national campaign aimed at modifying supermarket policies in relation to checkout confectionery displays and a campaign which aims to reduce the sale and use of sweetened baby drinks. Both approaches aim to modify physical and social environments which have a direct impact on oral health. The success of each approach is largely dependent upon securing and mobilizing the support and involvement of the public and a variety of non-health agencies such as the media and retail and manufacturing sectors. These campaigns therefore involve a very different type and style of working from traditional dental health education but have the potential to produce major oral health benefits within the wider community. Both campaigns have been led and directed by a multidisciplinary lobbying group, Action and Information on Sugars.

Baby drinks campaign

The consumption of sweetened baby drinks such as concentrated syrups, fruit juices, granulated herbal and chocolate bedtime drinks commonly result in nursing bottle caries in infants. This condition in many cases leads to dental pain and sepsis which ultimately result in the need for multiple tooth extractions under general anaesthesia, a traumatic and potentially dangerous procedure for a young child. In the early 1990s sales of sweetened baby drinks rose steadily in the UK, which prompted the formation of an alliance of organizations dedicated to combating this trend.

The campaign focused attention directly on the infant feeding industry, lobbying for the withdrawal of sweetened products, a switch in production to sugarless alternatives and improvements in the labelling of baby drinks. The campaign aimed to force structural change on the infant feeding industry to enable healthy choices to be the easier choices for mothers of infants. After a 2-year period major successes have been achieved. Sales of sweetened baby drinks have been reduced nationally in the UK by almost 25% with a corresponding dramatic rise in sales of sugarless alternatives. Labelling of these products has also been greatly improved.

How has such a major change been achieved? The creation of an alliance of nine organizations representing a range of health professionals directed pressure on the food industry about this issue. Of greater influence on the industry was undoubtedly the considerable media interest generated by the campaign. A host of local and national television and press reports generated national public awareness. Legal action against the sweetened drinks manufacturers by a group of parents of infants affected by nursing bottle caries has been another powerful force for change within the campaign (Winkler, 1993). Process evaluation of this campaign has consisted of monitoring media and press coverage, and outcome evaluation has so far included a detailed assessment of the food industry's response to the campaign in terms of product withdrawal or modification and the quality of labelling information presented to consumers. The long-term aim is to reduce the prevalence of nursing bottle caries as the sales of sugarless baby drinks come to dominate the market.

The success of this national campaign has been largely due to the effective mobilization of media interest and the subsequent public pressure that has been applied to the baby drinks manufacturers. The initial stages of the campaign comprised a centralized lobby of the manufacturers combined with a media awareness drive. Subsequent stages aim to support local action by developing an action pack to enable effective action and monitoring at the local level across the UK (Winkler, 1994).

Chuck sweets off checkout campaign

A second national campaign launched by Action and Information on Sugars has again focused attention on the need for structural changes within society. The aim of this campaign was to stop all major UK retailers' displaying confectionery at checkouts within stores. The success of this campaign has again been largely due to the multidisciplinary and collaborative approach adopted by the campaign in which a wide range of health professionals and community groups have joined together to press for a change in retailers' selling policies (Smeaton, 1993). The campaign consisted of two key approaches. At the national level pressure was applied directly to all the major food retailers, supported by a major media and press campaign in which over 1000 national and local media contacts were made. In addition to the national campaign, action at the local level was considered to be an essential element of the project. An action pack was therefore produced and circulated across the UK which provided local action groups with resources and information to support the campaign.

After 2 years, major changes have taken place within the UK retailing sector with several large retailers now no longer promoting confectionery at their checkouts. Such a change reduces pressure on parents of young children to purchase confectionery–clearly a beneficial outcome for oral health. The success of this project again has been largely due to the media interest, both national and local, generated by the campaign, together with the widespread supportive local action across the UK. Monitoring and evaluation of this campaign have been a central feature of the project. Process evaluation data collated included media coverage, local action group activities and views and responses of the food retailers to the campaign. In the second year of the project a detailed monitoring exercise was undertaken across the country to assess outcomes in terms of the extent of the retailers' support for the campaign.

Limitations of the media

It is a commonly held belief that national campaigns using the mass media are the most important part of health education. This is not so. A successful community programme incorporates mass media as a subsidiary but important element within the programme as a whole (Tones *et al.*, 1990). The likelihood of success of a mass media campaign can be increased through carrying out rigorous problem definition, creative development research,

pretesting and evaluation (Leather, 1988). However, many expensive media-based health education campaigns have shown little change in knowledge or attitude among the target group and no change at all in behaviour despite having followed this approach. Advertising formed part of a campaign to encourage dental attendance in a British town (Anderson and Morgan, 1992). The aim was to test the use of advertising to try to overcome some of the perceived barriers to dental care, and to increase the uptake of general dental practitioner services by those people who did not attend regularly. The message was 'dentistry is not what you think it is, it has changed in recent years'. The media campaign was intended to stimulate the public to visit the dentist for an update or discussion of any aspect of the service. Advertisements featuring a celebrity were piloted and placed on bus shelters, buses, in newspapers and on leaflets distributed to each household. The campaign was evaluated by patient attendance recorded at dentists, by the numbers attending the dentist for updates, by intercept interviews to assess awareness of the campaign, by qualitative interviews to establish attitude and behaviour shifts and by the number of dental treatments carried out over the campaign period compared with a control area. The system of recording new attenders at practices was discontinued as it did not work. Only 44 people attended for dental updates.

Awareness of the campaign was high; 6 out of 10 people had noticed at least one aspect of the campaign. Unfortunately the message received was simplified to 'visit your dentist'. The message offered by some of the posters was confusing or unintelligible and conveyed nothing about the dental update scheme, a concept which was widely misunderstood. Newspaper adverts were more successful, conveying in addition to the message 'visit your dentist' that dentists are friendly and there is no need to be frightened. In-depth interviews showed that the campaign only made an impact on those who already acknowledged the need for dental services and all the action and favourable comments came from this group. Although dental attendance did not improve in the test town, it fell less than in neighbouring districts during the campaign. Overall the evaluation highlighted that the campaign was both very expensive and ineffective.

This stringently evaluated campaign demonstrates the limitations of the media in terms of promoting behaviour change. However, as has been shown, the media can be used successfully to raise awareness of issues and to set the agenda. Developing a productive relationship with the local media by supplying regular and topical press releases is an important part of any oral health strategy.

Conclusion

If oral health is to improve it must be on the policy agenda of relevant organizations at every level of society. This requires those involved in oral health promotion to work in partnership with other agencies and with the public. Changes in legislation and policy, underpinned by educational initiatives, will improve the social and physical environment which will support and encourage healthy behaviours. The success of such a strategy is built upon the achievement of a range of defined short-term goals which together lead to long-term sustainable improvements in general and oral health.

References

Anderson, R.J. and Morgan, J.D. (1992) Marketing dentistry; a pilot study in Dudley. *Community Dental Health* 9 (suppl. 1): 69–126.

Baric, L. (1991) Health promoting schools–evaluation and auditing. *Journal of the Institute of Health Education* 29:114–120.

Baric, L. (1992) Health promoting hospitals. *Journal of the Institute of Health Education* 30:141–148.

Bentley, E.M. and Holloway, P.J. (1993) An evaluation of the role of health visitors in encouraging dental attendance of infants. *Community Dental Health* 10:243–249.

Bentley, E.M. and Mackie, I.C. (1993) A qualitative investigation into general practitioners' views on prescribing sugar-free medicines for children prior to a dental health education campaign. *Health Education Research* 4:519–524.

Bentley, E.M., Mackie, I.C. and Fuller, S.S. (1993) Pharmacists and the 'Smile for sugar-free medicines' campaign. *Pharmaceutical Journal* 251:606–607.

Blane, D. (1985) An Assessment of the Black Report's explanations of health inequalities. *Sociology of Health and Illness* 7:423–445.

Blinkhorn, A.S. (1978) Influence of social norms on toothbrushing behaviour of young children. *Community Dental and Oral Epidemiology* 6:222–226.

Blinkhorn, A.S. (1982) The caries experience and dietary habits of Edinburgh nursery school children. *British Dental Journal* 152:227–230.

Blinkhorn, A.S. (1989) Promoting dietary changes in order to control dietary caries. *Journal of the Institute of Health Education* 27:179–186.

Catford, J. (1983) *Healthy Living: Towards a National Strategy for Health Education and Health Promotion.* Health Education Council, London

Craft, M. and Holloway, P.J. (1983) A programme of dental health education. *Health Education Journal* 42:16–19.

Croucher, R.E. (1993) General dental practice, health education, and health promotion: a critical reappraisal. In: *Oral Health Promotion* (Schou, L. and Blinkhorn, A., eds), pp. 153–169. Oxford University Press, Oxford.

Croucher, R.E., Rodgers, A.I., Franklin, A.J. and Craft, M.H. (1985) Results and issues arising from an evaluation of community dental health education: the case of the Good Teeth Programme. *Community Dental Health* 2:89–97.

Department of Health (1994a) *An Oral Health Strategy for England.* HMSO, London.

Department of Health (1994b) *Weaning and the Weaning Diet. Report on Health and Social Subjects 44.* HMSO, London.

Ewles, L. and Simnett, I. (1992) *Promoting Health: A Practical Guide.* Scutari Press, London.

Grabauskas, V.J. (1987) Integrated programme for community health in non-communicable disease (Interhealth). In: *The Prevention of Non-communicable Diseases: Experiences and Prospects* (Leparski, E., ed.), pp. 85–310. World Health Organization Regional Office for Europe, Copenhagen.

Green, L.W., Krenter, M. and Deeds, S. (1980) *Health Education Planning: A Diagnostic Approach.* Mayfield Publishing, California.

Grossman, R. and Scala, K. (1994) *Health Promotion and Organisational Development: Developing Settings for Health.* World Health Organization Regional Office for Europe, Copenhagen.

Hamel, G. and Prahalad, C. (1989) Strategic intent. *Harvard Business Review* 67:63–76.

Hodge, H.C., Holloway, P.J. and Bell, C.R. (1982) Factors associated with toothbrushing behaviour in adolescents. *British Dental Journal* 152:49–51.

Hodge, H., Buchanan. M., O'Donnell, P. *et al.* (1987) The evaluation of the junior dental health education programme developed in Sefton, England. *Community Dental Health* 4:223–229.

Leather, D.S. (1988) The development and assessment of mass media campaigns. *Journal of the Institute of Health Education* 26:6–12.

McCarthy, M. (1982) *Epidemiology and Policies for Health Planning.* King Edward's Hospital Fund for London, London.

McKinlay, R. (1994) *A Study to Determine the Levels of Knowledge of the Infant Oral Situation in Teenagers and Young Mothers from Deprived Areas of Edinburgh; with Proposals for Appropriate Oral Health Promotion.* MDSc Thesis. University of Dundee.

Milio, N. (1986) *Promoting Health Through Public Policy.* Canadian Public Health Association, Ottawa.

Morrow, N.C. and Maguire, T.A. (1989) Dental health care as a focus for health promotion in community pharmacy practice. *Health Education Research* **4**:181–191.

Nadanovsky, P. and Sheiham, A. (1994) The relative contribution of dental services to the changes and geographical variations in caries of 5 and 12 year old children in England and Wales in the 1980s. *Community Dental Health* **11**:215–223.

Nettleton, S. (1986) Teach or treat? Questions posed by demands for prevention in dental consultations. *Health Education Journal* **45**:163–165.

North West Region Dental Public Health Resource Centre (1994) *Working Together to Promote Dental Health.* FDI World Dental Press, London.

Quinn, G. and Freeman, R. (1991) Health visitors as dental health educators: their knowledge, attitudes and behaviours. *Health Education Journal* **4**:191–194.

Rise, J. and Holund, U. (1990) Prediction of sugar behaviour. *Community Dental Health* **7**:267–272.

Rose, G. (1992) *The Strategy of Preventive Medicine.* Oxford University Press, Oxford.

Scottish Health Education Group (1989) *The Healthy School.* World Health Organization Report, SHEG, Edinburgh.

Shafford, A. and Sharpe, K. (1988) *The pharmacist as a Health Educator.* Research report no. 24. HEA, London.

Sheiham, A. and Joffe, M. (1991) Public dental health strategies for identifying and controlling dental caries in high and low risk populations. In: *Risk Markers for Oral Diseases. Volume 1: Dental Caries: Markers of High and Low Risk Groups and Individuals* (Johnson, N.W., ed.), pp. 445–483. Cambridge University Press, Cambridge.

Smeaton, I. (1993) *Chuck Sweets off the Checkout: Campaign Summary Report,* personal communication.

Tones, K. (1974) A systems approach to health education. *Community Health* **6**:34–39.

Tones, K., Tilford, S. and Robinson, Y. (1990) *Health Education Effectiveness and Efficiency.* Chapman and Hall, London.

Towner, E. (1984) The 'Gleam Team' programme: development and evaluation of a dental health education package for infant schools. *Community Dental Health* **1**:181–191.

Welsh Health Planning Forum (1992) *Oral Health–Protocol For Investment In Health Gain.* Welsh Office/NHS Directorate 1992, Cardiff.

Winkler, J. (1993) *First Annual Report. The Baby Drinks Campaign, Action and Information on Sugars,* Personal Communication.

Winkler, J. (1994) *Second Annual Report. The Baby Drinks Campaign, Action and Information on Sugars,* Personal Communication.

World Health Organization (1984) *Health Promotion. A Discussion Document on the Concept and Principles.* World Health Organization Regional Office for Europe, Copenhagen.

16

The principles of organization and models of delivery of oral health care

Helen C. Gift, Ronald M. Andersen and Meei-shia Chen

The purpose of this chapter is to review the principles of the organization of oral health care within a society in order to provide understanding of:

1 how different societies provide resources for oral health care delivery;
2 the potential for change in the organization to adapt to different needs and demands;
3 the impact of organization on oral health outcomes.

Social, economic, political and environmental conditions and prevalent morbidity and mortality influence the development and establishment of the health care system, public and professional values, beliefs and behaviours associated with care delivery and how oral health is integrated into the overall health care system.

The oral health care delivery system

A systems approach is valuable for examining the organization of oral health care delivery (Andersen *et al.*, 1995). A system is a set of elements, actively interrelated, which operates in a bounded unit (Baker, 1970). Oral health care systems work towards a goal such as freedom from diseases and impairments (Scott, 1987). They are influenced by society structure and cross-cutting social policies. The oral health care system should improve the quality of life of the population through research, education,

provision of services, and through the promotion of policies such as fluoridation. Oral health care is an open system composed of policy, organization and resources (Andersen *et al.*, 1995).

History of oral health care systems

Oral health care systems throughout the world have different historic roots. Dentistry as an established independent occupation was not widespread until the 19th century when oral health care became more organized with licensing and training in Europe and the USA (Young and Cohen, 1979; Davis, 1980; Cowell and Sheiham, 1981; Slack and Burt, 1981). School care systems began early in the 20th century in several countries, while other countries responded to children's oral health needs differently (Dunning, 1979). During the 20th century, there was a rapid increase in dental caries in industrialized countries as well as improvements in dental therapeutics, materials and equipment. These factors, combined with expectations of (and consequently education of) medical and dental professionals, influenced the organization of systems of care as well as the structure and process of dental practices (Gies, 1926; Dunning, 1979; Davis, 1980; Cowell and Sheiham, 1981; Slack and Burt, 1981).

In some developing countries, there is no unique, separate system of oral health care and community health care workers are trained to respond to a variety of social, medical and dental conditions. In many countries the oral health care system is an integral part of the medical system and may be perceived to be a subspecialty of medicine. In others, systems evolved separately from medicine and remain unique systems for only oral care. The historic roots also vary in terms of whether the system is integrated with social, educational and employment institutions in the society. Similarly, the organization of oral health education of the public has emerged uniquely in different countries in response to dominant societal pressures (Dunning, 1979; Davis, 1980; Cowell and Sheiham, 1981; Slack and Burt, 1981; Andersen *et al.*, 1995).

Oral health care systems have been dynamic, responding to changes in population demographics; patterns of oral diseases; impact of oral diseases in relation to other systemic diseases; and, most importantly, to changes in social, political or economic structure and societal norms as reflected in national policies, legislation, regulations and payment systems (Davis, 1980; Fredericks *et al.*, 1980; Slack and Burt, 1981; Schieber *et al.*, 1991; Inglehart, 1992a; Gift, 1993; Andersen *et al.*, 1995). Oral health care systems are integrally associated with other social systems, including housing, water, food and safety (Slack and Burt, 1981). Societal changes affect availability of resources to provide oral health care and, conversely, to pay for care received. The economic and governmental structures of a country are particularly influential. For example, dental care expenditures are more sensitive to changes in gross national product than are medical care expenditures (Yule and Parkin, 1985), and, generally, lower-income individuals are less likely than higher-income individuals to have comprehensive dental care irrespective of other influencing factors (Kudrie, 1981; Andersen *et al.*, 1995).

The outcome of the oral health care system is oral health status, with intermediate outcomes of oral health behaviours (Andersen *et al.*, 1995). Success is measured by improvements in intermediate and ultimate outcome measures. However, outcomes are not the result of the current system alone, but represent the cumulative process of years of transitions resulting from interactions among the socio-environmental, health care and oral health care delivery systems (Aday *et al.*, 1980, 1993; Gift *et al.*, 1990; Gift, 1993; Andersen *et al.*, 1995; Woseth and Chen, 1995).

System characteristics

Oral health care systems worldwide can be described by policy, organization, payment mechanisms and outcomes (Andersen *et al.*, 1970). They are characterized by the following parameters: who provides what services/functions for whom; in what locations; with what resources; by what payment mechanisms; and with what effects. These dimensions are illustrated simplistically in Figure 16.1. The complexity in comparing these systems becomes obvious in Table 16.1, which lists examples of key characteristics of existing systems. Oral health care systems respond to oral diseases and policies that focus on specific populations such as age groups (Dunning, 1979; Slack and Burt, 1981; Andersen *et al.*, 1995). A different system will develop in a nation that has stated objectives for school-age children than in a country that targets infants or no specific age group. Worldwide, systems differ in the focus placed on the range of functions. For example, many developing countries emphasize relief of pain and emergencies; some national health care systems traditionally have focused on treatment; and many nations have limited or no research, administration or policy functions in the oral health care system. The appropriateness of organizations to carry out system functions varies. For instance, hospitals are appropriate for managing emergencies but such facilities have a less obvious role in prevention. Schools offer opportunities to promote children's oral health education while industrial clinics may cover acute oral treatment needs as well as health promotion for employees. Universities and government are logical components of the system to carry out functions of administration, policy and research.

Often an oral health care system is described on the basis of only one or two characteristics, perhaps reflecting what is most unique to that country. For example, the New Zealand system is often characterized as a school-based system employing dental nurses; the British system is described as the National Health Service; and the USA often is described as a fee-for-service private practice system. However, each system should be understood for all its characteristics. Many of the current challenges to oral health care systems are based on incongruencies evolving between policy, organizational structures and resources. For example, oral health systems may espouse a policy of prevention, yet an investigation of the work of their oral health care personnel shows most practice time devoted to treatment (Andersen *et al.*, 1995).

Over the years, oral health care systems have been described and examined independently, from the perspective of specific countries or regions. During the past few decades, examinations of systems across countries have allowed a more global perspective with opportunities to consider conceptual issues (Arnljot *et al.*, 1985; Yule and Parkin, 1985; Andersen *et al.*, 1995; Woseth and Chen, 1995; Chen *et al.*, 1996).

Policies and objectives

At the very basis of the system of oral health care are the goals and objectives–the purposes and expected outcomes of care. Confusion regarding goals and objectives, or the potential for changes in these, is at the heart of many debates regarding oral health care reform as the end of the 20th century arrives. Some countries have neither clearly articulated oral health objectives nor a well-defined system of care (or have one but not the other); others have oral health objectives that appear to have been developed independently of the organization of care, with a system that is unresponsive to those objectives; yet others have clearly stated objectives and a system designed to respond to those objectives, both of which are

Policy

Oral health care delivery system		
Personnel	Target population	Financing
Functions	Structure	Reimbursement

Oral Health

Fig. 16.1 Overview of the oral health care delivery system.

Table 16.1 Taxonomy for systematic cross-national comparative analysis of oral health care systems*

Personnel	*Structure/location*	*Financing*
Dentist	Government facilities	General government revenue
Dental hygienist	Universities	Specific taxation, compulsory
Dental therapist	Worksites	insurance
Expanded-duty assistant	Hospitals, institutions	Insurance or prepayment supported
Dental assistant	Schools	by employers or individuals
Oral health (community) worker	Health and/or dental clinics	Direct payment from private income
Community worker	Mobile units	
Other health care professionals	Individual dental offices	*Reimbursement*
		Fee-for-service
Target populations		Capitation
Infants	*Functions*	Contract
Preschool children	Policy development and	Salary
School-age children	implementation	
Young adults	Administration	*With what effect (examples)*
Adults	Quality control	Appropriate dental care
Older adults	Research	Improved knowledge values,
Special care populations	Professional education	opinions and behaviours regarding
(e.g. nursing home residents)	Oral health education of the public	oral health
Identified occupational groups	Preventive services	Lower DMFS among youth
(e.g. military)	Emergency services	Reduced edentulousness among
Identified racial and income groups	Treatment services	older adults
(e.g. Native Americans in the USA)	Rehabilitative services	Improved oral health

*A comprehensive assessment of a national oral health care system minimally requires description of who provides what services/functions for whom in what locations with what resources by what payment mechanisms with what effect.
DMFS = Decayed, missing, filled surfaces.

outdated (Lennon, 1981; Jacob and Plamping, 1989; Andersen *et al.*, 1995). Often uncoordinated programmes and appearances of ambivalence about oral health care as a 'social good' result when there is no clearly articulated policy (Inglehart, 1992a).

Objectives of oral health care systems range from preventing future oral diseases, to treating existing diseases, to managing and eliminating emergencies, pain and trauma, or a combination of any of these. Similarly, objectives may range from finding new methods of preventing and treating oral diseases (research), improving the use of new and existing preventive and treatment approaches (education), and/or treating existing diseases and eliminating the progression of diseases through use of existing therapies. How these objectives are implemented varies. Systems vary by the extent to which oral health is considered a responsibility of the public sector, whether it is represented in national policies, and how that responsibility is implemented (Dunning, 1979; Davis, 1980; Slack and Burt, 1981; Cowell and Sheiham, 1981; Arnljot *et al.*, 1985; Jacob and Plamping, 1989; Andersen *et al.*, 1995; Chen *et al.*, 1996).

Systems of oral health care are influenced by societal policies and have policies of their own that affect the organization of the system and services provided. Policies, set for meeting the objectives of the oral health system, provide guidelines for securing and organizing resources and may be either explicit or implicit. Policies might be represented by national nutrition guidelines or mandated governmental sponsored research, provision of care, or school education and service programmes, among others. The facilities, types, numbers and distribution of personnel, sources of revenue and reimbursement procedures are representative of resources in the oral health care system that are influenced by policy (Gift, 1993; Andersen *et al.*, 1995).

National policies influence which age group are emphasized, what types of care are received, who provides the care and where the care is provided (Gift, 1993; Andersen *et al.*, 1995). For example, two countries both may have policies focusing on children but have different systems and outcomes depending on the nature of the policy. A preventive policy is observed in implementation of school fluoride programmes; policy focused on treatment results in programmes that emphasize extraction, fillings and education. For example, during Mao Tse-tung's era in the People's Republic of China, policy guidelines were observed in the implementation of an oral health programme through the provision of services such as fillings, extractions and stainless steel crowns to a range of workers, peasants and soldiers using the counterpart of barefoot doctors, dental health workers. Traditional Chinese medicine such as acupuncture and herbal medicine was integrated into dental treatment (Ingle, 1978).

Policies may focus on issues other than age. For example, for years the National Health Service for England and Wales had an explicit policy to increase the number of dentists as well as the amount of treatment provided. This policy directly influenced the organization of care (Lennon, 1981; Jacob and Plamping, 1989).

The actual system of care may have outcomes very different to those anticipated by policies, suggesting that policies and system outcomes need to be evaluated regularly to determine if they are on parallel paths. For example, evaluations have suggested that policies focusing on regular examinations and restorations for children in school-based settings do not necessarily result in lower levels of disease in adulthood and may not encourage orientations toward disease prevention and oral health promotion (Lennon, 1981; Jacob and Plamping, 1989; Arnljot *et al.*, 1985; Isman, 1994; Andersen *et al.*, 1995). In industrial countries, oral health care systems have evolved from a focus on removing and replacing teeth to restoring teeth to preventing oral diseases and conditions and now, envisioning oral health as part of general health. These changes in implicit policies have not yet been fully recognized in organizations of oral health care that still have predominantly technical and curative approaches to care (Andersen *et al.*, 1995; Gift *et al.*, 1990; Gift, 1993).

Organization

What the oral health care system does with resources established by policies results in a formal organization (Andersen *et al.*, 1970). This organization has a structure as well as coordination and quality control strategies for the various components such as research, education/training and care provision. For the purpose of this chapter, delivery of care is used to illustrate organization and payment mechanisms of the oral health care system. Generally, the organization of the delivery system has been described using a medical model, limited to the oral health care professionals associated with dental schools, clinics, individual dental practices and governmental components directly associated with policy, remuneration or delivery of oral health care (Jacob and Plamping, 1989). More recently, comprehensive community/public health models have gained favour over the medical model (Gift, 1993; Andersen *et al.*, 1995; Drury and Snowden, 1995; Woseth and Chen, 1995). Then, oral health care delivery includes activities at the community level such as implementation of policies related to promotion and consumption of sugar products; establishment of regulations and enforcement such as those related to tobacco consumption and cessation of community water fluoridation; oral health education and provision of fluoride therapies in prenatal clinics and well-baby clinics, among others. Using this expanded model, pharmacists, physicians, nurses, schoolteachers and water-work supervisors become part of the oral health care delivery system. Similarly, worksites, hospitals, nursing homes and institutions are appropriate facilities for care. Using this broader definition of the oral health care delivery system, however, illustrates how limited our ability is to describe, evaluate and improve the organization of care. Some of these wider matters are considered in Chapters 11 and 15 and the following description focuses on more traditional oral health care facilities and personnel.

Structure

Country level

At the national level, oral health care may be entirely centrally organized or all or part of the system may be decentralized. Oral health may be well-identified with defined structures and leadership, may be integrated with other medical services, or may not be acknowledged as part of a national agenda at all (Cohen, 1971; Cowell and Sheiham, 1981; Slack and Burt, 1981; Cohen and Bryant, 1984; Jacob and Plamping, 1989; Andersen *et al.*, 1995). The level of visibility and resources devoted to oral health have strong historic roots in most countries (Cowell and Sheiham, 1981; Davis, 1980). There are few examples of increasing focus; rather, in contrast,

oral health is receiving decreasing emphasis (White, 1994).

Since a large part of oral health care is provided within a dental operatory and these contain most of the essential equipment for providing comprehensive services, oral health care is often available in facilities located throughout communities, independent of hospitals and medical services (Dunning, 1979; Cowell and Sheiham, 1981; Slack and Burt, 1981; Jacob and Plamping, 1989; Gift, 1993; White, 1994; Gift and White, 1996). Most often, services are provided in dental clinics, independent dental practices or in schools. Dental and dental hygiene schools provide services in clinics as part of training oral health care professionals. The distribution, location and ownership of care-provision facilities vary by country as a result of national oral health care policies and subsequent targeting of specific populations. Hospitals and related health and social services facilities usually provide emergency care rather than general oral health services, except to some special care groups. Some countries are providing care where people are working or living–in factories, offices and other workplaces, and nursing homes–attempting to integrate oral health within general health services in neighbourhood or industrial clinics (Kostlan, 1978; Dunning, 1979; Gift, 1991). These efforts have been undertaken to address absenteeism, accidents and occupational hazards and to improve the health of employees or residents. Improvements in portable dental equipment enhance provision of oral health services, particularly for remote locations (Dunning, 1979; Cowell and Sheiham, 1981).

Practice level

The most frequently observed structures for delivery of oral health care are independent *practices* with one or more dentist (owners or employed associates) and clinics (public or private; Dunning, 1979; Cowell and Sheiham, 1981; Slack and Burt, 1981; Arnljot *et al.*, 1985; Jacob and Plamping, 1989; Neenan *et al.*, 1993; Andersen *et al.*, 1995). General dentistry group practices, multispecialty groups and dentists in group medical care settings are more complex forms of organization that also exist in some countries. Clinics and group practices imply a larger number of staff with specific duties, more administration and increased opportunity for consultation, referral, continuity of care, convenience and economy in purchasing. If the dentist owns the practice, as is the case in most private systems, increases in scale means moving from the combined role of health professional/ entrepreneur to that of a health professional/ business manager.

Clinics, it has been suggested, provide geographically centralized services that may be potentially more culturally sensitive based on location (Dunning, 1979). Clinics provide more opportunity for education and peer review; and can be more cost-efficient by the sharing of expenses among multiple programmes (Dunning, 1979; Cowell and Sheiham, 1981; Jacob and Plamping, 1989). Large group practices, as well as private and public clinics, in communities, worksites or schools appear to be responses to concerns for efficiency of location and economies of scale. In many countries, however, public clinics have become part of a two-tier system, and, while demonstrating some economies of scale, have not demonstrated completely any advantages in cultural sensitivity or quality enhancement attributes (Dunning, 1979; Gift, 1984, 1993). A two-tiered delivery system in which public and private patients predominantly use different parts of the oral health care organization may actually increase the gap in oral health between lower and upper socioeconomic level individuals (Gift, 1984; Gift *et al.*, 1990). Such systems may not only be available differentially to these groups; the policies and styles of practice and types of personnel may vary and affect care. For example, there may be fewer specialists in public clinics; public patients may not be referred to specialists.

Current care organizations have developed from the demands of treating caries and periodontal diseases (Davis, 1980; Slack and Burt, 1981). However, the structure of dental practices appears to be less suitable for many health promotion and disease prevention initiatives, particularly for people who do not routinely visit an oral health provider.

Oral health care personnel

Education and training

The education and training of oral health care personnel set the stage for the organization of the oral health care delivery system. The time devoted to education and training of dentists usually is more than that for other oral health personnel, and the system is organized through licensing and credentialing to represent this (Dunning, 1979; Chambers, 1994; Jeffcoat and Clark, 1995; Kress, 1995; Tedesco, 1995). In most countries dentists have an educational and training track that lasts from 2 to 4 years beyond secondary school; in some cases this dental training is in addition to a university degree in another academic area.

The education of many dental hygienists, dental therapists and expanded-duty auxiliaries is extensive. Education of dentists and dental hygienists may be integrated into a health professions school or isolated from other health care professionals and from each other (Tedesco, 1994, 1995; Kress, 1995). The amount of general education required prior to professional training varies and influences the interaction of these future oral health care personnel with other professionals. Worldwide, the education for dental hygienists ranges from 2 to 4 or more years. This education typically is received in specific educational programmes and, depending on the country's academic system, may result in a bachelor's or master's degree or certificate which can be supplemented with other courses to receive a degree in a related science. In most countries, dental hygienists are required to hold a licence to practise (Barmes, 1989). Many auxiliary and office personnel in dental practices worldwide, particularly in developing countries, receive on-the-job training or only attend short training courses. The training of dental assistants varies from formal college education, to targeted certificate programmes, to on-the-job training (Dunning, 1979; Elderton, 1981; Tedesco, 1994).

The nature of the education and training of all types of oral health personnel influences the organization and delivery of care in other ways. For example, in the USA, the training of dentists is provided almost exclusively in the dental school with few experiences in community settings and hospitals. Dentists are trained to provide all oral health services as general practitioners and only a small percentage obtain more in-depth education in specialty areas (Dunning, 1979; Gift *et al.*, 1990; Gift and White, 1996; Kress, 1995). Both of these processes encourage an independent rather than interactive and a stationary rather than flexible organization of care.

Furthermore, the guidelines and regulations established for education and licensing facilitate the maintenance of the system. Regulations for accreditation of schools, graduation of students and licensing of practitioners may be formulated by national public health agencies or by boards made up predominantly of individuals who have been trained and who practise in the existing system. Traditionally, examinations include little that evaluate behavioural competencies in patient care or practice management for health and social contingencies of today's patients (Cowell and Sheiham, 1981; Chambers, 1994; Tedesco, 1994; Gift and White, 1996; Kress, 1995). In the USA assessments are underway to determine if dental and dental hygiene schools can effect institutional changes to improve the training of dental and dental hygiene students, and ultimately, the responsiveness of the organization of oral health care delivery to the oral health needs of society (Gift *et al.*, 1990; Field, 1995).

Types of personnel

In all countries the dentist is the responsible individual, directly or indirectly overseeing or coordinating contributions from related personnel (Dunning, 1979; Cowell and Sheiham, 1981; Slack and Burt, 1981; Jacob and Plamping, 1989; Andersen *et al.*, 1995). A dental hygienist is a health professional who, through clinical services, education, consultative planning and evaluation endeavours, seeks to prevent oral diseases, provide treatment for existing diseases, and assist individual patients (public) in maintaining an optimum level of oral health (International Federation of Dental Hygienists, 1989).

Dental hygienists serve as primary prevention personnel in approximately 40 countries. Hygienists have direct patient contact and provide specific preventive services, such as fluorides, dental sealants, oral prophylaxis (including periodontal therapy), as well as oral health assessment and education. Additional services, such as local anaesthesia and nitrous oxide sedation, may be provided by dental hygienists if specified in the dental hygiene regulations (Barmes, 1989). Productivity of the oral health care delivery system increases with the appropriate use of dental hygienists (Walsh, 1987; Wang, 1994). Hygienists may work in settings such as schools, public health clinics, institutions or nursing homes with only general oversight or, in some cases, independently

(Dunning, 1979; Elderton, 1981; Barmes, 1989; Johnson and van Lierde, 1992).

Dental therapists (dental nurses and expanded duty auxiliaries) exist in over 50 countries (Barmes, 1989). These personnel operate under guidelines that allow them to provide specified services (such as restorative procedures and extraction of primary teeth) in schools or in remote rural areas. Therapists operate under the general supervision of a dental officer who, in some developing countries, may be geographically very remote. In New Zealand as well as in parts of the UK, Swedish and Canadian systems dental therapists provide specific services of comparable quality at lower costs than dentists (Lombardo, 1978; Dunning, 1979; Davis, 1980; Elderton, 1981; Kudrie, 1981; Barmes, 1989; Andersen *et al.*, 1995).

Other oral health personnel include dental assistants, who perform a variety of tasks in processing the patient through care provision. The employment of dental assistants increases the number of patients a dentist can provide care for in a specified period of time (Dunning, 1979; Elderton, 1981) and requires that the dentist has management and delegation skills. With assistants performing much of the technical work, the dentist should have more time to be responsive to the patient through diagnosis, treatment planning, counselling or training, but it is not clear that this outcome has been achieved. Public health clinics, large group practices, and orthodontists, specifically, have benefited from the employment of dental assistants through increased productivity (Dunning, 1979; Elderton, 1981). Other types of personnel, including oral health community workers, dental aides, school teachers and general community health aides provide oral health services, particularly in countries (including Venezuela, Cuba and Mexico) where there is a shortage of dentists or in remote rural areas. Services provided are usually education and preventive therapies, but may include other procedures, particularly those related to emergencies (Lombardo, 1978; Andersen *et al.*, 1995; Frazier and Horowitz, 1995).

Dental laboratory technicians are critical to the field of restorative dentistry, preparing prosthetic materials based on prescriptions from the dentist. Few dental laboratory technicians are employed in independent dental practices or small clinics. Rather, this profession is usually employed in laboratories in separate locations

(Dunning, 1979; Elderton, 1981). By law or regulation, in most countries, they have little or no direct contact with patients. However, in some states in the USA and in other countries, laboratory technicians (i.e. denturists) are licensed to provide dentures directly to patients.

Schoolteachers have been recognized in many oral health care delivery systems in their roles as educators and supervisors of fluoride mouthrinse programmes. In some industrial countries where dental caries rates are declining, the continuation of school oral health programmes is being challenged. The potential of other extenders of the oral health care delivery system, such as visiting nurses or caregivers for individuals in institutions, has not been examined fully, and it appears that they are ill-trained for the oral health functions they do perform in the absence of available oral health care personnel. Considerations of the role of health visitors in promoting oral health are described in more detail in Chapter 15. With increased focus on both age extremes, staff in prenatal and well-baby clinics as well as nursing homes may become more closely identified as oral health care personnel (Gift *et al.*, 1990; Gift, 1993). Considerably more attention needs to be given to articulating the appropriate roles of many of these extended oral health care workers in addressing the full range of oral health education and disease prevention activities (Inglehart, 1993).

Distribution of workforce

The distribution of personnel within an oral health care system reflects the emphasis of the system (Gift, 1984; van Amerongen and Kalff, 1984). For example, a high proportion of dental hygienists or preventive therapists may demonstrate a preventive philosophy or policy at the system level (Gift, 1984; Arnlijot *et al.*, 1985; Andersen *et al.*, 1995; Tedesco, 1995) The distribution of personnel in different geographical areas, measured by oral health care providers to population ratio, may demonstrate the various levels of availability and access to care in these areas. However, other factors, such as patients' characteristics, may play an important role in service utilization. For example, motivated individuals appear to seek care even in situations where the dentist-to-population ratio is low (Gift, 1984; Arnljot *et al.*, 1985); in contrast, individuals, due to various barriers, may fail to utilize oral health services even in areas where the dentist-to-population ratio is high. The likelihood of individuals seeking care is discussed in further detail in Chapter 12 which examines the principles of health behaviour.

Patients and services

Patients enter the system by meeting requirements and overcoming barriers such as transportation or cost. Providers and facilities influence the patient after gaining entry to the system. Transactions between the patient, oral health care professionals and related third parties (family members, consulting physicians, payment sources) are the social processes in the organization and are influential in determining the outcomes of the system (Andersen *et al.*, 1995; Grembowski *et al.*, 1989).

Oral health care personnel are critical gatekeepers with primary responsibility for transferring information and establishing the practice orientation, e.g. preventive versus curative. Communication style and orientation of the provider, as well as the availability of services, affect the outcome of the visit. For example, not all practices have a preventive orientation, nor do they provide preventive services to appropriate age or risk groups (Gift, 1993; Andersen *et al.*, 1995; Frazier and Horowitz, 1995). When dental hygienists are not employed, the dental practice appears to be placing less focus on prevention and health promotion tending to reduce the provision of dental sealants, dietary fluorides and oral health education. Some oral health promotion strategies, such as counselling about nutrition or smoking, have been met with resistance and have not been built into the culture of the dental practice (Gift, 1984, 1993).

The organization of services influences individual care-seeking behaviour. If these are established early in childhood, they appear to carry on through to adulthood. In open (unrestricted), unstructured systems (such as in the USA) individual motivation appears to be a reason for dental utilization more than in other systems, and unmet need appears to be greater among children than in a structured system. In systems that are structured and closed for (restricted to) school-age children and unstructured and open during adulthood (for example, New Zealand), there is some evidence that socialization for care-seeking behaviour does not occur, e.g. oral health care programmes targeting young age groups do not necessarily result in routine care-seeking behaviour or improved oral health among adults (Gift, 1984, 1993; Arnljot *et al.*, 1985; Andersen *et al.*, 1995; Woseth and Chen, 1995).

Interpersonal relationships, as well as bureaucratic and administrative incentives or barriers, vary among countries and may differ in public and private sector delivery systems within a single country (Gift, 1993). In studying patterns of dental utilization or prevalence of oral diseases, system characteristics are often assessed only implicitly, if at all. When they are examined, all too often system characteristics are interpreted as individual enabling characteristics. Such an approach directs health promotion initiatives towards individual behaviour change rather than alterations in social, community or delivery system characteristics. For example, addressing an individual's income, employment or geographic location leads to discussions of discretionary activities with limited budgets and problems in getting to a dental office. These same factors–cost of oral health care, hours of operation and distribution of oral health care facilities–envisioned at the system level result in debates about alterations in policies, organizational structure and financing mechanisms.

The populations or groups who are most in need of oral health care often have limited access to the organization of oral health care or do not avail themselves of the system (Aday *et al.*, 1980, 1993; Gift, 1984, 1993; Cockerham *et al.*, 1988; Jacob and Plamping, 1989; Gift *et al.*, 1990; Andersen *et al.*, 1995; Woseth and Chen, 1995). Additionally, some characteristics of oral health care delivery systems have been observed to be culturally inappropriate (e.g. similar languages are not spoken, organizational structures are unfamiliar to the client, etc.) for many racial and ethnic minorities resulting in differential health outcomes for these individuals (Chen, 1995).

From the public health model perspective, the focus on social, cultural, economic, structural and delivery system influences on care seeking and care receipt becomes as important as people's individual characteristics. The possibility of altering system level factors to improve oral health need to be considered in lieu of or in addition to a singular focus on changing individual behaviours. Moving a step further, beyond the public health model that emphasizes doing something to the people, a community model that involves the population in decisions about their lives and health also enhances the likelihood of oral health promotion (Drury and Snowden, 1995). Involvement of communities and individuals in oral health care increases the potential for change in the organization of care.

Financing, reimbursement and remuneration

Financing reflects how the money gets into the system, the most common approaches being general government revenues or specific taxation, insurance or prepayment premiums paid by individuals and/or employers, and out-of-pocket direct payment by individuals. Reimbursement, including remuneration, is the mechanism for payment for services, e.g. fee-for-service, capitation, contract or salary. Financing and reimbursement, while different concepts, are integrally related to each other in describing oral health care delivery systems. The influence of financing mechanisms is so pronounced that financial terms are used to describe the organization of oral health care delivery rather than structural terms. For example, oral health care systems can be categorized into those that are financed with a social security system, those in which the state is directly responsible for provision of services, and those characterized by private financing (Yule and Parkin, 1986; Andersen *et al.*, 1995). Financing systems range from market-based to centralized tax-financed national health services systems with mixed systems in between the two extremes (Evans, 1981).

Remuneration and reimbursement mechanisms involve third parties such as family members, government, employers, an operating agency and programme manager for payment (either public or private) for services provided in the system of care delivery However, the term third party is generally used in reference to formal payment organizations other than family. In most countries, reimbursement mechanisms are integrally associated with the organizational structure of the oral health care delivery system, as well as with its utilization and accessibility. Although variable throughout the world, the structures of payment plans affect the quantity and quality of oral health services, as well as their costs (Andersen and Newman, 1973; Dunning, 1979; Davis, 1980; Cowell and Sheiham, 1981; Slack and Burt, 1981; Gift, 1984, 1993; Jacob and Plamping, 1989; Gift *et al.*, 1981, 1990; Andersen *et al.*, 1995). The flow of funds is altered with the introduction of a third-party financing system. In the absence of a formal third party the individual or family pays or the care is provided free. With a third party, the dentist may receive a salary to provide care for the patient who does not pay, the care may be provided under contract to the dentist with no payment from the patient, or the dentist may be reimbursed directly or indirectly for services provided for the patient through private or public prepayment or insurance plans that pay in full or in part based on deductible and coinsurance schedules (Evans, 1981).

Managed care is an example of a mechanism for providing care within a specified reimbursement approach (Inglehart, 1992b). Managed care includes closed panels with arrangements for care delivery based on the purchase of dental care for groups of people, often at specific locations such as schools or worksites. Examples are health maintenance organizations (HMOs) which offer an agreed set of services by a specified group of oral health care professionals, with prenegotiated and fixed payment, for a voluntarily enrolled group of people, often at a central location in a geographic area. Managed care approaches are often viewed as restrictive by dentists, particularly by those in traditionally market-based systems. While dentists feel driven towards managed care arrangements to secure their income and access to patients, requirements of managed care and other third-party mechanisms have been viewed by dentists as interference in the professional–patient decision process.

Dentists traditionally have demanded the right to appraise the quality of the work they themselves do, the time they spend on services, and the fee charged (Freidson, 1972; Dunning, 1979; Reisine and Bailit, 1980; Gift *et al.*, 1990). Third-party agents concerned with payment (whether public or private), in combination with growing consumerism, change this independence and authority. With third parties, organizations and individuals (other than the dentist and patient) have responsibilities in such matters as scope and quality of care, time per operation, fees and facilities to be furnished (Dunning, 1979; Gift, 1984; Gift *et al.*, 1990). Third-

party involvement introduces processes and expectations (such as capitation, fee schedules, peer review, record review, profile studies, production standards, prior approval, cost-effectiveness analysis and cost–benefit analysis) into organizations previously functioning independently and in isolation (Dunning, 1979).

Responses to these changes have varied. For example, some practitioners have withdrawn from a third-party reimbursement system; dental professional associations have retained authority by forming their own dental service corporations in which the dentists act as administrators controlling quality assurance and peer review (Dunning, 1979). It is not unusual for dentists to resist changes in the delivery system, as observed in the USA in the 1970s with the introduction of prepayment review systems, involvement of the Federal Trade Commission in fee and advertising issues, or requirements of informed consent. Today, dentists remain cautious about changing reimbursement mechanisms such as managed care and decreases in professional autonomy (Jerrold, 1988; Romberg and Cohen, 1990; Gunn *et al.*, 1992; McCulloch, 1994; Gift and White, 1996), as well as regulations affecting how they deliver care (Verrusio *et al.*, 1989).

The nature of financing in a system, the mechanism of reimbursement (e.g. salaries, contracts, fee-for-service) and its specific characteristics (e.g. eligibility, degree of cost sharing) interact with individual socioeconomic status and influence equity and efficiency of the system (Aday *et al.*, 1980, 1993; Gift, 1984, 1993; Cockerham *et al.*, 1988; Andersen *et al.*, 1995). Cost of care influences demand for services and consequently affects the system (Manning *et al.*, 1985; Coventry *et al.*, 1989). Data from the Rand Health Insurance Experiment in the USA showed that reducing the level of cost sharing significantly increased the demand for dental services (Manning *et al.*, 1985). Assistance with payment, when associated with appropriate services (e.g. prevention versus treatment, restoration versus extraction), appears to increase the number of visits, comprehensiveness of services received and satisfaction with care (Gift, 1993). As is the case with other payment assistance, dental prepayment and insurance often most influence those who are already predisposed to visit a dentist more regularly (Gift, 1984, 1993; Arinen and Sintonen, 1994; Andersen *et al.*, 1995). Depending on the nature of health system financing and reimbursement mechanisms, the impact of socioeconomic factors will be different. For example, in a relatively market-based delivery system, individual socioeconomic factors will have more direct impact on use of services than in a system that has a more centralized, tax-financed national health services system, essentially free from direct out-of-pocket costs to all residents (Gift, 1993; Andersen *et al.*, 1995; Chen, 1995; Woseth and Chen, 1995).

The interaction of the financial system and reimbursement mechanisms with other dimensions of the oral health care system is well-illustrated in countries where public funds are available for care in the private sector. For example, in the USA, children in poverty covered by state-based Medicaid plans visit the dentist less than other children. This outcome appears to result from the lack of reimbursement for comprehensive services at usual and customary fees of the private dentists, unwillingness of dentists to provide care to Medicaid patients, lack of potential clients' awareness of coverage for dental services under Medicaid, and different cultural orientations of the provider and the patient which affect follow-through and compliance (Lang and Weintraub, 1986; Office of Technology Assessment, 1990; Gift, 1993).

The nature of the financing and reimbursement can influence whether oral health policies are realized. For example, if a policy states a goal of disease prevention but only treatment services are paid for in the payment assistance programme, then it is unlikely that the goal will be achieved. Payment assistance programmes have met with varying degrees of success in reducing oral diseases, in part because appropriate services may not always be matched with needs of specific target groups, or sufficient resources may not be available to sustain mandated and appropriate services. For example, payment assistance programmes have traditionally encouraged services for diseases that are visible by examination or in records, and have discouraged those services that are difficult to observe or measure (e.g. sealants or oral health education). Also, payment policies may deny the services that have the longest-term benefits for tooth retention (restorations rather than dentures). It appears that there may be insufficient recognition of the complexity of the interacting biological, individual, professional, social and cultural determinants of oral health

outcomes in the design and implementation of financing systems and reimbursement mechanisms (Lennon, 1981; Jacob and Plamping, 1989; Gift, 1993; Andersen *et al.*, 1995).

Policy, organization, financing and reimbursement of the oral health care delivery system in the context of social systems

Oral health care systems can be characterized by a country's level of economic development (e.g. industrialized, middle-income developing, and low-income developing), degree of market intervention (non-market-based and market-based), the financing system, and whether it is public or private (Evans, 1981; Chen, 1995). Oral health care systems in countries with a non-market-based system (e.g. China and former GDR) are usually government-run systems, similar to their general health care systems. Health care systems in countries with a market-based general economic system include national health systems (e.g. the UK); national health insurance systems (e.g. Canada), fee-for-service systems (e.g. USA) and various combinations of these types (e.g. Denmark, Finland, New Zealand; Hurst, 1991; Chen, 1995). Further descriptions are given in the following chapter and examples below illustrate the complex interactions of oral health care with the overall sociopolitical system.

The former GDR had an oral health care delivery system that had centrally coordinated management and control functions, was public, socialist and financed through social insurance (mandatory monthly contribution from employees and employers) and government subsidies from general revenues. The system was almost exclusively free to the public with care provided through centres, large group practices and hospitals. The state's responsibility included examining and providing care for children with a focus on fluoride, nutrition and education in addition to care (Nippert, 1992; Andersen *et al.*, 1995). After unification of West and East Germany, the former socialist oral health care system was transformed to one with decentralized planning and predominantly private practices. This transformation presents a rare natural experiment for assessing the impact of two very different oral health care systems.

In contrast, the Japanese system can be described as welfare-oriented and funded by a national health insurance. Fees are determined by a government schedule and recipients are responsible for copayments specified by their own insurance programme. Almost all care is provided in clinics and hospitals under private ownership and control with very limited government regulation (Andersen *et al.*, 1995; Woseth and Chen, 1995). Children are required to receive an oral examination annually by a school dentist who is a private practitioner in the community, and treatment is referred via the child's parents to a private dentist (Woseth and Chen, 1995). Japan, like other countries, is a system under stress with health care expenditures rising at a more rapid rate than other goods and services and growing concern regarding government involvement (Inglehart, 1988).

In describing any one country's oral health care system according to prevailing policy, organization, financing, reimbursement and social systems, one has to acknowledge that internal variations in environmental and population factors can lead to different outcomes for segments of the population. For example, while the USA has a predominantly private practice system (94% of dentists are in private practice and 95% of the care is paid from the private sector; Neenan *et al.*, 1993), local variation in water fluoridation, income levels, insurance coverage or ethnic mix may lead to large discrepancies in services received and oral health status (Andersen *et al.*, 1995; Woseth and Chen, 1995). The findings from the Second International Collaborative Study (ICS II), particularly from the former GDR, Poland and the Indian Health Service sites (Andersen *et al.*, 1995; Woseth and Chen, 1995; Chen *et al.*, 1996), help illustrate the complex interactions of social systems with oral health care delivery systems and oral health status. With dramatic changes in national demarcations, forms of government and other global changes at the sociopolitical levels, the next decade will be a very fluid situation for the organization of health and oral health care in many countries.

Potential for change and evaluation of opportunities

Many sociopolitical changes are occurring globally, notably major social upheavals such as observed during this decade in eastern Europe. As part of these large-scale sociopolitical changes, questions are raised about the effectiveness, efficiency and appropriateness of the oral health care system (Inglehart, 1990, 1991; Hurst, 1991). Often there is no systemic information to address these questions. While experiments with alternatives to traditional system characteristics have been tested in many countries, little exists in the way of longitudinal or cross-sectional comparisons of different approaches to organization. Different responsibilities of oral health personnel, office locations, payment for services and sizes of practice have been examined with varying degrees of success. Few large-scale evaluations of major alterations in an oral health care system have been conducted–perhaps, in part, due to potential difficulty in implementing any proposed changes because of the large investment in the existing physical facilities and educational systems, and the presence of deeply entrenched cultural norms affecting care provision (Perry *et al.*, 1994).

Opportunity for change is different at each level of the organization. The choice of where to practise and with whom usually remains within the factors the dentists can control. However, broader system financing and reimbursement arrangements do not, and it is these that have the potential to result in more far-reaching changes in any country. In the mid 1990s, it seems that both extremes of financing systems are converging. This evolution may tend to combine the advantages of managed care and fee-for-service, i.e. public and private financing. Third-party payment (private or public, central or decentralized) has become integral to most oral health care systems. Consequently, alterations in government policies, mandates or consumer interests that influence financing and reimbursement arrangements hold the most potential for changes in organization of care through effects on where providers practise, the levels of services provided and patients' access to care (Inglehart, 1990).

Outlook

The organization of oral health care affects access, quality, costs and outcome of oral health services. Considerable research has been conducted over the years on structure and function of the oral health care delivery system as it relates to use of oral health care personnel, productivity, quality and cost of care, and patient and health care provider satisfaction (Schieber *et al.*, 1991). Much of the research on the oral health care delivery system in industrialized countries was conducted in the time period of increasing supply of dentists, expected growth of prepayment and little recognition of changing patterns of oral diseases. Since the 1980s the environment has changed: there was a decreasing entry supply of dentists; questions were raised about employee or public benefit plans in times of limited resources; there was increased evidence of changes in patterns of oral diseases; and more evidence of need for integration of oral health care with the medical care delivery system. In the 1990s massive changes in sociopolitical systems and evaluations of national economic security worldwide have introduced even more need to evaluate systems and institutions, such as oral health care, for effectiveness, efficiency and appropriateness in meeting national goals.

There have been numerous improvements in the delivery and organization of oral health care. Disease rates and total tooth loss are declining in many countries and people are increasingly engaged in preventive behaviours. Advances in dental restorative materials and dental equipment make the receipt of dental care a very different experience to what it was several decades ago. Emerging technology and a community focus favour expanding organizations of care (Inglehart, 1993). Yet, despite these improvements and advances, there are large segments of the population worldwide who do not benefit from the simplest kinds of preventive care or restorative services. An increased life expectancy and tooth retention place many people at risk for oral diseases for more years. There are special categories of patients such as the geographically remote, those living in substandard conditions for food, water or housing; and the aged, medically physically, or mentally challenged for whom access to and availability of oral health care system are critical barriers (Gift, 1993; Gift and White, 1996). Artificial barriers to integrating oral health services, into health and social services, particularly preventive services must be eliminated. If people who have most of the oral diseases are the ones not receiving services from the current oral health care delivery systems, these systems may be more in need of change than the people. How can we adjust and alter the oral health care delivery systems to be more responsive to a wider range of populations who live in a variety of situations? How can we reach out to where the people are rather than wait for them to come into the current system (Inglehart, 1993)?

Oral health does not occur in isolation from general health or social services. Opportunities may exist to expand the concept of the organization of oral health care within the context of general health and social services. Research needs to be conducted to investigate the roles oral health care systems play in promoting health directly: predisposing and enabling the population to improve health, encouraging the external environment to enhance health, facilitating appropriate personal health practices, and emphasizing efficient and effective means of achieving positive health outcomes. The oral health care delivery system and the policy-level, administrative, research and care-providing professionals in it are influenced by a complex web of sociopolitical, scientific, epidemiological, administrative and legal forces. These forces need to be recognized in the curriculum for all oral health care personnel if oral health care systems are to become responsive to population needs over the next decades. Oral health care professionals need to study and understand people's risk behaviours, multiple diseases, time and cost of care, and how these factors should be considered in organizing services. Acknowledging these issues points to more collaboration and outreach with a multidisciplinary approach involving health care professionals from diverse backgrounds as well as the community at all levels.

References

Aday, L.A., Andersen, R.A. and Fleming, G.V. (1980) *Health Care in the USA: Equitable for Whom?* Sage Publications, Beverly Hills, CA.

Aday, L.A., Begley, C.E., Lairson, D.R. and Slater, C.H. (1993) *Evaluating the Medical Care System: Effectiveness, Efficiency and Equity.* pp. 6–16. Health Administration Press, Ann Arbor, MI.

Andersen, R.A. and Newman, J.F. (1973) Societal and individual determinants of medical care utilization in the United States. *Milbank Memorial Fund Quarterly: Health and Society* 51:95–124.

Andersen, R.A., Smedby, B. and Anderson, O.W. (1970) *Medical Care Use in Sweden and the United States: A Comparative Analysis of Systems and Behaviour. Research Series 27*, pp. 28–41, Center for Health Administration Studies, Chicago, ILL.

Andersen, R., Marcus, M. and Mahshigan, M. (1995) A comparative systems perspective on oral health promotion and disease prevention. In: *Oral Health Promotion: Socio-dental Sciences in Action* (Cohen, L.K. and Gift, H.C., eds), pp. 307–340. Munksgaard International Publishers, Copenhagen.

Arinen, S-S. and Sintonen, H. (1994) The choice of dental care sector by young adults before and after subsidisation reform in Finland. *Social Science Medicine* **39**:291–297.

Arnljot, H.A., Barmes, D.E., Cohen, L.K. *et al.* (eds). (1985) *Oral Health Care Systems: An International Collaborative Study.* Quintessence, London.

Baker, F. (1970) General system theory, research and medical care. In: *Systems and Medical Care* (Sheldon, A., Baker, F. and McLaughlin, C., eds), pp. 4–5. MIT Press, Boston, MA.

Barmes, D.E. (1989) Dental hygienists as health care providers. In: *Proceedings of the 11th International Symposium on Dental Hygiene*, Canadian Dental Hygienists' Association, Ottawa.

Chambers, D.W. (1994) Competencies: a new view of becoming a dentist. *Journal of Dental Education* **58**:342–345.

Chen, M.-s. (1995) Oral health of disadvantaged populations. In: *Oral Health Promotion: Socio-dental Sciences in Action* (Cohen, L.K. and Gift, H.C., eds), pp. 153–212. Munksgaard International Publishers, Copenhagen.

Chen, M.-s., Andersen, R.M., Barnes, D.E. *et al.* (1966) *Comparing Oral Health Care Systems: Second International Collaborative Study.* World Health Organization, Geneva (in press).

Cockerham, W.C., Kunz, G. and Lueschen, G. (1988) Social stratification and health lifestyles to two systems of health care delivery: a comparison of the United States and West Germany. *Journal of Health and Social Behavior* **29**:113–126.

Cohen, L.K. and Bryant, P.S. (eds). (1984) *Social Sciences in Dentistry: A Critical Bibliography*, vol. II. Quintessence Publishing Company for the Fédération Dentaire Internationale, London.

Coventry, P., Holloway, P.J., Lennon, M.A. *et al.* (1989) Trial of a capitation system of payment for the treatment of children in the general dental service. *Community Dental Health* **6** (suppl.):1–62.

Cowell, C.R. and Sheiham, A. (1981) *Promoting Dental Health.* King Edward's Hospital Fund for London, London.

Davis, P. (1980) *The Social Context of Dentistry.* Croom Helm, London.

Drury, T.F. and Snowden, C.B. (1995) Community oral health promotion: organizational, methodological, and statistical issues. In: *Oral Health Promotion: Socio-Dental Sciences in Action* (Cohen, L.K. and Gift, H.C., eds), pp. 505–584. Munksgaard International Publishers, Copenhagen.

Dunning, J.M. (1979) *Principles of Dental Public Health.* Harvard University Press, Cambridge, MA.

Elderton, R.J. (1981), Dental ancillaries. In: *Dental Public Health: An Introduction to Community Dental Health*, pp. 201–220. John Wright, Bristol.

Evans, R.G. (1981) Incomplete vertical integration: the distinctive structure of the health care industry. In: *Health Economics, and Health Economies: Proceedings for the World Congress on Health Economics* (van der Gaag, J. and Perlman, M., eds), pp. 329–354. Leiden.

Field, M. (1995) *Dental Education at the Cross Roads: Challenges and Change.* National Academy Press, Washington, DC.

Frazier, P.J. and Horowitz, A.M. (1995) Prevention: a public health perspective. In: *Oral Health Promotion: Socio-Dental Sciences in Action* (Cohen, L.K. and Gift, H.C., eds), pp. 109–143. Munksgaard International Publishers, Copenhagen.

Fredericks, M.A., Lobene, R.R. and Mundy, P. (1980) *Dental Care in Society: The Sociology of Dental Health.* McFarland, Jefferson, NC.

Freidson, E. (1972) *Profession of Medicine.* Dodd, Mead, New York.

Gies, W.J. (1926) *Dental Education in the USA and Canada: A Report to the Carnegie Foundation for the Advancement of Teaching.* The Carnegie Foundation for the Advancement of Teaching, New York.

Gift, H.C. (1984) Utilization of professional dental services. In: *Social Sciences in Dentistry: A Critical Bibliography*, Vol. II (Cohen, L.K. and Bryant, P.S., eds), pp. 202–266. Quintessence Publishing Company for the Fédération Dentaire Internationale, London.

Gift, H.C. (1991) Prevention of oral diseases and oral health promotion. *Current Opininion in Dentistry* **1**:337–347.

Gift, H.C. (1993) Social factors in oral health promotion. In: *Oral Health Promotion* (Schou, L. and Blinkhorn, A.S., eds), pp. 65–102. Oxford University Press, Oxford.

Gift, H.C. and White, B.A. (1996) Health behavior research and oral health. In: *Handbook of Health Behavior Research* (Gochman, D.S., ed.). Plenum, New York.

Gift, H.C., Newman, J.F. and Loewy, S.B. (1981) Attempts to control dental health care costs: the US experience. *Social Science Medicine* **15A**(6):767–780.

Gift, H.C., Gerbert, B., Kress, G.C. and Reisine, S.T. (1990) Social, economic and professional dimensions of the oral health care delivery system. *Annals of Behavioral Medicine* **12**:161–169.

Grembowski, D., Andersen, R.M. and Chen, M. (1989) A public health model of the dental care process. *Medical Care Review* **46**:439–496.

Gunn, S.M., Maxson, B.B. and Woolfolk, M.W. (1992) Mean career satisfaction and optimism scores among women. *Journal of the American College of Dentistry* **59**:35–38.

Hurst, J.W. (1991) Reforming health care in seven European nations. *Health Affairs* **10**(3):7–21.

Ingle, J.I. (1978) Dental care delivery in the People's Republic of China. In: *International Dental Care Delivery Systems* (Ingle, J.I. and Blair, P., eds), pp. 151–159. Ballinger, Cambridge, MA.

Inglehart, J.K. (1988) Japan's medical care system–Part II. *New England Journal of Medicine* **319**:1166–1172.

Inglehart, J.K. (1990) Canada's health care system faces its problems. *New England Journal of Medicine* **322**:562–568.

Inglehart, J.K. (1991) Germany's health care system–Part I. *New England Journal of Medicine* **324**:503–508.

Inglehart, J.K. (1992a) The American health care system: introduction. *New England Journal of Medicine* **326**:926–967.

Inglehart, J.K. (1992b), The American health care system: managed care. *New England Journal of Medicine* **327**:742–747.

Inglehart, J.K. (1993) The American health care system: community hospitals. *New England Journal of Medicine* **329**:372–376.

International Federation of Dental Hygienists (1989) Synopsis of the International Federation of Dental Hygienists board of directors' meeting. In: *Proceedings of the 11th International Symposium on Dental Hygiene*, 11, Canadian Dental Hygienists' Assoc., Ottawa.

Isman, R. (1994) Implications for state and local dental programs and relationships between public and private dental practice. *Journal of Dental Education* **58**:307–312.

Jacob, M.C. and Plamping, D. (1989) *The Practice of Primary Dental Care*. Butterworth, London.

Jeffcoat, M.K. and Clark, W.B. (1995) Research, technology transfer, and dentistry. *Journal of Dental Education* **59**:169–184.

Jerrold, L. (1988) Informed consent and orthodontics. *American Journal of Orthodontics Dentofacial Orthopedics* **93**:251– 258.

Johnson, P.M. and van Lierde, L.L. (1992) *International profile of dental hygiene*. International Dental Hygienists Federation, London.

Kostlan, J. (1978) Dental care delivery in Czechoslovakia. In: *International Dental Care Delivery Systems* (Ingle, J.I. and Blair, P., eds), pp. 114–118. Ballinger, Cambridge, MA.

Kress, G.C. (1995) Dental education in transition. In: *Oral Health Promotion: Socio-Dental Sciences in Action* (Cohen, L.K. and Gift, H.C., eds), pp. 387–425. Munksgaard International, Copenhagen.

Kudrie, R.T. (1981) The implications of foreign dental coverage for US national health insurance. *Journal of Health Politics and Policy Law* **5**:653–689.

Lang, W.P. and Weintraub, J.A. (1986) Comparison of Medicaid and non-Medicaid dental providers. *Journal of Public Health Dentistry* **46**:207–211.

Lennon, M.A. (1981) The organization of dental services in the United Kingdom. In: *Dental Public Health: An Introduction of Community Dental Health*, pp. 119–132. John Wright, Bristol.

Lombardo, G.B.D. (1978) Dental care delivery in the state of Mexico. In: *International Dental Care Delivery Systems* (Ingle, J.I. and Blair, P., eds), pp. 66–67. Ballinger, Cambridge, MA.

McCulloch, C.A.G. (1994) Can evidence-based dental health care assure quality? *Journal of Dental Education* **58**:654–656.

Manning, W.G., Bailit, H.L., Benjamin, B. and Newhouse, J.P. (1985) The demand for dental care: evidence from a randomized trial in health insurance. *Journal of American Dental Association* **110**:895–902.

Neenan, M.E., Paunovich, E., Soloman, E.S. and Watkins, R.T. (1993) The primary dental care workforce. *Journal of Dental Education* **57**:863–875.

Nippert, R.P. (1992) The development and practice of social dentistry in Germany. *Journal of Public Health Dentistry* **52**:312–316.

Office of Technology Assessment (OTA) (1990) *Children's Dental Services under the Medicaid Program-Background Paper*. OTA-BP-H-78, US Government Printing Office, Washington, DC.

Perry, D.A., Freed, J.R. and Kushman, J.E. (1994) The California demonstration project in independent practice. *Journal of Dental Hygiene* **68**:137–142.

Reisine, S.T. and Bailit, H.L. (1980) History and organization of pretreatment review, a dental utilization review system. *Public Health Report* **95**:282–290.

Richards, N.D. and Cohen, L.K. (eds) (1971) *Social Sciences in Dentistry: A Critical Bibliography*. A. Sijthoff, for the Fédération Dentaire Internationale, The Hague.

Romberg, E. and Cohen, L. (1990) Dentists' outlook toward their profession. *Journal of Dental Practice and Administration* **7**:39–43.

Schieber, G.J., Poullier, J-P. and Greenwald, L.M. (1991) Health care systems in twenty-four countries. *Health Affairs* **10**(3):22–38.

Scott, W.R. (1987) *Organizations: Rational, Natural and Open Systems*. Prentice Hall, Englewood Cliffs, NJ.

Slack, G.L. and Burt, B.A. (eds) (1981) *Dental Public Health: An Introduction to Community Dental Health*. John Wright, Bristol.

Tedesco, L.A. (1994) Competencies and access to integration: summary comments to curriculum forum II. *Journal of Dental Education* **58**:359–360.

Tedesco, L.A. (1995) Issues in dental curriculum development and change. *Journal of Dental Education* **59**:97–147.

van Amerongen, B.M. and Kalff, D.J.A. (1984) Dental care expenditures in the Netherlands and the USA: a design for historical and international comparison. *Community Dental and Oral Epidemiology* **12**:237–242.

Verrusio, A.C., Neidle, E.A., Nash, K.D. *et al.* (1989) The dentist and infectious diseases: a national survey of attitudes and behavior. *Journal of the American Dental Association* **118**:553–562.

Walsh, M.M. (1987) The economic contribution of dental hygienists' activities to dental practice: review of literature. *Journal of Public Health Dentistry* **47**:193–197.

Wang, N.J. (1994) *Efficiency in the Public Dental Service for Children in Norway: Change in Use of Dental Hygienists and Recall Intervals*. Thesis. University of Oslo.

White, B.A. (1994) An overview of oral health status, resources, and care delivery. *Journal of Dental Education* **58**:285–290.

Woseth, D. and Chen, M.-s. (1995) Socioenvironmental characteristics and oral health systems. In: *Oral Health Care Systems: Second International Collaborative Study* (Chen, M.-s., Andersen, R.M., Barmes, D.E. *et al.*, eds). World Health Organization (in press).

Young, W.O. and Cohen, L.K. (1979) The nature and organization of dental practice. In: *Handbook of Medical Sociology* (Freeman, H.E., Levine, S. and Reeder, L.G., eds), pp. 193–208. Prentice-Hall, Englewood Cliffs, NJ.

Yule, B. and Parkin, D. (1985) The demand for dental care: an assessment. *Social Science Medicine* **21**:753–760.

Yule, B. and Parkin, D. (1986) *Financing of Dental Care in Europe-Part 1*. World Health Organization Regional Office for Europe, Geneva.

17

Delivery of oral health care and implications for future planning

In the UK

Gillian Bradnock and Cynthia M. Pine

Summary

By the millennium, the UK will have a population of about 57 million, around 30 000 dentists registered to practise, complemented by almost 40 000 dental ancillaries, and standards of oral health which have changed dramatically over the preceding 30 years. The forces that have driven those changes were not predicted and scientific reasoning may well continue to be a very unreliable tool to predict oral health needs for the long-term future. The crystal ball may continue to dominate our planning to a greater degree than we might wish. Delivery of oral health care should be dependent on need, demand and supply underpinned by the principle of equity. However, it is dominated by economic and political forces which tend to view oral health from a distance. It is the role of public health planners to influence those forces to support the development of a health-led rather than disease-based service via the utilization of up-to-date scientific evidence.

Introduction

A thorough exposition of the epidemiological data describing trends in oral health in the UK has been provided in Chapter 8 of this book and for completeness it is advised to read that chapter first. In this section, the delivery of oral health care and some considerations in future planning will be addressed. In the UK, as in many other developed countries, the oral health care system evolved along a somewhat separate route to the rest of health care; this has led to some successes but also to marked limitations. In simplistic terms, National Health Service (NHS) dentistry has produced one of the most cost-efficient treatment delivery systems in the world, but it is also responsible for its greatest limitation, in providing small independent units operating outside the main NHS administration. They are ill-equipped to support the growth of oral health and are oriented to the treatment of disease. The first part of this section will briefly describe the UK NHS and the organization of the oral care system. The second part examines some of the present dilemmas and challenges.

The changing nature of dental services in the UK

The stated aim of the 1946 National Health Service Act was to provide a comprehensive health service for all individuals in the community, free at the point of use. In 1948, compared to other western states 'Britain possessed fewer dentists, a smaller proportion of qualified dentists, a poorer service and lower expectations among the public' (Webster, 1988). Dentists entering the new general dental service scheme had resisted successfully, government attempts to house them in health centres and employ them as salaried staff. The resultant system, whereby general dental practitioners were given independent contracts and remuneration by 'item of service' provided, was accepted by 95% of dentists (Webster, 1988). From then on, these practitioners have provided the vast majority of primary dental care. Data from the time shows that during the first 9 months of the scheme 4.2 million teeth were filled, 4.5 million were extracted and 33.4 million sets of dentures were provided. Once the backlog of oral sepsis was cleared, the provision of dental care moved into one dominated by restorations. This phase moved on in the 1980s to one in which diagnosis and scale and polish became the most common course of treatment in younger adults. Figure 17.1 depicts the full history of extractions of permanent teeth provided in the NHS under fee-for-item since the inception of the service until 1989 (in 1990 a new contract was introduced). This figure depicts the proportion of patients attending for a dental examination and who received extractions in their course of treatment. This has reduced dramatically. In Figure 17.2, the mean number of extractions per course of treatment with extractions has also reduced, such that patients attending in 1949 had

an average of between 5 and 6 teeth extracted and this has fallen away to single extractions being the norm by the end of the 1980s. Figure 17.3 denotes the number of fillings through the 1950s with high figures in the 1960s falling away in the 1970s and 1980s.

Despite the original intention of the Act, dental care for adults has not been totally 'free at the point of use' (Ministry of Health, 1946) since charges for dentures were introduced in 1951. Furthermore, since 1988 charges for treatment levied on adult patients, who are not exempt on social grounds, have been proportionate to the total cost of the treatment. Dental care for children has been and remains free under the NHS, as does the care of other vulnerable groups–expectant and nursing mothers and those with state-supported incomes. The School Dental Service was established under the 1944 Education Act; however it was poorly thought of and understaffed. Under the Act, the service extended its dental inspection role in schools that had been present since 1907,

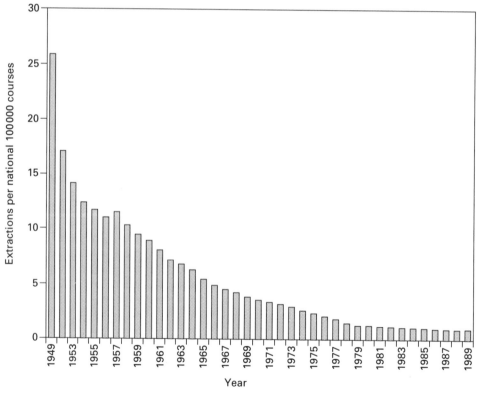

Fig. 17.1 The number of extractions of permanent teeth per notional 100 000 courses of treatment in England and Wales in the National Health Service general dental service annually from 1949 to 1989. A course of treatment is defined as one involving an examination of a child or adult. Data from the Dental Practice Board, Eastbourne.

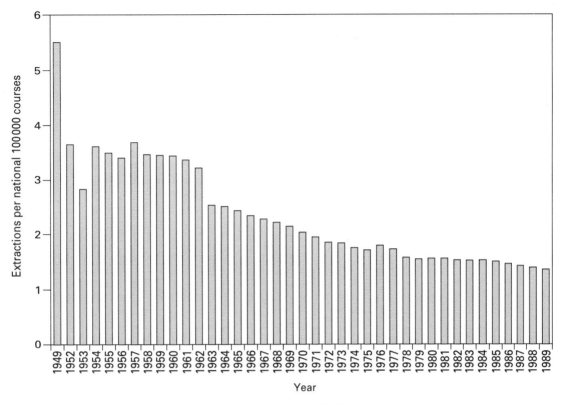

Fig. 17.2 The number of extractions of permanent teeth per notional 100 000 courses of treatment involving extractions in England and Wales in the National Health Service general dental service annually from 1949 to 1989. A course of treatment is defined as one involving an examination and a permanent tooth extraction for a child or adult. Data from the Dental Practice Board, Eastbourne.

to become that of the provision of treatment to all children in state-maintained schools. In the Interim Dental Report of 1944, the Chairman, Lord Teviot, noted that 'the dull, routine work of school clinics would never attract competent dentists' (Ministry of Health, 1944). Webster (1988) reports that between 1948 and 1951 numbers of dental officers had fallen by 25%. In this climate it is unlikely that levels of untreated dental disease would be monitored by the services providing care. There was little local epidemiological evidence available and the first national epidemiological surveys of adult and child dental health were not undertaken until 1968 and 1973, respectively (Gray *et al.*, 1970; Todd, 1975).

The current structure of the oral health care system within the UK NHS is shown schematically in Figure 17.4. There are four Health Departments–the largest is in England and headed by the Secretary of State for

Health. Scotland, Wales and Northern Ireland, sometimes called the territories, have separate administration and these Departments of Health may be part of a joint department with additional home or social services responsibilities. There are eight regional offices in England and each territory has its own central office in its capital. Administration and delivery of health care services is divided into those that purchase health care and those that provide care. Local commissioning authorities are principally Family Health Service Authorities (FHSAs) in England, in some cases coterminous with one or more District Health Authorities which, until recent mergers, were the original smaller, local administrative units. In Scotland, Wales and Northern Ireland, the local commissioning authorities are health boards. Under the general medical services, a small number of large general medical practices hold their own budget and are fundholders, so avoiding local commissioning

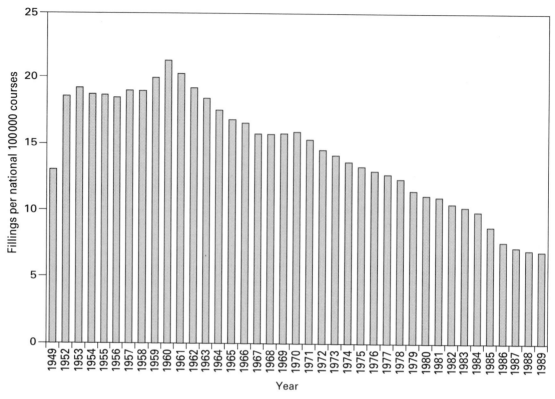

Fig. 17.3 The number of fillings of permanent teeth per notional 100 000 courses of treatment in England and Wales in the National Health Service general dental service annually from 1949 to 1989. A course of treatment is defined as one involving an examination of a child or adult. Data from the Dental Practice Board, Eastbourne.

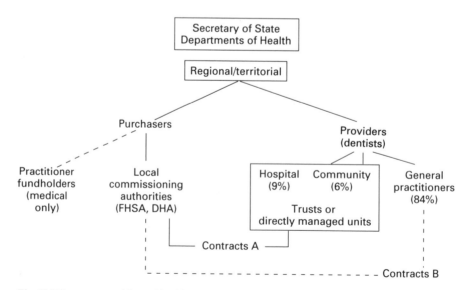

Fig. 17.4 The structure of the oral health care system in the UK 1995/96. Contracts A = for specific structures with strict quality and cost parameters; Contracts B = nationally agreed contracts: principally administrative related to registration, complaints, administering, remuneration. FHSA = Family Health Service Authorities; DHA = District Health Authorities.

control. This facility is not available to general dental practitioners. On the provider side of the figure, only the disposition of dentists is shown for simplicity. Approximately 9% of dentists are working in secondary care in hospital practice. In general hospitals, the dentists are providing specialist oral surgery, orthodontics or restorative care. In dental hospitals, some primary care is provided, within the context of undergraduate training, as well as specialist services. Around 6% of dentists are in the Community Dental Service (CDS). This service was formed from the School Dental Service but now has a different remit in forming a 'safety net' treatment service for those who are unable or unwilling to access care within the general dental service. In addition to this role, the CDS monitors the oral health needs of the population through screening of children in schools and regular epidemiological surveys. This latter function has been described in more detail in Chapter 8. In addition, the CDS has a health promotion role and provides a specialist referral service for general practice, principally for the provision of general anaesthesia and orthodontics.

As can be seen in Figure 17.4, both the hospital dental service and the CDS are administered within trusts or directly managed units of the local commissioning authority. As such, these two services are under strict contractual arrangements with the commissioning authorities for the provision of specific services with preset quality and cost parameters. Consultants in dental public health are employed by the commissioning authorities to advise on the purchase of appropriate oral health care services and the monitoring of oral health. In this respect, this 16% of dental workforce provides services under the same contractual arrangements as that of other parts of the NHS. However, the vast majority of dentists–84%–are outside these contractual arrangements. They operate within the NHS as independent practitioners and the contracts they have with the local commissioning authorities are essentially administrative. They are related to registration with the authority as working within their geographic boundaries, they enter a dental list and need to specify their arrangements for emergency care. Under these arrangements, they are accountable for complaints connected to work conducted under the NHS and the FHSA assists locally in the disbursement of remuneration which is calculated centrally within Dental Practice Boards. However, the local commissioning authority has no power to specify the type, quantity, cost or to whom the general dental practitioners provide dental care. Practitioners registered to work within the NHS are entirely free to undertake private practice. In fact, the number of dentists registered with the FHSA or health board does not directly equate with NHS treatment provision, as many may be selective in the services they will provide under the NHS. This selective approach has grown considerably in some areas, particularly parts of London, such that some adults have encountered difficulties in being able to register for NHS care in their locality. At the same time, there has been a growth in private dental insurance companies.

Although the system of oral health care delivery did not change in real terms between 1948 and the 1990s, the NHS has been subject to constant reorganization since 1974. A more detailed account of these reforms can be found elsewhere (Gelbier, 1994). Subsequent changes in the structure of the NHS during the 1980s focused on improving the efficiency of the service (Department of Health, 1984). These political influences affected the CDS, and to a lesser extent the hospital dental service, but had little impact on the general dental services until 1990. The change in the contracts of dentists working in the general dental services (1990) was part of the government programme for improving primary health care (*Promoting Better Health*; Department of Health, 1987). *Promoting Better Health*, and two other White Papers, *Working for Patients* (Department of Health, 1989a) and *Caring for People* (Department of Health, 1989b) formed the basis of the NHS and Community Care Act 1990. The reforms incorporated in this Act have been called the most fundamental changes experienced by the NHS since its inception in 1948 (Ham, 1991). Ham maintains that the proposals laid out in the White Papers would have a major impact on the delivery of services to patients, although the government had emphasized that the basic principles on which the NHS was founded–'health services, available to all, irrespective of means, on the basis of need'–would not be undermined by the reforms.

Dental services through the NHS have been available to all, although for many, not easily. However the general dental service has always been demand-led. The remuneration of dentists from Treasury funds has been increasingly subsidized by the charges laid on the public for dental services. The system of payment for general dental practitioners had not been addressed for 40 years. It is the very nature of the system that generations of general dental practitioners have known no alternative. Any changes proposed by government which would potentially alter the working practices of around 18 000 professional people was bound to be subject to some disquiet. The present remuneration system and the crisis precipitated by the new dental contract are examined in the next section.

Provision of oral health care through the general dental services

The payment to dentists for each item of treatment provided is essentially a piecework system, which for many years fulfilled the role for which the piecework philosophy is designed– the harder you work, the more you receive. In the early days of the service, there was clearly a backlog of disease and insufficient dentists to meet the need (Gelbier, 1980). This was addressed in two ways, by increasing the number of dentists in training and by encouraging dentists in practice to increase their workload. By the 1980s a number of changes had occurred. Dental caries levels had reduced (Anderson, 1981), dental workforce levels had increased and practitioners were beginning to have space in their waiting rooms. Representations from general dental practitioners that their job security was under threat from the oversupply of dentists, were being made to the Review Body on Doctors' and Dentists' Remuneration (DDRB, 1988) from the early 1980s. There was some questioning that the provision of primary dental services should be reorganized in some way (Dental Strategy Review Group, 1981). Although the basis of the remuneration system was questioned and some modification suggested, no plans were announced to make any fundamental changes.

The *remuneration system* of dentists is designed to establish what an average dentist might earn through item of service after meeting practice expenses, but before income tax has been levied. For each year a target average net income (TANI) is then determined by the review body (which is an independent panel set up by the Health Departments). Most dentists will of course earn something around the average depending on the amount and type of work that they undertake within the NHS. After the review body has established the target net income, the Dental Rates Study Group sets fees per item of service, based on the earnings and output of those general dental services (GDS) dentists who have been in practice throughout the previous financial year. The government can either accept the recommendations of the review body, i.e. the recommended target net income for dentists, or can request modifications. The payment of fees is administered by three Dental Practice Boards.

Currently, patients pay 75% of the actual cost of their course of treatment up to a prescribed maximum charge of £225, with priority groups exempted. In 1991–92 charges to patients thus enabled the recovery of 33.7% of the gross fee costs in England and Wales (Bloomfield, 1992). Although research has shown that dental costs have been and remain a barrier to attendance at the dentist, it is the uncertainty about costs and the complicated manner in which they are presented to potential patients that is of greater concern to the public (Anderson and Morgan, 1992). Prior to establishment of the new dental contract in 1990 the contract between dental practitioner and individual patient lasted for one course of treatment and was completed when the patient was rendered 'dentally fit'. Although in reality most patients returned to their chosen practitioners at regular intervals, there was no mechanism whereby the practitioner could maintain a list of patients, parallel to their colleagues in general medical practice.

The new dental contract

The changes in the dental contract of dentists working in the general dental services did not affect the fundamental basis of the remuneration system of payment for item of service undertaken, reviewed annually. The new contract aimed 'to improve the oral health of the nation by encouraging patients to visit their dentists regularly, and dentists to practise preventive care' (Department of Health, 1994a). The mechanism determined to achieve this aim was the introduction of continuing contracts between dentists and their patients. Adult patients sign on for a 2-year rolling contract and dentists in addition are given a 'continuing care' payment to enable them to undertake basic preventive work with their patients. Dentists are also given a capitation fee for each child registered plus an entry fee to undertake any initial restorative work. It is estimated that capitation fees amount to 20% of the annual income of an average dental practitioner (Bloomfield, 1992). A summary of the financing, reimbursement and fees to the patient is shown in Table 17.1. Where the provider is within the hospital dental service or CDS, the care is financed through the NHS. Specifically, all adults in work have compulsory deductions from their wage to contribute to the health and social services provision. Each employer has to make a contribution for each employee in addition, the employer's amount being the greater. In addition, it is possible that some funding will come from general taxation. Dentists in these services are reimbursed by salaries. In contrast, the general practitioner may be working under any one of three financing arrangements. The vast majority of work is still conducted under the NHS with increasing growth of private third-party funders.

The problem of an oversupply of dentists was addressed by establishing a compulsory retirement age of 70 and the closure and amalgamation of dental schools. Workforce levels are gradually slowing down, three dental schools have been closed in the last decade and the annual addition to the dental register has reduced by a third in that time.

Dental policy in the 1990s

As shown in Chapter 8, dental need has reduced in the young over the past 20 years whilst more middle-aged adults are retaining their teeth. Dental demand has increased slowly over that period of time alongside staffing levels. A policy document issued by the Dental Strategy Review Group, DSRG (an *ad hoc* professional group set up by the Secretary of State in 1981) reviewed the role of primary dental services and questioned the way in which services to children were provided. In particular it recommended that as far as possible children should be treated in the general dental service, as opposed to the CDS. As such it was felt that the system of remuneration in operation whereby dentists were paid by the item of treatment provided may be inappropriate. A system of capitation which would enhance a preventive approach to child dental health was seen to be more appropriate. The DSRG recommended that a pilot study be undertaken to test the effectiveness of the capitation system first suggested in the Court Report, *Fit for the Future* (1976). In the event a capitation system of remuneration was implemented despite the findings of the clinical trial that the dental health of children treated under capitation was not significantly different from those experiencing treatment under the item of service system which had been operating since 1948 (Coventry *et al.*, 1989). The Dental Practice Board bulletins showed that the numbers of patients being signed up to the new system increased steadily. However, a cash shortage in 1992 occurred due to an 'inaccurate forecast' by the review body which resulted in 'dentists grossing an average of some £12 500 each more than intended for that one year alone,

Table 17.1 Financing, Reimbursement and Charges paid by patients

Provider	Financing		Reimbursement	Charges paid by patient at the point of delivery of the service	
Hospital* ——————— Community	General taxation National Insurance (employer employee)	} NHS	Salary	None	
General Practitioner	NHS (most care is provided under the NHS)		Capitation + Fee-for-item	Children	None
				Low income adults, Pregnant, Nursing }	None
				Employed adults	Pay $\frac{4}{5}$ up to set amount (£300)
	Private Third Party Insurance		Capitation/ fee-for item	Monthly amount (dependent on age/disease level)	
	Direct Payment		Fee-for-item	Full costs-no nationally agreed parameters	

*Some services are provided under private contract, often involving insurers.

at a total gross cost of some £200 million' (Department of Health, 1994). Following the 1992–93 review body report, dentists' income was reduced by 7%. The general dental practitioners demanded and got an independent inquiry led by Sir Kenneth Bloomfield.

Bloomfield (1992) was able to show that fees for many items had reduced considerably since 1950, e.g. using present-day figures, the fee paid to the dentist for a one-surface amalgam filling had fallen from £13.38 to £5 in 1992. Furthermore, courses of treatment had increased rapidly (Fig. 17.5). He recommended several options, some building on the existing system with more radical options including a more locally sensitive system of administration. A government consultative document (Department of Health, 1994) responded by suggesting two changes to the system: first to pay dentists on a sessional basis for the patients they treated under the NHS, which would give dentists opportunity to 'place a high premium on preventive work' and eliminate the fear of a treadmill. Second, if the government was to build on the existing fee scale, a move away from TANI and the 'average dentist' was recommended. Following the

consultation period the sessional fees were dropped in the final package of reforms, announced in April 1995 (*Improving NHS Dentistry*, 1995), which included the following:

to improve the capitation system currently in place for the care of children by relating payments to dentists to disease levels; to introduce more rigorous prior approval procedures for monitoring treatment to ensure that the general dental service provides only those treatments which are clinically essential and for which there is no clinically acceptable, less costly, alternative; to develop the Community Dental Services to meet the needs of patients in areas of the country where there is difficulty obtaining NHS treatment under the General Dental Service.

In the short term, dental services for those not wishing or able to avail themselves of private dental care have been supported in some locations by salaried dentists employed by the FHSAs. The intention to strengthen the safety-net role of the CDS underlines the pessimism of the government that many of the disenchanted dentists will not return to the fold.

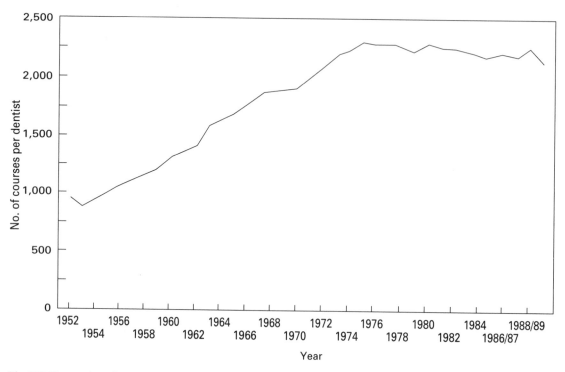

Fig. 17.5 The number of courses of treatment per dentist undertaken between 1952 and 1989–90. From Bloomfield (1992), with permission.

The 1990 NHS and Community Care Act

The health service reforms of the early 1990s had been predicted by policy analysts more than a decade previously. Gradual changes strengthening the role of management and increasing accountability were introduced throughout the 1980s, notably the implementation of the Griffiths Report proposals in 1984 introducing general managers responsible for budgets of defined health units (Department of Health, 1984). Meanwhile, the Secretary of State for Health warned that 'every nation must adjust to the economic realities of the time ... the NHS is not immune from these realities' (Harrison, 1988). In such an environment the dental services were to be made aware of the financial restraints under which they were to operate and the limited power they had to implement their plans. Thus, when the document which heralded the 1990 act was published, *Working for Patients* (Department of Health, 1989a), those involved in health care management were somewhat prepared for the 'market orientation' of the new proposals. Essentially health authorities would decide which services were required to be provided and purchase them from provider units which would be organized into independent trusts. This potentially affected dentistry in two ways: first, purchasers might decide they did not wish to buy certain items of dental care, and the more private dentistry flourished, the more likely they were to consider it inessential. Consequently trusts would not be able to maintain services which would not be used. The essential focus of the purchaser–provider split was to relate need to the provision of service through contracts and hence develop competition. Purchasers could and should buy services from the provider who offered the best programme on cost and quality, not simply the trust that covered the same geographical locality. Health commissions have a larger role than purchasing health services from year to year; they have also taken on the policy-implementing and planning function.

There are substantial groups within the population with high dental need and without adequate access to or uptake of NHS dentistry. The inverse care law (Tudor-Hart, 1971)–those most in need of care are those least likely to receive it–is still active. Oral health care for priority groups is presently purchased from the CDS. These services are managed by dentists with training in public health. The proposed changes in legislation indicate that the CDS should have an expanded role in the provision of health care. Given the vagaries of the NHS policy-making machinery, it could be that the CDS is particularly well-placed to play an important part in the future planning and provision of oral health care.

Policy towards the millennium

In 1994, the Department of Health published an oral health strategy which determines desired levels of health. The Oral Health Strategy, which has set such targets as 'by the year 2003 70 per cent of 5-year-old children should have had no caries experience', is indicative of the approach developed to increase accountability of health care workers in the NHS in the 1990s (Department of Health, 1994b). Oral health targets have particular feasibility problems, however, because general dental practitioners are only able to provide care on the basis of expressed need, i.e. demand, and can have little other impact on normative need. The epidemiological evidence relating to dental need demonstrates that need is lower and dental attendance higher in the south of England than elsewhere in the UK. Staffing ratios have understandably correlated more closely with high levels of demand than high levels of need. This dental scenario is historical but continues to persist following 50 years of a state-organized and dominated system of delivery.

In order to attempt to predict the style of dental provision in the future it is useful to identify any issues of policy and culture which appear to be prevalent at the time of writing. Policy-making in the UK of the 1990s can be seen to be dominated by the desire to curb, or at least control, public spending, complemented by the belief that the market will decide what services it does and does not require. Market approaches have been hampered in the past by the gatekeepers of those services, the health professionals. The 1980s witnessed direct challenges to professional autonomy which in the case of health professionals was determined by the introduction of executive management by Griffiths (1984). Although the professionals responded and are still responding to this attack on their autonomy and in some instances supremacy, a cultural movement to reassess the monopolies enjoyed by certain professions has taken hold. In the western world a salutary example was the deregulation of dentistry in New Zealand. In the last decade of the 20th century alternative practitioners, professions allied to medicine and nurses are challenging the monopoly of orthodox medicine.

In dentistry there has been a rekindling of interest in the role of ancillaries as a possible way of providing services. This has been complemented by general pressure to deregulate the professions. New grades of ancillaries might evolve to challenge the monopoly of the general dental practitioners to provide what is seen to be routine dental care and emergency dental treatment. The Nuffield report into the *Education and Training of Personnel Auxiliary to Dentistry* (1993) outlined a number of areas in which ancillary provision of care might develop. A growth in ancillary care would certainly be supported by the change in oral health care provision. For example, 43% of the courses of dental treatment undertaken in England and Wales in the year ending March 1994 were for non-operative treatment. Many of the procedures could be delegated to ancillary staff but would require legislative amendments to current practice laws which currently require a dentist to see the patient first. However, even with legislative amendments, a change in practice structures would be needed to achieve optimum ancillary use, as few single-handed practitioners would be able to pass this work on to ancillaries.

The purchaser–provider split is an attempt by government to limit both the supply and the demand of health care. In the 1990s, financial incentives were offered to general medical practitioners to enable and encourage them to be more critical in the use of resources in secondary care through becoming fundholders of their own budgets, general dental practitioners, although gatekeepers for orthodontics and oral surgery, do not have major drug-prescribing expenses to the NHS. Neither do they have, on an individual basis at any rate, significant expenditure identified within the secondary care services. It is likely that the further development of purchaser–provider in the general dental services will be limited to a more active role for commissioners of general dental services in attempts to curb unnecessary expenditure within the orthodontic and oral surgery services. It is unlikely that full fundhold-ing is feasible for financial and organizational reasons for dentistry alone. Fundholding general medical practitioners might become gatekeepers for secondary dental services. Such an outcome would be fiercely opposed by the dental profession. Other European countries are observing the UK experience on purchaser–provider closely, as recounted in the section on Nordic countries later in this chapter.

The NHS provided an efficient mechanism for the treatment of dental disease and led to dentists becoming established as small businessmen. General debates within the profession centre on the relative merits of different funding mechanisms for these small businesses to continue producing the same product–treatment of disease. Once this introspective phase has passed, it is hoped the profession will emerge and lead the broader debate of how the needs of those accessing the service has changed and how they can organize their businesses to meet the new challenge of promoting the growth in oral health. It is the responsibility of public health planners to consider mechanisms to support equality in both access and uptake of oral health care in its broadest definition.

References

Anderson, R.J. (1981) *Changes in the Dental Health of School Children after an Interval of 15 years.* DDS thesis, University of Birmingham.

Anderson, R.J. and Morgan, J.D. (1992) Marketing dentistry: a pilot study in Dudley. *Community Dental Health* **9** (suppl.).

The Bloomfield Report (1992) *Fundamental Review of Dental Remuneration.* London.

Coventry, P., Holloway, P.J., Lennon, M.A. *et al.* (1989) A trial of a capitation system of payment for the treatment of children in the general dental service. *Community Dental Health* **6** (suppl.).

Dental Strategy Review Group (1981) *Towards better Dental Health.* DHSS, London.

Department of Health (1984) *Implementation of the NHS Management Inquiry (Griffiths report).* HC(84)13, HMSO, London.

Department of Health (1987) *Promoting Better Health.* CM249. HMSO, London.

Department of Health (1989a) *Working for Patients.* CM555. HMSO, London.

Department of Health (1989b) *Caring for People.* CM849. HMSO, London.

Department of Health (1994a) *Improving NHS Dentistry.* CM2625. HMSO, London.

Department of Health (1994b) *An Oral Health Strategy for England.* HMSO, London.

Education and Training of Personnel Auxiliary to Dentistry (1993) The Nuffield Foundation, London.

Gelbier, S. (1980) *Dentists, Dentistry and the NHS: A Study of their Interaction.* PhD thesis, University of London.

Gelbier, S. (1994) Where have we come from? In: *Introduction to Dental Public Health.* (Downer, M.C., Gelbier, S. and Gibbons, D.E., eds) FDI World Press, London.

Gray, P.G., Todd, J.E., Slack, G.L. *et al.* (1970) *Adult Dental Health in England and Wales in 1968.* HMSO, London.

Ham, C. (1991) *The New NHS Organisation and Management.* Radcliffe Medical Press, Oxford.

Harrison, S. (1988) *Managing the NHS. Shifting the Frontier.* Chapman Hall, London.

Improving NHS Dentistry (1995) Ministerial letter. FHSL(95)22.

Ministry of Health (1944) *Interim Report of the Inter-Departmental Committee on Dentistry (Teviot Report).* Cmd. 6565. HMSO, London.

Ministry of Health (1946) *NHS Bill. Summary of the Proposed New Service.* Cmd, 6761. HMSO, London.

Review Body on Doctors' and Dentists' Remuneration 18th Report (1988) CM358. HMSO, London.

Todd, J.E. (1975) *Children's Dental Health in England and Wales 1973.* HMSO, London.

Tudor-Hart, J. (1971) Inverse care law. *Lancet* **1**:405–412.

Webster, C. (1988) *The Health Services since the War,* vol. 1. HMSO, London.

In the Netherlands

Gert-Jan Truin and Ewald Bronkhorst

A global sketch of oral health and dental attendance

Changes in oral health

The oral health of young people in the Netherlands has improved spectacularly in the past 20 years. Some 65% of children aged 5–6 and 45% of 12-year-olds have sound deciduous teeth and permanent teeth, 1993b). The oral health of 12-year-olds compares favourably with that in most other European Union (EU) countries (Marthaler *et al.*, 1990). There is a tendency towards lower caries prevalence among young people (20–25-year-olds) compared to 10–20 years ago (Truin *et al.*, 1993a). Until 1986, no national data on the prevalence of dental caries or periodontal diseases in adults were available. In 1985, a comprehensive oral survey took place in a single town (van Rossum and Kalsbeek, 1985), followed in 1986 by the first nationwide survey of adults in the Netherlands (Kalsbeek *et al.*, 1991; van't Hof *et al.*, 1991). Unfortunately, this lack of representative studies among adults makes it impossible to be exact about trends in dental caries and periodontal diseases. However, using cross-sectional studies conducted on selected as well as representative adult populations between 1970 and 1989, the data suggest that the average decayed, missing, filled teeth (DMFT) score in

the older age groups has hardly changed (Truin *et al.*, 1993a, 1993b). However, due to improvements in oral hygiene, it is assumed that the prevalence of periodontal disorders will be lower now than it was 20 years ago, as has been found in the USA (Burt, 1988).

In the Netherlands, the percentage of toothless people remained constant during the 70s: about 32% of those aged over 16 were edentulous (Bouma, 1987, 1989). From a 1984 survey in the EU countries, the percentage of edentulous people (people with a set of full dentures) was highest in the Netherlands (Dowell and Scarrot, 1985). Data from CBS, the Dutch Government Statistical Unit, shows a changed pattern after 1980. Between 1981 and 1987, the percentage dropped in the 16–44-year age group from 9.4 to 5.5%, in the 45–64 age group from 54.3 to 44.1% and in the age group over 64 from 77.6 to 74.7%. From recent CBS statistics, 1988–1990, 24.4% of those aged over 16 had full dentures for both upper and lower jaws (CBS, 1992).

Factors relating to changes in oral conditions

Data taken from various sources show that the Dutch population clean their teeth more frequently now than 20 years ago. In 1989, twice as much toothpaste was sold than in 1975 (Westrate, 1991); the frequency with which young people brush their teeth every day seems to be on the increase (Kalsbeek *et al.*, 1992); and the amount of dental plaque is much lower than was found in a survey of young adults at the end of the 1960s (Kalsbeek *et al.*, 1992). Possible reasons include: the higher standard of living and education; the growing awareness of body hygiene in general; and an increased interest in a healthy appearance. Oral health information on caries prevention and commercial advertising for toothpastes and tooth-brushes may have contributed to improved oral hygiene.

The consumption of sugars (mono- and disaccharides) in the Netherlands amounts to more than 50 kg per person each year (König, 1990). Most of this sugar is incorporated in industrially prepared foods and drinks. It is those products which are consumed between meals which are particularly responsible for the occurrence of caries. The extent to which the consumption of snacks has increased or decreased over the years is hard to assess. In spite of the increasing use of sugar substitutes, for instance in chewing gum, the total consumption of sugar has increased over the past decades. In spite of this, the incidence of caries has decreased, attributed to the increased use of fluoride (Marthaler *et al.*, 1990). Over 95% of the toothpaste sold in the Netherlands now contains fluoride (Westrate, 1991). This makes toothpaste the main source of fluoride.

The decision to have full dentures is not only determined by the condition of the remaining teeth but also by sociopsychological factors (Bouma, 1987). Changed public attitudes towards full dentures, in addition to advances in treatment, have probably played an important part in the relative decrease in the number of people with a set of full dentures in the Netherlands.

Changes in dental attendance

In recent decades, considerable attention has been given in the Netherlands to (dental) health education and information, both on a collective and an individual level. In parallel, there was a realignment of the strongly conservative orientation of the dental profession such that applied prevention was integrated into patient treatment. In 1988–1990, 85% of the dentate Dutch visited the dentist each year. The average annual number of dentist contacts per patient amounted to 2.4 (CBS, 1992). Ten years ago, only 77% visited the dentist at least once a year (CBS,

1989). In the Netherlands, the average annual dentist contact figure per person is higher than in countries such as Belgium or France (1.3 and 1.0, respectively; van Amerongen *et al.*, 1993) and is now similar to that in the USA.

Developments in the supply of dentists and dental hygienists

Up to the middle of the 70s, there was a shortage of dentists in the Netherlands. This was one of the reasons why the number of students was increased to a maximum inflow of 465 new first-year students per year in the 60s. This quickly eased the shortage of dentists, but also led to tension in the labour market for dentists at the end of the 70s. In January 1984, the Dutch National Health Insurance (NHI) funds were authorized (on the basis of section 47 para. 3 of the Medical Insurance Decree) to reject contracts for new dentists' practices, if in a certain region, the dentist–inhabitant ratio of 1 to 3250 had been reached. The closure of the Utrecht faculty and the consolidation of the two Amsterdam faculties reduced the number of places for students to 280. According to many people, the new enrolment capacity would still result in a substantial reservoir of unemployed dentists (AOT, 1985). Therefore, the Minister of Education decided to reduce the enrolment capacity for dentists to only 120 students a year. In 1990, 4 years after the decision to reduce the number of first-year dental students to 120, this figure was gradually increased to 210 in 1995.

The policy regarding dental auxiliaries was influenced, among other things, by the developments in the pool of dentists over the past two decades. In 1968 the first training centre for dental hygienists started at the University of Utrecht, followed by training centres at the University of Amsterdam, the Catholic University of Nijmegen and the Free University of Amsterdam in 1971, 1972 and 1974, respectively. In addition, experiments with auxiliaries with restorative duties (for instance, dental auxiliaries for children and dental hygienists with more extended duties) started at the beginning of the 70s. These experimental training courses were closed down a decade later, partly as a result of the increased pool of dentists. In 1980, some 90 new students were admitted to the training courses for dental hygienists each year. In 1988 the annual inflow of first-year dental hygiene students was increased to 120 in

1992, to 144 and 174 per year in 1992 and 1995 respectively. By 1991 the dentist–population ratio in the Netherlands was 1:1900. In that year the total number of registered dentists and dental hygienists amounted to 7900 and 900, respectively. The dentist–population ratios in other European countries generally turn out to be much lower. In 1989, for instance, the dentist–population ratios in Belgium, Germany, France and Sweden were 1:1380, 1:1522, 1:1500 and 1:900, respectively (van Amerongen *et al.*, 1992).

Cost of dental care

In 1989 the cost of medical care in the Netherlands amounted to 8% of the gross national product or GNP (van Amerongen *et al.*, 1991). In the same year the cost of dental care amounted to 0.4% of the GNP, just like in the preceding years (van Amerongen *et al.*, 1992). Table 17.2 provides an international comparison of these percentages for 1987. This table also includes the GNP, the cost of medical care and the cost of dental care per inhabitant in US dollars. In a comparison of nine highly industrialized countries in 1987, the cost of dental care per inhabitant was the lowest in the Netherlands, with the exception of the UK. The total cost of dental care (general dental practitioner plus specialists) in the Netherlands was NLG 2089 million. The cost of care provided by general dental practitioners was 87% of the total cost of dental health care (NLG 1809 million). Medical insurances compensated 57% (NLG 1026 million) of the costs for the general dental practitioners. Of this NLG 1026 million,

the Dutch NHI accounted for NLG 714 million (40% of all treatment costs in general dentists' practices). These statistics relate to 1989 and are based on data from the Federation of NHI funds. This means that 43% of the total costs of the general dental practitioners are not compensated by any form of insurance; in short, the Dutch population paid dentists NLG 783 million directly out of their own pockets.

Until 1994, 62% of the Dutch population was compulsorily insured with NHI. Patients within the system (who visit the dentist twice a year and who also have a dental insurance card) did not need to pay for most of the dental services. Their insurance covered all regular check-ups, preventive and restorative treatments and most prosthetic treatment. In 1995, the government introduced a new system of insurance for dental care. The NHI now includes only preventive treatments (check-ups, oral hygiene instruction and scaling). Young patients up to 19 years of age still have the right to full dental care. Adults have to pay for dental care not covered by the new system themselves or to arrange privately a supplementary insurance. This radical change in the National Health system makes it very difficult to assess implications for future developments in the Dutch dental health care.

Dutch dental health care in the future

In the preceding paragraph information is given on the current state of the Dutch dental health care system. Trying to see where, starting from this state, current developments will lead is

Table 17.2 The cost of medical care and cost of dental care as a percentage of the gross national product (GNP), the GNP, the cost of medical care and the cost of dental care in 1987 in various countries

Country	GNP on medical care (%)	GNP on dental care (%)	GNP per capita (US$)	Cost of medical care per capita (US$)	Cost of dental care per capita (US$)
Netherlands	8.3	0.4	12121	1007	49
FRG	8.7	1.0	13141	1137	127
France	8.5	0.5	12769	1088	69
Finland	7.4	0.4	12703	940	56
UK	5.9	0.2	12502	733	27
USA	11.1	0.6	17670	1961	108
Japan	6.8	0.5	13354	907	71
Australia	7.9	0.4	13401	1054	50
Canada	8.8	0.5	17186	1507	82

From van Amerongen *et al* (1992), with permission.

extremely difficult. For instance, on one hand, it can be expected that the improvement in oral health seen in the younger part of the population will work through as those people age. On the other hand, the general ageing of the Dutch population combined with the fact that more and more people retain their natural teeth far longer than a few decades ago might have serious implications on the demand for dental care. For the Netherlands a simulation model has been developed which enables health politicians to go beyond subjective qualitative reasoning (Bronkhorst *et al.*, 1994; Bronkhorst, 1995). This simulation model comprises the most important causal relations which influence the Dutch dental health care system. In the model, knowledge from scientific disciplines such as demography, psychology, economy and oral pathology is brought together in one framework. The model allows predictions over a 15-year period and the main object is to give health politicians a tool with which they can analyse their policy options. The model can be fed with interventions or scenarios that the health politician is considering and then simulates the consequences from this intervention for the oral health status of the Dutch population; the cost of the dental health care system; the treatment profiles applied; the utilization level of dental practices. Generally, these results are compared with the base run. The base run can be regarded as the neutral policy experiment, that is, a simulation of developments assuming that no changes occur in the factors that influence dental health care in the Netherlands. For instance, the incidence of caries or gingivitis is assumed to be maintained at its current values and the number of students allowed to enter a dental school is fixed at the current enrolment capacity. A comparison of the results of a scenario with the base run facilitates the interpretation of changes that are the result of a certain change in policy. In this section some results from the base run, regarding the oral health status of the Dutch population, the financing of the system and the workload of dentists are presented. For a full overview of the assumptions underlying the base run one is referred to Bronkhorst (1995).

Predicted developments in oral health for the period 1990–2020

Each age group in the Dutch population will show a rapid decline of the prevalence of toothlessness. In the age group 45–64 for instance, in the period 1990–2020 the prevalence will fall from 39% to 9%. The age group 65+ will show a decline from 71% to 37%. For the entire population aged 16 years or older the decline is less pronounced due to the ageing of the population. For this group the prevalence of toothlessness will drop from 25% in 1990 to 12% in 2020. Improvements in the DMFT index will be most visible in the age groups 19–29, 30–44 and, to a lesser extent, 45–64. In the younger age groups, the rather steep decline in caries experience of the past decades has led to a level from which further improvement is difficult. In the oldest age groups, the fact that more people will retain their natural teeth will have a stabilizing effect on oral status of dentate adults. In other words, for these age groups, the improvement in oral health is mainly visible in the decline of toothlessness. In the age group 19–29, the number of sound teeth per person increases from about 16 in 1990 to 20 in 2020. The number of filled teeth decreases from 8 to 4. The number of decayed teeth and the number of missing teeth will be more or less stable at 2–2.5 decayed teeth and about 1.5 missing teeth. (Missing teeth is used here to indicate *all* missing teeth, not only teeth missing due to caries.) In the age group 30–44 the number of sound teeth also increases from 11 in 1990 to 18 in 2020. The number of filled teeth decreases from 10 to 5, and missing teeth from 4 in 1990 to 3 in 2020. The number of decayed teeth is fairly stable at 2–2.5 decayed teeth. In the age group 45–64 the number of sound teeth per person increases from 9 to 14. The number of filled teeth decreases from 9 to 7, but now the number of missing teeth shows a major decrease from 8 in 1990 to 5 in 2020. The number of decayed teeth is stable at 2 teeth during the 1990–2020 period.

Developments in financing the system

Financing of the Dutch dental health care system has been altered drastically, as described. Figure 17.6 shows what changes will occur due to this change in the amounts paid from various sources. The graph clearly shows that, as a consequence of the changes, NHI patients have to pay far larger contributions out of their own pockets: increased from nearly 300 million NLG to about 750 million NLG in the new system. The amount covered by the NHI decreases by 300 million NLG from a little

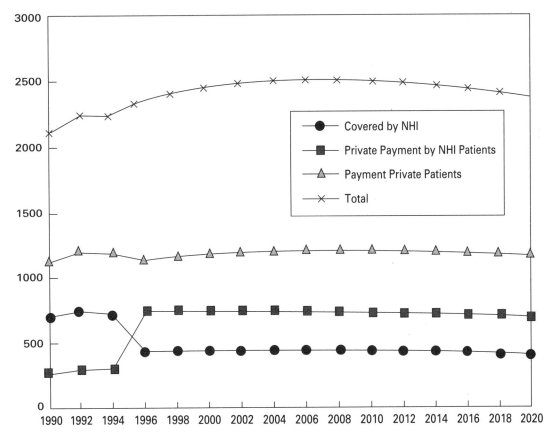

Fig. 17.6 Predictions of the relative contributions of National Health Insurance (NHI) and private payments in financing the Dutch dental health care system, 1990–2020.

over 700 million NLG to 400 million NLG. Privately insured patients benefit, since the fees for dental treatments were more expensive for private patients than for NHI patients and these have been harmonized in the new system. The boundary condition of the change in the financing of the system was the impact on the overall costs of the dental health care system. It can be concluded that the results comply quite well with this condition. The long-term development of the total costs is very moderate, certainly when the increase of the Dutch dentate population in the period 1990–2020 by 24% is taken into account. However, it is questionable whether this fact is due to the financing system.

The simulation model is capable of calculating the workload of dentists. If there is no change in the current policy, dentists will become gradually overloaded. This is a direct consequence of the growth of the dentate population and a more or less stable supply of the working potential of dentists and oral hygienists. To reduce this overload, dentists respond by working more hours, taking less time for treatments and adapting their treatment pattern towards simpler treatments. This explains the reduction of the cost development to be expected when considering the growth of the dentate population. In other words, if no steps are undertaken to increase the working potential of dentists and oral hygienists, it will be impossible to maintain the current level of health care.

The simulation model can be used to analyse which enrolment capacity for dental schools results in an equilibrium between supply and demand for dental care. The resulting enrolment capacity is 300, as compared to a capacity of 210 in 1995. This might seem a large increase, but one has to remember that in the 70s this capacity had been 480. If an enrolment capacity of 300 is realized, this will have its own effect on the dental health care by 270 million NLG (an 11% increase). However, expressed as the average cost per dentate patient, in this scenario the costs will remain more or less stable, whereas this figure would gradually decline in the base run due to the increasing discrepancy between demand and supply. The equilibrium obtained also results in a reduction of the number of people becoming edentulous by up to 2400 per year (a decrease of 8%).

Naturally, increasing the enrolment capacity of dental schools is not the only option to increase the supply of care to reach an equilibrium. A simultaneous increase of both the supply of dentists and dental hygienists is just as viable for this purpose, so the results from the simulation model should not be interpreted as simply a plea for more dentists. What it does demonstrate is that, due to the rapid increase in the dentate population (which, in itself, can be considered a consequence of the progress made in prevention and treatment of dental diseases) the dental care system is becoming overloaded. Whether this overload becomes a major problem in the next decades is still to be seen. But, unless there is a major drop in demand for dental care, for instance, due to a breakthrough in the prevention of periodontal diseases or as a consequence of a deep economic recession, the current level of health care in the Netherlands cannot be maintained without increasing the supply of dental care in the near future.

References

AOT (1985) *Eindrapport Adviescommissie Opleiding Tandarts, Volksgezondheidsreeks VR 85/22*, Den Haag.

Bouma, J. (1987) *On becoming edentulous. An investigation into the dental and behavioral reasons for full mouth extractions*. Academic Dissertation Rijksuniversiteit Groningen.

Bouma, J., Westert, G., Schaub, R.M.H. and Poel, F. van de (1987). Decision process preceding full mouth extractions. *Community Dental and Oral Epidemiology* 15:268–272.

Bouma, J. (1989) De zorg voor de edentate oudere. *Ned Tijdschir Tandheelkd* 96:344–345.

Bronkhurst, E.M. (1995) Modelling the Dutch dental health care system; a comprehensive system dynamic approach. PHD Thesis. University of Nigmegen.

Bronkhurst, E.M., Truin, G.J. and Burgersdijk, R.C.W.

(1994) STG-report. *Future scenarios dental health care; a reconnaissance of the period 1990–2020*. Bohn, Scheltema & Holkema, Rijswijk.

Burt, B.A. (1988) The status of epidemiologic data on periodontal diseases. In: *Periodontology Today*. Guggenheim B. (ed), pp. 68–76. Basel, S Karger AG.

Central Office of Statistics (CBS) (1989) *Maandbericht Gezondhd* 9:15–17.

Central Office of Statistics (CBS) (1989) *Maandbereicht Gezondhd* 17:24–25.

Central Office of Statistics (CBS) (1992) *Statitisch Jaarboek* 1992. 's-Gravenhage; SBU, CBS-publicaties.

Dowell, T.B. and Scarrot, D.M. (1985) *Dental manpower in Member Countries of the European Regional Organisation* (ERO) in the FDI. London, ERO.

Kalsbeek, H., Kwant, G.W., Groeneveld *et al.* (1992) Stopzetting van drinkwaterfluoridering. Resultaten van het cariesonderzoek in Tiel en Culemborg in de periode 1968–1988. *Ned Tijdschr Tandheelkd* 99:4–8.

Kalsbeek, H. and Verrips, G.H.W. (1990) Dental caries prevalence and the use of fluorides in different European countries. *Journal of Dental Research* 69(Spec Iss):728–732.

Kalsbeek, H., Truin, G.J., Burgersdijk, R.C.W. and Hof, M.A. van 't (1991) Dental caries in Dutch adults. *Community Dental and Oral Epidemiology* 19:201–204.

Kalsbeek, H., Truin, G.J. and Verrips, G.H. (1992) Epidemiologie van tandcariës in Nederland. *Ned Tijdschir Tandheelkd* 99:204–208.

König, K.G. (1990) Changes in the prevalence of dental caries: How much can be attributed to changes in diet? *Caries Research* 24(suppl):16–18.

Marthaler, T.M. *et al.* (1990) Caries status in Europe and predictions of future trends. *Caries Research* 24:381–396.

Truin G.J., van't Hof, M.A. Kalsbeek, H. *et al.* (1993a) Meta-analysis of caries surveys amongst 6- and 12-yr-old children in the Netherlands. *Community Dental and Oral Epidemiology* 21:249–252.

Truin, G.J., König, K.G. and Kalsbeek, H. (1993b) Trends in dental caries in the Netherlands. *Advances in Dental Research* 7:15–18.

van Amerongen, B.M., Schutte, G.J.B. and Alpherts W.C.J. (1993) *International Dental Key Figures: A Dynamic and Relational Data Base Analyzing Oral Health Care*. Key Figure, Amsterdam.

van Rossum, G. and Kalsbeek, H. (1985) *Tandartsbezoek en Mondgezondheid. Een Sociaal-wetenschappelijk/tandheelkundig Onderzoek*. Basisrapport. Instituut voor Toegepaste Sociologie, Nijmegen.

van't Hof, M.A. Truin, G.J., Kalsbeek, H. *et al.* (1991) The Dutch national dental survey; the problem of participation. *Community Dental and Oral Epidemiology* 19:57–60.

Westrate, J. (1991) (Kortman Intradal, Amersfoort) Personal communication.

In the Nordic countries

Dorthe Holst

The Nordic countries share a common cultural basis and are often looked upon as one single unity. Traditionally the Nordic countries have had an eye on each other and learned from each other's experience. The countries have used each other to justify references and for the introduction/refusal of new ideas or for the implementation of specific policies. After World War II closer formal cooperation was instituted at the top political and administrative levels. Ties were established which not only furthered the coordination of public policies on a number of topics, but which contributed and still contribute to the development of similar policies within each of the national territories (Kuhnle, 1978). Not since the period 1389–1520 have the Nordic countries made up one political administrative unit. The area is split into five different national units, each of which has had, to a large but varying extent, its own unique history.

Although it is fair to talk about a Nordic welfare state tradition, there are differences between the Nordic countries with regard to when major welfare policies were introduced and chosen tools for implementation (Kuhnle, 1978). These differences can to a certain extent also be identified along the chain of policy decisions related to development of oral health care services throughout the century. The focus of this part of the chapter will nevertheless be on the common features of oral health care, as they appear in the wake of the first steps of welfare policies towards development of the welfare state in Denmark, Norway, Sweden and Finland. The linkage is felt a necessity in order to provide a platform for interpreting why the services developed as they did. From this it can be extrapolated that the authors assume that the future of the organization and financing of oral health services in these countries to a large extent will follow in the footsteps of the changing welfare society (Holst, 1989, 1991).

The development of the welfare state

It is generally accepted that the modern welfare state is a European invention (Flora and Heidenheimer, 1981). The origins of the western European welfare states reach back to the 19th century, some of their present institutional features predating the first World War. Industrialization and urbanization, accompanied by a competitive market economy, were unable to eliminate poverty and extreme differences in resources. Governments were also unable to create social justice and human dignity across groups of citizens. However, the market as an organizational form could be used by governments. It could be planned, regulated or replaced by governments based on an evaluation as to how it contributed to the common good. Fundamentally, welfare rights were seen as functional to economic efficiency (Olsen, 1992).

The boundaries of the welfare state have been questioned. The definition of a welfare state by Wilensky (1975) is compatible with the welfare politics and the common-sense opinion in the Nordic countries: 'The essence of the welfare state is a government-protected minimum standard of income, nutrition, health, housing and education, assured to every citizen as a right, not charity'. However, the definition by Wilensky provides no indication of how far the expected government protection should go in terms of level of protection and in terms of equality.

In short, it is justified to describe four periods in the development of the welfare idea in the Nordic countries (Heclo, 1981; Holst, 1991). This represents a simplification of processes in social security. It should not mislead anyone to believe that the welfare state was planned right from the beginning. In fact, the concept of social welfare was first introduced during the Second World War (Flora and Heidenheimer, 1981). Shortly before the turn of the century the 'poor law legislation' period was replaced by elements of social security legislation. An average of 20% of the employed population was covered by accident insurance and slightly more by sickness insurance in 1910 (Kuhnle, 1978). Gradually initiatives were taken to protect the working classes against the danger of losing their income due to industrial injuries, unemployment, sickness and old age. However, the basic premises of government action were open to a relatively great deal of wide-ranging argument (Heclo, 1981). Questions were asked about legitimacy of government programmes and about the boundaries of a public programme. Benefits and eligibility went up and down.

The first legislative initiatives in the Nordic countries were partly triggered by German legislation during the Bismarck era (Kuhnle, 1978). The first period can best be described as an era of *experimentation* which lasted to the beginning of the 1930s (Heclo, 1981). Through the interwar period, the social forces most relevant to the welfare state development were those of the working class. During the Second World War and immediately after, the social security system was further developed towards the principles of the welfare state characterized by three cornerstones: a broad coordinated system of social security; universal eligibility; and minimum standards of services and contributions. The benefits of both social insurance and social services were extended on a massive scale to increasing proportions of middle classes. The social insurance mechanisms had by the 1950s become institutionalized. While it can be said that the Nordic countries inherited the social state from Germany, the welfare state principles were inspired from the UK. While the security during the experimentation was selective, the principles of welfare were considered a right and were meant to secure everybody against the consequences of accidents and old age, loss of income and job, and to secure necessary treatment during illness. From approximately 1930 to 1955 the welfare principles were *consolidated* (Table 17.3).

During the 1960s and 1970s there was an unprecedented growth in the public sector in many western democracies (Olsen, 1992). Economic growth led to expansion both in kind and in cash. Thus, while the economies from 1950 to 1970 grew by 3–4%, the average growth of social expenditure was about 6.5%. It is therefore appropriate to call this a period of *expansion*. Extensive reforms multiplied as government intervened against the hazards of modern society by creating new individual as well as collective welfare rights and services. The economic crisis in the world economy of the 1970s had two obvious consequences for the welfare states: it reduced revenues and increased expenditures, creating a structural deficit of the

public households (Flora, 1986). The problems were increased by the high birth rates of the 1950s and by high numbers of women entering the labour market. This situation called for a *reorientation* of the welfare state.

Compared to the development of the welfare legislation in other European countries, the following elements can be said to be typical for the Nordic model (Kuhnle, 1978): *a greater government involvement* in both financing and delivery of services; *a high proportion of public employment* in education and in health and social services; policies and services are *universal* and not selective; the eligibility is based on *rights* related to citizenship and is to a small extent earned by employment and other merit; the political aims are to a larger extent a *redistribution* of wealth.

The oral health services and the welfare concept

The public dental service

At the turn of the century epidemiological surveys in all Nordic countries drew professional and political attention to the dental health of schoolchildren (Friis-Hasche, 1994). An alarming number of these children were found to experience dental disease to a degree which affected their school attention and their general well-being. As most welfare services originated at the local level, dental care for children was also first organized out of charity by individual private dentists at the municipal level. However, this was not sufficient either in financial resources or in organizational structures. There was a growing political awareness about the need for *improved accessibility* of dental care for children (Table 17.3). As a consequence the responsibility of dental care for children was moved from the private market to the arena of public politics, i.e. public school dental clinics initiated by urban municipalities. In Norway, this was formalized as part of the School Law in 1917. This law stated that if resources were available the schools should provide dental service for the children and the municipality would be reimbursed by 25% of the costs by the state. Similar initiatives were taken in Sweden and Finland. In Denmark an application was sent to Parliament in 1913 about the need for inspection of schoolchildren's teeth. It was not until 1972 that this principle was integrated in

Table 17.3 Development of the public dental service and the stages of the welfare state

Stages of the welfare state	Dental care	
	Legislation	*Aims*
1900	N(1917): School dental service	Improved access
Experimentation		
1925	S(1938): The public dental service: *Folktandvården*	
Consolidation	N(1949): The public dental service: *Folketannrøkta*	
1955	F(1956): School dental care: *Folkskoletandvården*	
	DK(1972): The children's dental care act: *Børnetandplejen*	Equal access
Expansion	F(1972): Act on Public Health Care: *Folkhälsolagen*	
1980	N(1984): Act on dental care: *Lov om tannhelsetjenesten*	
	S(1986): Act on dental care: *Tandvårsdslagen*	Equality of oral health
Reorientation	DK(1987): Act on dental care: *Tandplejeloven*	
2000		?

N = Norway; S = Sweden; F = Finland; DK = Denmark.

the first act of the school dental service. In 1966, 50% of schoolchildren in Denmark were covered by the public school dental service (Ministry of Internal Affairs, 1966). Some municipalities in Denmark had introduced a free school dental service for schoolchildren while the rest of the children had their dental care expenditure reimbursed by the general sickness scheme. This points to a very important debate from 1910 to 1920 which took place in Norway and in Denmark in the national dental associations. The question was whether children's dental treatment should be reimbursed by some third-party agency, for example, health insurance or whether dental care services should be delivered by public clinics (Erichsen, 1990). The public service model was chosen in Norway while the reimbursement principle lasted until 1972 in Denmark.

During the first third of the century the Nordic municipalities introduced school dental services slowly and primarily in the urban municipalities. There was a constant lack of dentists and the municipalities had no duty to start a school dentist service except in Norway. The inadequacy of the services, the observed inequality between children covered and not

covered by systematic dental care and the dawning understanding of the preventive perspective led to a new wave of professional and political interest into finding better solutions to the dental care of children. In fact, in 1935, the principle of a public dental service for all children and some adults had been proposed by a Swedish departmental committee (Ministry of Social Affairs, 1935). The public service Folktandvården started in 1938. The same political process was found in Norway, leading to a report in 1946 to the government on a public dental service (Ministry of Social Affairs, 1946) which actually started in 1951. In Finland, the municipalities became responsible for providing tax-financed dental services for all primary schoolchildren in 1957 (Sintonen and Sirkkasisko, 1993). In Denmark, a commission for children's dental care was appointed by the government in 1959. The commission's report came out in 1966 (Ministry of Internal Affairs, 1966) and the Act of Child Oral Health Care *Børnetandplejen* came into force in 1972 (Table 17.3).

The fundamental principles laid down in these acts were *universalism, national responsibility, free care* and *total coverage* with regard to the age groups specified in the acts. These were schoolchildren (6–7 to 16–18 years old). In Norway and Sweden the public dental service was also supposed to render services to adults primarily in remote areas if resources were sufficient. Adults were otherwise supposed to demand services from private practitioners. It is easy to see that the fundamental principles of the welfare ideology had broken through in oral health care for children. The nature of the oral diseases at the time was interpreted in terms of lifelong incidence of irreversible lesions. This interpretation formed the basis for an outreach delivery system with emphasis on short intervals between examinations in order to prevent further development of cavities combined with some prevention and health education.

In all the Nordic countries the undersupply of dentists postponed the fulfilment of the intentions of the dental care acts belonging to the consolidation period. Increased numbers of graduates from the dental schools in the 1970s, however, improved the situation, though the geographical distribution was still unsatisfactory. The increased availability of dentistry made it possible for some municipalities to include preschoolchildren in their programmes. As a consequence of the expanding social and health care services to new groups, budgets grew. Political desires to control budgets and to use resources efficiently led to the appointment of new committees, some of which looked into the total use of oral health care resources. The rather sharp division of tasks between the public and the private services created inflexibility in both rural and urban districts. The dental services had developed into a fragmented, patchwork population carpet. Though late in the expansion period of the welfare state, the governmental committees could combine the still prevailing expansion ideology with early signs of what soon became the fourth step of the welfare state development: the *reorientation* or *revision period*.

The expansion of the public dental services culminated with the new Oral Health Acts in Norway in 1984, in Sweden in 1986 and in Denmark in 1987 (Table 17.3). Common to the three acts was: expansion to include *all children* aged 0–18 (Denmark), 0–18 (Norway) and 0–19 (Sweden), and to provide free systematic preventive services and comprehensive treatment; a *total population perspective* and responsibility; and *flexibility* with regard to a *coordinated and*

efficient use of public and private resources. In Norway and Sweden new groups of priority, i.e. disadvantaged, handicapped and institutionalized old-age people were included as target groups of the public dental service. As a crown of achievement of the public dental services, the prime intentions and objectives of the public services were stated in terms of *equity of results*, i.e. equal lifelong oral health potential. Within health care, oral health care seemed to have adopted the most radical interpretation of equality. In the welfare literature the concept of equality of opportunity is juxtaposed with equality of results (Wagstaff *et al.*, 1991; Williams, 1993). The interpretation differs between countries, political parties, and between health care, education and other social security systems. The success of prevention in oral health care and the professional recognition of the full potential of fluorides and health promotion provided the public dental service with a legitimate role to work towards equal oral health results.

The milestone in Finland was partly the enacting of the Primary Health Care (PHC) Act already in 1972 and the proposal for oral health services for adults to be reimbursed by the National Health Insurance in 1992. The structural principles of the PHC Act 1972 were to integrate public services that were run separately (dental care, school health care, local hospitals) under locally integrated management and planning through a network of health centres. In addition, a uniform government subsidy system was created in order to increase resources in primary care (Sintonen and Sirkkasisko, 1993). Though reimbursement of dental treatment for the adult population by the National Health Insurance had been decided by the government, the reform came too late. The economic crisis in Finland in the beginning of the 1990s stopped all proposals resulting in increased public spending.

By 1990 the public dental services for some time had offered full coverage for all children and adolescents in all the Nordic countries. Annual and biannual examinations had been the rule. The recall intervals are in many places extended to more than 12 months. This creates some difficulties as to interpretation of services statistics, since long intervals reduce the percentage treated yearly. It has therefore been necessary to draw a distinction between percentage being *monitored* and *treated* in the public service (Table 17.4). Moreover, the focus was directed towards prevention and health promotion and the oral health results were very promising (Table 17.3). Service statistics showed that the percentage of children free of caries had increased and the mean number of DMFT was low. The statistics could also demonstrate improved efficiency of the services. A study making use of national survey data in Norway showed that equity of treatment access was reached (Rossow and Holst, 1991). However, the public dental health service cannot rest on its laurels long. Despite and because of the promising results, the public dental services were faced with budget cuts and demands for further improvements in efficiency. A study showed that two-thirds of the DMF reduction among 15-year-olds could be explained as an effect of change in treatment criteria (Gimmestad and Fylkesnes, 1994). The incidence of oral diseases had changed from epidemic to episodic (Holst, 1989), which raised the question whether the prevailing preventive population-based strategies should be changed to risk strategies.

The private sector

The adult populations of the Nordic countries demand oral health care primarily from private practitioners. In Sweden, Finland and Norway (not in Denmark), the public service is dimensioned to provide services to the adult population on demand, particularly in districts where there is no or low availability of private practitioners. In Sweden, Finland and Norway, 21% (Sundberg, 1995), 30% (Utriaininen and Widstrom, 1990) and 9% (Ellingsaeter, 1992) of the adult population demand their service from the public dental services (Table 17.4). The private and the public sector were not meant to compete but to complement each other. Yet, as a consequence of the high dentist–population ratio, some competition has developed, mostly in the big cities. In order to increase accessibility of the services the National Health Insurances (in Sweden since 1974 and in Denmark since 1959) have reimbursed part of the expenditure for dental care. In Norway, only emergency care and some surgical care has been reimbursed, and in Finland expenditure for health care including oral health was tax-deductible up to 1992. During the 1980s the patient charges in Sweden and Denmark increased from 30-40% to 60-70% of the cost (Holst, 1989). Despite the variations in reimbursement from the National Health Insurances, the demand for services is high by the adult non-institutionalized population (Table 17.4). In Denmark, Sweden and Norway, the percentage of the adult population who visited the dentist within the last year is 70–75%, while it is somewhat lower in Finland.

At present, the role of the health insurance in oral health care is being reconsidered. The function seems to be more budgeting than insurance with a limited potential of oral health gain (Holst, 1982). The empirical evidence of

Table 17.4 Workforce, annual visits and oral health indicators

	Denmark (1993)	Finland (1993)	Norway (1993)	Sweden (1994)
Number of dentists	5100	5566	3480	9900
Number of dental hygienists	360	1003	381	1800
Number of dental assistants	6700	6501	3600	14 000
Number of dental technicians	800	469	700	2000
Number of denturists	550	338		
Dentist:population ratio	1:1050	1:1098	1:1250	1:900
Dental care during last 12 months 0–18/19 years	All are entitled to systematic care: 80–100% are seen annually			
>20 years	70	52	77	79
Per cent caries-free (12 years)	50	30	36	48
DMFT (12 years)	1.1	1.2	2.1	1.4
Per cent caries-free (18–19 years)	17	13	10	13
DMFT (18–19 years)	4.8	4.5	6.8	5.2
Per cent edentulous	13	15	8	

DMFT = Decayed, missing, filled teeth.

supplier inducement in the delivery of services in the dental care market (Grytten, 1991), which hampers a geographical distribution of dentists and an efficient use of resources combined with strict budget control, may lead to a changed position of the National Health Insurances. Homebound, elderly, institutionalized and handicapped persons are offered a mix of institutional, outreach and private arrangements for their oral health care. In Finland and Norway the Public Dental Services are supposed to provide the necessary services. In 1994, it became mandatory for the Public Oral Health Service in Denmark to do the same. From an oral health perspective, the situation is judged to be unsatisfactory by the professions (Vigild, 1992). However, a large part of this population group lost their natural teeth early in life. The expectations of oral health are considerably lower in this age cohort than in the cohorts to come (Ettinger, 1992). The senior citizens to come will to a large extent keep their natural teeth and the need and demand for prevention, functional and aesthetic dentistry will be obvious. This will also affect the expectations of oral health care for other dependent groups.

The oral health service faces the reorientation of the welfare state

When the acts of oral health care came into force the reorientation of the welfare state was already apparent. Table 17.5 provides an overview of health care resources by 1992. At present the political goals are still the same, but the instruments are changing. The state is becoming a little less involved, the individual responsibility

is more clearly expressed. Elected leaders have argued that government cannot solve social and economic problems and that politics should have a more modest role in society (Olsen, 1992). The predominant agenda has for some time been flavoured by a renewed faith in the vision of a society built on decentralized decision-making, a society with a privileged status to private property rights, free enterprise, consumer sovereignty, markets, prices, private incentives and competition. The state should be less active, the public sector smaller, and there should be less redistribution across social groups. The business firm appears as a model for the state, the markets the arena for politics and businessmen models for politicians and public servants. Two interpretations of the changes and reform efforts of the 1980s have been of special importance. One describes the reorientation as an economic necessity and the other focuses on the political mandate, according to which the welfare state is discredited by experimental learning and the changes based on rational adaptation (Olsen, 1992). Some tentative observations seem to show that the new political rhetoric is far in advance of both public opinion and political institutions. People resist cuts in services and examples of privatization, yet also express wishes for lower taxes and improved control of abuse of the system. The actual pattern of policy change is a mixed one. During the 1980s the welfare state reforms came to a halt (Flora, 1986). However, aggregate public spending did not change much, though some cuts were made.

In the 1990s the social democratic parties are back in power in the Nordic countries. The first wave of dismantling of the welfare state has cooled. Yet, health services have not been

Table 17.5 Social security expenditures in the Nordic countries (millions of national currency units)

	Denmark	Finland	Norway	Sweden
Population	5 189 378	5 066 447	4 311 991	8 718 561
Total health care	51 555	38 612	56 650	131 123
Dental care	2104	1093	1154	7214
Social security	212 862	109 343	146 862	399 553
GNP	873 237	480 470	733 664	1 442 181
Total health care as a percentage of GNP	5.9	8.0	7.7	9.1
Dental care as a percentage of total health care	4.1	2.8	2.0	5.5

GNP = Gross national product.
From Yearbook of Nordic Statistics (1995), with permission.

exempted from the *reorientation* of the welfare state. New structures are being built into the delivery systems of oral health care, though the goals are the same. Adolescents (16–17 years) in Denmark and children (0–19 years) in some counties in Sweden are offered a free choice between oral health care in private practice or the public service. The principle of creating internal markets within the public provision, i.e. the split of the purchaser and the provider role in the public service, has been introduced in at least three counties in Sweden. A prerequisite for this arrangement is a capitation payment known as 'the payment follows the patient'. From this follows that a public service cannot be financed through budgets. Instead, the income must come from the consumers who choose to demand its services. In order to increase efficiency of the services, the intervals between children's regular examinations are extended and individualized. Dental hygienists are to a greater extent given a first-line role comprising practical responsibility for the oral health examinations and appropriate prevention (Petersen, 1993; Wang, 1994).

At the political level the welfare *state* expression is being exchanged by the welfare *society concept*. This indicates a reorganization and a redefinition of the appropriateness of different institutions. Flora (1986) states that the reorientation turbulence has brought to the surface basic challenges which will require long and complex processes of institutional adaptation. Three such challenges are the ageing of the population and the necessity of a new contract between generations; the changing sexual division of labour and the necessity of a new contract between the sexes; and the change of values and the necessity of a new contract between the state and the citizens. The organization of the health services and the oral health services will find its place within the new contracts. The welfare state was a response to history-specific problems of harmonizing production of wealth with its production. It was a compromise, not to remove the market, but to modify some of its effects. Western democracies may be ready for a new round of social, economic and political experiments (Myles, 1988).

The reorientation of the institutional welfare has not resulted in clear political signals yet. Two observations believed to be important for the future structure of oral health care services can be offered:

1 A strong belief in *competition* and *incentives*, both of which to a large extent have been absent in the public health care system. As a consequence and very much inspired by the Enthovian thinking (Enthoven, 1986) and the reforms in the UK and the Netherlands, a possible organizational model for the public dental services may appear, as shown in Figure 17.7). The responsibility for the oral health services will still rest with the political institutions which will decide on objectives, eligibility and budgets. Health care will be a public responsibility. Within these frames, purchasing bodies will be established. The purchaser role will be to negotiate with providers (both public and private) on type, amount, price and quality of services. The consumers will to a large extent be given freedom of choice (where a real choice exists). In order to perform adequately, the purchasing body will need and therefore demand data on oral health needs, preferences and outcome. An independent information system will provide the purchasing bodies and the political institutions with necessary data for monitoring resources and outcome, and also provide the purchasers with information on production, costs and quality. Adequate incentives can be integrated at consumer, purchaser and provider levels. The purchasing body may well operate at the local level, and will by doing so also reinforce another contemporary tendency to move from *macro-* to *micromanagement*.

2 The second observation relates to *method of payment*. The principle of a fee-for-service payment system has been the dominating

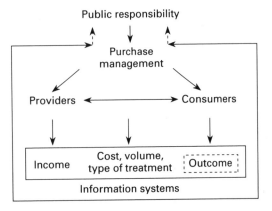

Fig. 17.7 Structure of oral health care.

system in private practice in the Nordic countries. A fee-for-service payment system is expected to create adequate incentives in times with an undersupply of dentists and a backlog of unmet treatment need. The situation is different in the Nordic countries today. There is little backlog of unmet treatment need and there is a sufficient number of dentists. Therefore, an adequate incentive structure would focus on the maintenance of oral health, prevention and health promotion. A recent Swedish committee (Socialdepartementet, 1993) had proposed a change from fee-for-service to a three-level capitation system, according to which the dentist and the adult patient together decide within which of the three premium levels all necessary treatment 1 year ahead should be given.

Though each of the Nordic countries seems to be too small to take advantage of the models of managed markets and internal markets, it is expected that elements of these principles will be included in the delivery system. As for the Organization for Economic Cooperation and Development (OECD) countries (*The Reform of Health Care*, 1992), the Nordic health care is searching for a system with some of the competitive advantages of the market combined with a public governance of resources and a targeted distributive regulation of personnel and resources.

Concluding remarks

In the Nordic countries, considerable political attention has been given to oral health care during the 20th century. Attention moved from an altruistic feeling of charity for children with bad teeth, through improved access, to total solidarity and the principle of universal access to a free public dental service. In the adult population, better access was secured by increasing the number of dental personnel, reducing economic barriers and some regulation of the geographical availability. If the success continues, less political attention may be expected after the turn of the century. It could therefore be important for the dental professions to secure alliances with the populations in order to maintain well-informed consumer groups.

References

Ellingsaeter, B.E. (1992) *Oral Health Services in Norway.* Report no. 7. Directorate of Health, Oslo.

Enthoven, A. (1986) Managed competition in health care and the unfinished agenda. *Health Care Financing Review* (suppl.):105–119.

Erichsen, V. (1990) *Professionalisation and Public Variations. The Case of Dental Care in Britain and Norway.* Thesis. University of Bergen, Norway.

Ettinger, R.L. (1992) Attitudes and values concerning oral health and utilization of services among the elderly. *International Dental Journal* 42:373–384.

Flora, P. (ed.) (1986) *Growth to Limits. The Western European Welfare States since World War II*, vol. 1. Walter de Gruyter, Berlin.

Flora, P. and Heidenheimer, A.H. (1981) The historical core and changing boundaries of the welfare state. In: *The Development of Welfare States in Europe and America.* (Flora, P. and Heidenheimer, A.H., eds), pp. 17–34. Transaction Books, New Brunswick, NJ.

Friis-Hasche, E. (ed) (1994) *Child Oral Health Care in Denmark.* Copenhagen University Press, Copenhagen.

Gimmestad, A.L. and Fylkesnes, K. (1994) Endringer i sykdomsprogresjon og kreterier for behandling av primaer karies. *Den Norske Tannlegeforenings Tidende* 104:360–364.

Grytten, J. (1991) The effect of supplier inducement on Norwegian dental services, some empirical findings based on a theoretical model. *Community Dental Health* 8:221–231.

Heclo, H. (1981) Towards a new welfare state. In: *The Development of Welfare States in Europe and America* (Flora, P. and Heidenheimer, A.H., eds), pp. 17–34. Transaction Books, New Brunswick, NJ.

Holst, D. (1982) *Third Party Payment in Dentistry.* Thesis. University of Oslo, Oslo, Norway.

Holst, D. (1989) Tandplejen i Norden. *Tandlaegebladet* 93:112–118.

Holst, D. (1991) Health care–plan or market? Markedsbaserte tannhelsetjenester-Studier av fordelingsvirkninger og kostnader. In: *Helsevesenet i Knipe* (Piene, H., ed.), pp. 135–148. Ad Notam, Oslo.

Kuhnle, S. (1978) The beginnings of the Nordic welfare states: similarities and differences. *Acta Sociologica* 21 (suppl.):9–32.

Ministry of Internal Affairs (1966) *Betaenkning om Offentlig Bornetandpleje*, no. 427, Statens tryksakskontor, Copenhagen.

Ministry of Social Affairs (1935) *Betankande Angående Folktandvarden.* Statens Sjükvärdskommitté, Stockholm.

Ministry of Social Affairs (1946) *Instilling fra Komite til a Utrede Sporsmalet om en Landsplan for Offentlig Tannrokt.* Ministry of Social Affairs, Oslo.

Myles, J. (1988) Decline of impasse? The current state of the welfare state. *Studies in Political Economy* 26:73–107.

Olsen, J.P. (1992) Rethinking and reforming the public sector. In: *Staat und Demokratie in Europe* (Kohler-Koch, B., ed.), pp. 175–278. Leske and Budrich, Opladen.

Petersen, P.E. (ed.) (1993) *En Beskrivelse af Tandplejens Opgaver i de Kommende 10-20 ar.* The National Board of Health, Copenhagen.

Rossow, I. and Holst, D. (1991) Legislation and reality in public dental services in Norway: dental health services for children and adolescents in 1975 and 1985. *Journal of Public Health Dentistry* **51**:152–157.

Sintonen, H. and Sirkkasisko, A. (1993) The dental care system in Finland. In: *Dental Care Systems in Europe* (Arvidsson G. and Jonsson, B., eds), pp. 5–22. SNS, Stockholm.

Socialdepartementet (1993) *Premietandvärd–En Effektivere Tandvärdsförsäkring.* Stockholm.

Sundberg, H. (1995) Folktandvarden 1993–verksamhetsstatistik for distriktstandvard og specialisttandvard. Socialstyrelsen, Meddelandeblad, no. 11.

The Reform of Health Care (1992) A comparative analysis of seven OECD countries. Series OECD Policy Studies, Paris.

Utriaininen, P. and Widstrom, E. (1990) Economic aspects of dental care in Finnish health centres. *Community Dental and Oral Epidemiology* **18**:235–238.

Vigild, M. (1992) Oral health programmes for the elderly in Scandinavia. *International Dental Journal* **42**:323–329.

Wagstaff, A., van Doorslaer, E. and Pac, P. (1991) Equity in the financing and the delivery of health care: some tentative cross-country comparisons. In: *Providing Health Care. The Economics of Alternative Systems of Finance and Delivery.* (McGuire, A., Fenn, P. and Maghen, K., eds), Oxford University Press, Oxford.

Wang, N. (1994) *Efficiency in the Public Dental Service for Children in Norway. Change in Use of Dental Hygienists and Recall Intervals.* Thesis, Oslo.

Wilensky, H. (1975) *The Welfare State and Equality.* University of California Press, Los Angeles, CA.

Williams, A. (1993) Equity in health care. In: *Equity in the Finance and Delivery of Health Care. An International Perspective.* (Doorslaer, E.v., Wagstaff, A. and Rutten, F., eds), pp. 287–319. Oxford Medical Publications,

Yearbook of Nordic Statistics (1995) Nordic Statistical Secretariat, Nord. Vol. 33.

In Latin America

Hamilton Bellini and Victor Gomes Pinto

The region

Health care, including oral health, is closely related to the social and economic situation of each country or region, particularly in Latin America. Although Spanish is a common language to all countries but Brazil, a few Caribbean islands and the Guyanas, homogeneity is not a characteristic of the region. Actually, enormous differences between countries are common and huge contrasts are also found within each country, both regionally and socioeconomically (Table 17.6). The region is strongly sensitive to the recessive impact of the economic macro policies carried out in the last decades. Lack of statistical data is a common feature for the region. Thus, even when mentioning existing data, one should be aware of the limitations of averages and of the data *per se*.

The estimated population is 460 million people–a little over 8% of the world's population–in an area of 2 million km². Its GNP per capita is around US$2650, a sixth of that in developed countries (comparative figures are given in the section on the Netherlands in this chapter). The real average buying power is approximately US$4490 (real per capita GNP). However, the region consumes only 6% of the world's products. Latin America is in an intermediate position, between the high standards of the industrialized nations, and the crude reality of some economically critical areas in Asia and in Africa (Table 17.6; Comisión Económica para América Latina, 1993; United Nations Organization, 1993; World Bank, 1994; Fédération Dentaire Internationale, 1993).

The pattern of economic development that has ruled the region since the last World War gave clear signs of deterioration by the late 1970s and early 1980s. The 1980s were characterized by the aggravation of poverty rates, as well as by a rise in the number of poor and indigent people, a phenomenon witnessed, above all, in the most populous countries. Nowadays, 2 out of 5 urban inhabitants are poor, whereas in the rural areas the ratio is 3 to 5 (Fédération Dentaire Internationale, 1993; Pinto, 1994). The intense urbanization undergone by the region in the last three decades has imposed severe penalties on those who have remained in the countryside, making them even poorer. On the other hand, a set of unquestionable and fast-paced changes also characterized Latin America in this period. A fast-growing industrialization process led to clear improvements in productivity and modernization in several regions. In politics, there were improvements in democratic rules in some countries, as well as more consolidated democracy in others. Governments based on armed power are now an exception. The massive development in means of communication, the general increase in the percentage of children at school and the decrease in infant mortality represent, also, positive points which cannot be overlooked.

Oral health epidemiology and related conditions

World Health Organization epidemiological data, as well as local data in several countries, indicate that both in children and adolescents the most critical conditions for caries can be found in Latin America. In fact, only Latin America presents high scores for DMFT up to the age of 19. In contrast, in Asia and Africa the DMFT at the age of 12 has kept to their traditional low levels, and the industrialized nations are proud of their data showing decreases in the caries index. However, in Latin America, epidemiological data have not shown any such impressive changes.

Table 17.6 shows DMFT data at the age of 12 for 32 Latin American countries, together with some global data from other large regions, for comparison. These data are also related to GNP per capita and average daily sugar consumption. Besides these figures, the population for each country is presented for a better evaluation of the size of the challenge. The average DMFT of 4.7 at the age of 12 is 260% higher than in Africa, 163% higher than in Asia, 79% higher than in the industrialized countries and 28% higher than in Eastern Europe. Fourteen out of the 19 countries where the DMFT at 12 is considered high (5.0 or above) are situated in Latin America. In spite of that, it seems that some countries have managed to have some reductions, with Cuba probably achieving the highest reduction. In Brazil, the DMFT at the age of 12 was reduced from 6.7 in 1986 to 4.9 in 1993 (Pinto and Lima, 1995). In Colombia, the reduction was around 43% in the 5–14-year-old children and 25% in the 15–19-year-olds, after 15 years (Bojanini, 1995). Some countries like Mexico and Argentina report acceptable levels for the region, with DMFT of 3.9 and 3.4 respectively, at the age of 12 (World Health Organization, 1994a).

When looking at the caries situation in Latin America, its leading position may be attributed to the high level of sugar consumption. Brazil, Cuba and Mexico together produce annually about 19 million tons of sugar, which represents around 17% of the global production and 26% of the total sugar from sugar cane. While qualitative changes in habits of sugar intake may be observed in industrialized countries, in Latin America sugar is consumed in the refined form, as a cultural value and a must, both in social events and after meals (Pinto, 1990; International Sugar Organization, 1993, 1994). As a result, many of the adult population in Latin America are edentulous following treatment for caries and periodontal disease (Pinto, 1990; World Health Organization, 1994a, 1994b), with high prevalences of full and partial denture wearers (Ferraz and Bellini, 1983). In Brazil, for instance, in the 35–44-year-old group, the mean DMFT is 22.5 with 67% of the teeth comprising the M component. In Colombia, the same analysis shows DMFT of 20.2 with 74% in the M component. Comparable data for periodontal diseases are lacking. One of the scattered surveys on a national basis was performed in Brazil in 1986 using the Community Periodontal Index of Treatment Needs (CPITN): health sextants were recorded in only 30% of the 15–19-year-old group and 12% for the 35–44-year-old group (Pinto, 1990).

The proportion of the indigenous Indian population relative to the total population varies enormously from country to country. In the South Cone countries, those groups represent quite a small percentage of the population, whereas for Andean countries they may represent a significant part of the total population. Data on their oral health are lacking, but it seems that the Indians living isolated from the dominant culture (which is mainly Caucasian) experience a lower DMFT than the average for the countries. However, caries are often diagnosed, mainly in the Amazonian Indians (Neumann and DiSalvo, 1958; De Smet, 1966).

Table 17.6 Population, decayed, missing, filled teeth (DMFT) at 12 years, per capita gross national product (GNP) and sugar consumption in Latin America and other world regions in 1993

Country	Population 1993 (million)	DMFT 12 years	GNP per capita in US$	Sugar consumption (g/per capita per day)
Argentina	33.50	3.40	6050	98
Bahamas	0.30	1.60	12070	97
Barbados	0.30	4.40	6540	116
Belize	0.20	4.00	2220	155
Bolivia	7.70	7.60	680	71
Brazil	156.60	4.90	2770	132
Chile	13.80	5.30	2730	119
Colombia	34.00	4.80	1330	93
Costa Rica	3.30	5.50	1960	158
Cuba	10.90	2.90	1170	200
Dominica	0.10	2.50	2520	
Ecuador	11.30	4.90	1070	88
El Salvador	5.50	5.10	1170	82
Granada	0.10	5.50	2310	
Guatemala	10.00	8.10	980	107
Guyana	0.80	2.70	330	75
Haiti	6.90	3.20	370	34
Honduras	5.60	6.40	580	86
Jamaica	2.50	6.70	1340	50
Martinique	0.30	6.30	5525	134
Mexico	90.00	3.90	3470	137
Nicaragua	4.10	5.90	340	100
Panama	2.60	4.20	2420	100
Paraguay	4.60	5.90	1380	60
Peru	22.90	7.00	950	81
Dominican Republic	7.60	6.00	1050	104
S. Kitts and Nevis	0.04	5.50	3990	108
S. Vincent and Granada	0.10	3.20	1990	
Surinam	0.40	4.90	4280	92
Trinidad and Tobago	1.30	3.90	3940	123
Uruguay	3.20	4.10	3340	81
Venezuela	20.60	3.60	2910	96
Latin America	461.14	4.74	2653	117
Africa	673.10	1.31	639	37
Asia	3147.73	1.80	751	32
Industrialized countries	812.63	2.65	22251	94
East Europe	358.20	3.71	2057	97

Oral cancer seems to be a rare condition, but it represents about 4% of the total of cancer cases, resulting in a mortality rate of approximately 3%, according to recent information about regional conditions of oral health (Pan American Health Organization, 1994). However, it is estimated that $1\frac{1}{2}$ million adults in Latin America were human immunodeficiency virus (HIV)-positive in 1993, constituting a total of 250 000 cases of acquired immune deficiency syndrome (AIDS). In many instances, oral manifestations associated with HIV infection have been reported: oral mycosis, leukoplasia, acute necrotizing gingivitis and periodontitis and, particularly, Kaposis' sarcoma. These oral manifestations may be one of the first signs of the disease (Pan American Health Organization, 1994).

Oral health care systems

All Latin countries have some sort of organized oral health care system. Its offer and delivery can be grouped into public and private sectors and their degree of planning and organization considered. For these purposes, the sum of all oral health services (private and/or public), plus all the measures implemented for promoting health or preventing and treating diseases are called the oral health system, independent of their degree of organization or effectiveness. On the other hand, when a country tries to organize the system, on a global basis, setting up priorities, goals and backing it up with human resources and financial support, one can consider such countries as having a national oral health programme.

Taking into account the individual average income in Latin America and the limitations of the national budgets, access to the oral health systems for all is far from reality. Even some global measures like fluoridation are available for only a minority of the population. Trying to present an average for all of Latin America may lead to entirely false conclusions, due to the marked contrast between countries. In 1993 the number of dentists reached approximately 251 500 with a projection of 317 000 for the year 2000 (Pan American Health Organization, 1986; Fédération Dentaire Internationale, 1990, 1993; _Dental Guide to the Americas_, 1994). This places the dentist : population ratio amongst the highest in the world at 1 : 1837 in 1993, with the projection of 1 : 1672 at the turn of the century. However, looking at specific countries the ratio is 1 : 13 529 in Haiti, in contrast to 1 : 748 in Uruguay (Fédération Dentaire Internationale, 1993; _Dental Guide to the Americas_, 1994).

In view of these considerations, in order to achieve a clearer understanding of the oral health situation in Latin America and its systems, comparable data for 25 countries were divided into three regions:

1 the Caribbean islands zone, Mexico, Central America and Panama;
2 the Andean region;
3 the South Cone (Tables 17.7–17.8).

For each country, the available data are classified trying to evidence the main characteristics of the oral health system or of the national oral health programme. The dentist : population ratio is also given. Existence of any systemic fluoride is tabulated where available, as well as the mean DMFT at the age of 12.

The oral health system in all countries but Cuba is predominantly on a private basis and only about 30% of the population have access to dentists, mainly because of economic limitations. This means that 70% of the Latin American population rely mostly on public services which employ only 25% of the dentists. In spite of this, public services are poorly structured, offer limited services and usually, their population coverage is low (Tables 17.7–17.8). For the adult population, tooth extraction is the main procedure. Some countries (Table 17.7a) are trying to organize a system for schoolchildren, educating different types of personnel with varying duties. In this connection, auxiliary personnel have not always followed regular courses, but in some countries participate in preventive programmes and clinical work, mainly for schoolchildren. Other countries, like Mexico, Venezuela, Jamaica, Bahamas, Barbados, Colombia, Haiti, Nicaragua, Panama and Guatemala started regular courses for dental nurses and/or dental technicians. Brazil has some scattered experiences with dental hygienists and dental hygienic technicians mainly aiming at increasing production in the public services in some municipalities. Brazil, Argentina and Mexico have all together 188 000 dentists, which represents 16–19% of the total number of dentists in the world (Fédération Dentaire Internationale, 1990, 1993; Pinto, 1990). Each year, the region receives between 9000 and 10 500 newly graduated dentists, coming out of 207 dental schools.

At the end of the 1980s to early 1990s, there were particular changes in the classical public health services, though the trends were different from country to country. Brazil set out to integrate the social security and health services, proposing a unified health system decentralizing the services to a municipal (local) level but under a centralized budget. Under today's economic policy of privatization, the system is struggling more for its survival rather than for improving its services. On the other hand, Chile privatized social security under its model of open economy whereby the state should intervene and/or participate only minimally. Nevertheless, in most countries dental care is still mainly on a private basis (Tables 17.7–17.8).

Private services are financed mainly by means of direct payment to the dentists, but through the 1980s there was a significant rise in private dental insurances, mainly in the most industrialized areas and richest countries. In Latin America, governmental services are usually exempt from direct taxation, but with very low coverage, in spite of the fact that taxes have systematically increased both in number

Table 17.7a The Caribbean zone

Country	Oral health system	Main characteristics	Dentist/population	Systemic fluoride	DMFT 12-year-olds
Cuba	National oral health programme	Comprehensive and universal	1/1730	W <	2.0–4.0
Haiti	NA	NA	1/13 529	No	2.0–4.0
Dominican Republic	Mainly on private basis	Schoolchildren	1/5588	W <	>6.0
Jamaica	Organized public system for children	Schoolchildren	1/20 200*	No	>6.0
Trinidad and Tobago and other islands	Organized public system for children	Schoolchildren	1/14 240*	W NA	2.0–4.0
Bahamas	NA	NA	1/6800*	W NA	1.0–2.0
Barbados	Organized public system for children	Schoolchildren	1/10 600*	No	4.0–6.0

*Data from the 1980s.
DMFT = Decayed, missing, filled teeth; NA = not available; W = water fluoridation–population coverage (< less than 20%).

Table 17.7b Mexico, Central America and Panama

Country	Oral health system	Main characteristics	Dentist/ population	Systemic fluoride	DMFT 12-year-olds
Panama	Scattered public services	Low coverage	1/2780	W >	4.0–6.0
Costa Rica	Orgaized public system	Children education, low coverage	1/2308	S NA	4.0–6.0
Nicaragua	Public system	Lack of material, low coverage	1/4362	No	4.0–6.0
Honduras	Mainly on private basis	Incipient	1/9655	W <	>6.0
El Salvador	Mainly on private basis	Incipient	1/6322	No	4.0–6.0
Guatemala	Scattered public services, mainly on private basis	Incipient	1/10 000	W NA	>6.0
Belize	NA	NA	NA	NA	2.0–4.0
Mexico	Uncoordinated public sector, mainly on private basis	Low coverage	1/2275	W < and S	2.0–4.0

DMFT = Decayed, missing, filled teeth; NA = not available; S = salt fluoridation; W = water fluoridation–population coverage (<less than 20%, > more than 20%).

Table 17.8a The Andean region

Country	Oral health system	Main characteristics	Dentist/ population	Systemic fluoride	DMFT 12-year-olds
Venezuela	Scattered and uncoordinated services, mainly on private basis	Decline after oil boom, low coverage	1/2627	W >	2.0–4.0
Colombia	Public system, mainly on private basis	First in the region	1/3393	S	4.0–6.0
Ecuador	Scattered and uncoordinated services, mainly on private basis	To be implemented	1/983	S	4.0–6.0
Peru	Scattered and uncoordinated services, mainly on private basis	To be implemented	1/3693	No	>6.0
Bolivia	Scattered and uncoordinated services, mainly on private basis	Incipient	1/3249	No	>6.0
Chile	Mainly on private basis	Extremely low covarage	1/2339	W <	4.0–6.0

DMFT = Decayed, missing, filled teeth; S = salt fluoridation; W = water fluoridation–population coverage (< less than 20%, > more than 20%).

Table 17.8b The south cone

Country	Oral health system	Main characteristics	Dentist/ population	Systemic fluoride	DMFT 12-year-olds
Brazil	Uncoordinated public system/ mainly on private basis	Low coverage, private services hired	1/1316	W >	4.0–6.0
Uruguay	Mainly on private basis	Private services hired	1/748	W < and S	4.0–6.0
Paraguay	Mainly on private basis	Extremely low coverage	1/3740	W <	4.0–6.0
Argentina	Uncoordinated public system/ mainly on private basis	Private services hired	1/1142	W >	2.0–4.0

DMFT = Decayed, missing, filled teeth; W = water fluoridation (< less than 20%, > more than 20%); S = salt fluoridation.

and in percentage in the period covering the 1980s and the 1990s. Preventive programmes on a population level are few. Even systemic fluoride measures are scarce (Tables 17.7–17.8). The stated coverage is certainly optimistic, considering lack of regularity in the programmes. Water fluoridation covers more than 30% in Argentina, Brazil and Panama and less than that in Venezuela, Chile, Paraguay, Uruguay, Honduras, Mexico, Cuba and the Dominican Republic. Recently, five countries started salt fluoridation–Columbia, Costa Rica, Jamaica, Mexico and Uruguay (Tables 17.7–17.8). Topical fluoride programmes either with fluoride mouth-rinses or fluoride gels have been introduced to schoolchildren in Brazil, Colombia, Ecuador and the Dominican Republic, but with low coverage and lack of continuity. Fluoride varnish (locally produced) was introduced in Cuba (Pinto, 1990; Pan American Health Organization, 1994) for children and seems to be a common practice.

Fluoridated dentifrices introduced in the 1950s (Inacio, 1982) had achieved only 11–12% of the total sales of toothpaste in Brazil by 1981 (Inacio, 1982). Now, in the 1990s its use has reached a high percentage, mainly in the most populated countries. In Brazil, a recent survey in a poor urban area in an industrial city showed that all houses visited had at least one tube of fluoridated dentifrice (Bellini *et al.*, 1995). Actually, about 99% of the marketed dentifrices are fluoridated.

The dental industry in Brazil and Argentina (Pan American Health Organization, 1986) is important, with Brazil being one of the largest producers of dental equipment in the world. Countries like Mexico, Venezuela, Paraguay and Brazil are also producing less expensive and unsophisticated equipment (called appropriate-

technology equipments), attempting to use fewer resources in order to increase population coverage. However, from current knowledge, the problem of dealing with oral care is much more one of oral health promotion, including prevention and early diagnosis, than one of new technology for conventional treatment.

Implications for future planning

The high prevalence of oral diseases in Latin America, in all age groups, supports the call for increased levels of health promotion for the prevention of caries and periodontal diseases, reduction of oral cancer and early treatment and the reduction of malocclusion. We may need to question why with such a favourable dentist-to-population ratio we continue to have high levels of disease.

Effectiveness can be enhanced with improved knowledge on environmental factors, especially social ones. Coverage can be increased by implementing coordinated actions, mainly having oral health programmes associated with general health programmes. Resources could be optimized with improved management, priorities defined according to the target community and effectiveness evaluated by the results in health improvement and not by the amount of services delivered.

Future outlook

The trends for the end of the century are not encouraging. The present unequal system of mainly private practice directed to a minority of the population and based on reparative services seems to continue. There is no sign of changes in the model of high production of dentists (trained mainly for reparative services) for facing high prevalence of diseases.

Increasing difficulties in finding jobs may lead to a lower demand for places in dental schools in the near future. Organized oral health promotion, including prevention, has had a nominal role to date. Nevertheless, it is expected that there will be a decline in caries incidence due to a wider use of fluoride by means of water and salt fluoridation, fluoridated dentifrice and a more regular use of other forms of topical fluoride. A significant improvement in oral health of the adult population, however, cannot be expected until the younger cohort ages.

In general, there is a tendency for a gradual improvement in the Latin American economy, reflecting an expanding dental industry, dental dealers and dental insurances. The public sector, which tries to cover the low-income population, may remain close to what it is today. Largely, this is due to the model adopted by the majority of the governments in the region, which follows a neoliberal economy, implementing privatization and trying to reduce state participation in the economy. The lack of humanistic education, of tradition in social services and weak judiciary systems (impunity for political, financial and social crimes) leads to a lack of assistance, mainly for the low-income groups. The state is unable to compensate for the gap, unable to reduce the differences, even to the extremes. Such a future outlook makes international support to national initiatives in public health tremendously important. Population strategies need to be implemented, in order to reverse the negative trends prevailing today.

References

Bellini, H.T., Denardi, J.L., Martins, T.P.C. *et al.* (1995) Some housing conditions and oral habits among a group of Brazilian school children from Jundiai–Abstract. WCPD'95 Abstracts April 27–30, Sao Paulo. p. 87.

Bojanini, N.J. (1995) Salud oral para todos en el año 2000 en Colombia. Bogota. In manus.

Comisión Económica para América Latina (1993) *Panorama Social de America Latina, CEPAL*, Santiago, p. 129. Chile.

Dental Guide to the Americas (1994) Panorama Suvision, 10 13–26. Rome.

De Smet, R.M. (1966) Observations anthropologiques sur la denture des Indiens Xingu (Brésil). *Bull.Group.Int.Rech.Sc. Stomat.* 9:401–414.

Fédération Dentaire Internationale (1990) *FDI Basic Facts 1990, Dentistry around the World.* FDI, London.

Fédération Dentaire Internationale (1993) *FDI Basic Sheets, for Latin America Countries (1992).* FDI, London.

Ferraz, C. and Bellini, H.T. (1983) Condicoes dentarias de um grupo de trabalhadores adultos em Jundiai. *Rev. Assoc. Paulista de Cir. Dent.* 37:330–335.

Inacio, F. (1982) Mercado de creme dental e o segmento fluor. In: *Seminario de Prevencao da Carie e Doencas da Gengiva.* Jundiai, S.P. pp. 50–51.

International Sugar Organization (1993) *Sugar Yearbook 1993.* ISO, London.

International Sugar Organization (1994) *Examen Trimestral del Mercado.* ISO, London.

Neumann, H.H. and DiSalvo, N.A. (1958) Caries in Indians of the Mexican Cordillera, the Peruvian Andes and at the Amazon Headwaters. *British Dental Journal* 104:13–16.

Pan American Health Organization (1986) *Informacion dental sobre America Latina. Informe Tecnico 27.* Grupo de Trabajo Mixto no. 7. PAHO, WHO and FDI, Washington.

Pan American Health Organization (1994) *Regional Oral Health Strategy for the 1990s.* PAHO/HSS/94.14, by Estupinan-Day, S. p. 44. Washington.

Pinto, V.G. (1990) *Saude Bucal: Panorama International*, p. 257. Ministerio da Saude, Brasilia, Brazil.

Pinto, V.G. (1994) Solutions to fight poverty. Paper presented to the 26th International Conference of ICSW, workshop on "economic solutions to fight poverty", p. 18. Tampere, Finland.

Pinto, V.G. and Lima, M.P. (1995) Reducao de carie dental no Brasil: o estudo do SESI. Abstract Congresso Internacional de Saude Bucal. Associacao Brasileira de Odontologia. Brazilia, Brazil.

United Nations Organization (1993) *Human Development Report*, p. 249. NUDP, Madrid.

World Bank (1994) *World Development Report*, p. 267. Oxford University Press, New York.

World Health Organization (1994a) *Dental Caries Level at 12 Years.* WHO Oral Health/ORH, Geneva.

World Health Organization (1994b) *Periodontal Profiles, an Overview of CPITN Data in the WHO Global Oral Data Bank*, p. 43. WHO Oral Health, Geneva.

In developing countries

Martin Hobdell

Introduction

The concept of developing countries grew out of the concept of the Third World–a term often used interchangeably with that of developing countries. The Third World was a term that arose out of the language of the immediate post World War II period. The First World was the two superpowers (the USA and the Soviet Union); the Second World was the satellite nations of these two superpowers; and the Third World was the rest, or what are called today the developing countries. These countries were non-aligned politically (usually members of the Non-aligned Movement). This meant that they neither supported nor rejected the political orientation of either East or West, but were willing to work with both. As more and more countries gained their independence from western colonial powers during the 1950s and 1960s the focus of concern of the Non-aligned Movement, and that of its constituent member states, changed, from that of independence to development, in order to improve the lot of their people. For many newly independent states, the welfare state, as exemplified by the education and health policies in the UK and the Nordic countries, became models on which to base their new government's policies. For those countries which looked more to the East than the West, then the Soviet Union became the model for the achievement of social justice. Some countries attempted to develop their own models of a socially just society. However, whichever route was taken, the new leaders were faced with the legacy of the colonial past which was almost invariably typified by non-industrialization, dependence on single, often unpredictable cash crops, poor literacy levels and widespread poverty. Some governmental regimes that developed were dictatorial or undemocratic; marginalization and dependence on aid from the developed world became a recurring profile. The way forward for many countries is not clear, as despite their efforts, many face servicing the debt of aid, given as loans, for many years, so taking away a significant part of their GNP. There is a growing body of evidence that at least as much money is returned by developing countries to banks in the developed world, in the form of interest and debt repayments, as is given in aid (Denham, 1991). So there is little or no net financial gain.

The developing countries are the most numerous and poorest countries in the world. They include the most populous nations on earth. They are also the ones whose populations are, for understandable reasons, increasing most rapidly. Currently there are 48 out of roughly 150 developing countries which are classified as the *least developed* countries. Of these, 32 are to be found in the African continent. There are between 5000 and 6000 million people in the world today, of whom somewhere in the region of 75–80% live in the developing world. Therefore, the developed, industrialized world has around 1000 million people. This latter figure is of significance because it roughly equals the number of people who, it is estimated, live in extreme poverty in the least developed countries of the world.

The gap between rich and poor people in the world is increasing and extreme poverty is the world's biggest killer, with diseases linked to poverty increasing (World Health Organization, 1995). The gaps between the developing and least developed countries have widened in the last 10 years in respect of life expectancy at birth and infant mortality rates (Subramian, 1995). A person in one of the least developed countries has a life expectancy of 43 years, while life expectancy in developed countries is as high as 78 years. This effect of poverty on life expectancy, though less extreme, is shared by the growing number of disadvantaged and deprived population groups within industrialized countries (Davey Smith *et al.*, 1990). In some developing countries, rapid urbanization has further marginalized the urban poor. For some, this is complicated by war and its aftermath. The number of international refugees and internally displaced people increased by 40% between 1990 and 1993 from 30 million to 43 million, the majority of whom were in developing countries. Such immense dislocations in communities have profound implications for the management of health and welfare services.

Health care systems in developing countries

Many developing countries, unsurprisingly, opted to develop health care systems based on the social welfare models emanating from Europe at the time of their independence. This meant that they chose centrally organized programmes of planning, administration, provision and evaluation, with the government being sometimes the sole agent responsible for all of these activities. However, in most cases there was also a private sector of care provision, the size of which varied from country to country. In some, for example, private practice was explicitly forbidden. This private sector has been of two distinct types. There are those care-providers who have been trained through some type of individual apprenticeship under the tutelage of a traditional healer. Then there are those who have trained in formal educational institutions either in their own country or abroad. Commonly government and private systems, and traditionally and formally trained personnel all work in parallel with little coordination between them, although parts of the Indian subcontinent and China are perhaps unique in the way in which traditional medicine has been officially supported and incorporated into the national health care system.

Patients usually have to choose where they go. Social factors primarily influence people as to whether they go to the traditional healer first or to the formal government sector, with choice being finally determined by wealth in most cases. There have been some suggestions for collaboration between traditional healers and the formal health care system (Ademuwagun, 1969; Mshiu and Chhabra, 1982; Akerele, 1987). In Africa this has largely been unsuccessful (Kale, 1995). However, a greater understanding is being shown in some areas of conventional medicine and the recognition of alternative methods may increase. A traditional healer is a person with no formal training, but who is recognized by the community in which he or she lives as competent to provide health care by using vegetable, animal and mineral substances and certain other methods in treating disease and disability (Ngilisho *et al.*, 1994). There have been few

studies reporting on the efficacy of traditional remedies, although a recent study has reported on comparative dental care (Ngilisho *et al.*, 1994). In this study conducted in Tanzania, villagers in a rural region were interviewed, as were 73 traditional healers. Half of the 408 villagers interviewed had experienced toothache and 60% of those who had experienced toothache in the last 2 years had sought treatment from traditional healers. They had all been treated with local herbs. As has been found elsewhere and supporting the premise of a parallel service, the establishment of modern emergency oral care in rural health centres and dispensaries did not influence the villagers' use of the traditional healers (Ngilisho *et al.*, 1994). dispensaries did not influence the villagers' use of the traditional healers (Ngilisho *et al.*, 1994).

In establishing health systems, apart from the dearth of material resources, many new governments were faced with low levels of education and very limited numbers of trained personnel. This was exacerbated by the need to demonstrate rapid improvements in the health services. One way forward was to train intermediate-level health care workers. Therefore, initially some strong public health programmes were started in developing countries, like those, for example in Malaysia and Sri Lanka, and previously in a more modest way in Mozambique and Tanzania. For many countries, external political constraints have further hindered economic development and impinged on internal political structures. These factors have combined to undermine these public health programmes, inevitably resulting in the growth of private medicine for the few and gross inequity for the many. Mozambique provides an example of this change and the effects of the interplay of macro political, economic and social changes on the organization of health services in a developing country. To follow its complex history, readers are referred to other texts (Hobdell, 1980; Hanlon, 1986, 1991; Minter, 1994).

In the face of limited resources and the inappropriateness of high-technology curative-based approaches of western medicine, some countries have tried to base their health care systems on the primary health care approach or PHCA (WHO/UNICEF, 1978). The principles are described in detail in Chapter 2 of this book. Nigeria has attempted to follow this approach.

However, in a recent appraisal of Nigeria's primary health care system, several problems were identified (Onoja, 1995). Clearly, some of the problems were not only due to financial constraints but also to poor management of the meagre resources available. The population of Nigeria is over 30 million and 47% of the population is below 15 years. The number of cities with populations over 0.5 million people and the proportion of the population living in cities is growing (Federal Office of Statistics, 1985; Economist Intelligence Unit, 1990). Between 1974 and 1980, only around 1% of the country's GNP was allocated to health. All these features would be common in many developing countries. The World Health Organization recommends that at least 5% of GNP be allocated to the health system and, as can be seen in tables in previous sections of this chapter, these percentages range from 5 to 11%. Another prominent feature of the health services in Nigeria, again common elsewhere, is an uneven distribution of resources. There is general neglect of the rural population (Onoja, 1995). Health resources and facilities are concentrated in the urban areas and are oriented to middle- and upper-income groups. The doctor–population ratio is 1:12 500; this figure appears close to the World Health Organization's recommendation of 1:10 000 in developing countries. However, it hides a chronic maldistribution, since in the rural areas of Nigeria, the ratio would range from 1:40 000 up to 1:200 000. It is salutary to realize that in the least developed areas of the western world the ratio is 1:520.

Another problem is in implementation of the fifth concept of the PHCA, that of community participation in funding the health system. This has been interpreted by the Federal Authority such that much of the financial burden is being shifted to the community (Onoja, 1995). This problem was recognized some years ago by Stinson (1984), who contended that reliance on community financing often fails to achieve targets in health matters. Onoja (1995) makes several recommendations to improve primary health care in Nigeria. These centre on the need to improve living conditions through health education. He recommends a reversal of the present trend, where most of the effort is towards late intervention with curative measures, and that much greater efforts should be directed towards preventive measures in line with the concept of primary care. He considers that

policy-makers should be educated in the values of preventive measures as a means of problem-solving, enabling them to change their attitudes and perception of health and plan appropriate health care programmes.

A further recommendation is improved general education for all people. Much ill health arises from poor living conditions compounded by low levels of education. This latter leads to a lowered awareness of healthy practices and superstition of modern medical facilities. Incentive schemes could encourage health workers to accept positions in rural areas. The training of health workers needs to be addressed as the majority of their training is still geared to curative methods. Interestingly, one of his final recommendations is the integration of traditional health care into the modern system of health care. This would allow traditional practitioners to feel valued while, at the same time, encouraging improvements in hygiene (Onoja, 1995).

Vietnam is facing similar problems, but compounded by the effects of nearly 30 years of war which devastated the health services. In re-evaluating the health system, it was clear that the city health facilities tended to model themselves on modern hospitals in more developed countries, partly because of the influence of doctors who had been educated in those countries and because of the desire for state-of-the-art technology (Anh and Tram, 1995). The government has attempted to reorganize the health system, focusing on a primary health care policy and a complete subsidy principle. Anh and Tram (1995) describe the effects of introducing the primary health care concepts into a paediatric hospital in Ho Chi Minh City. The hospital has supported dramatic improvements in health in the 5 years since the policy was introduced. Through its involvement in community outreach, the staff have substantially reduced the number of admissions and seen dramatic improvements in mortality rates. There has been on-site health education for the child's carers and community-based rather than hospital-based nutritional rehabilitation. One factor in the financing mechanism may account for its success in contrast to the Nigerian experience. The government's contribution is 60% of the total budget and the proportion contributed by the patient, at around 20–30%, has not risen under the new system. Those patients who can afford to contribute pay daily charges rather than fees-for-service. The equity principle is the guideline for all financial changes.

Oral health care systems

To a large extent, the conflicts of transposing a western medical model-based system in general health care to developing countries have been echoed in oral health care systems. The fact that over 80% of all oral health personnel (particularly dentists) train and work in the developed, industrialized world, reflects the much greater wealth of these countries. But more particularly it reflects the history of the commercial production of sugar, which is so much bound up with the European Industrial Revolution, colonial expansion and the slave trade (Davidson, 1980; Olbrich, 1989). These events are mirrored in the global history of dental caries, particularly since the development and use of the centrifuge in the commercial production of sugar in the 1850s (Corbet and Moore, 1976; Marthaler, 1990), which made it so much more readily available to industrial populations. As a result of this history the bulk of dental disease, in the form of dental caries, and therefore oral health services developed in the developed world. This has inevitably led to dentistry and oral health services taking on a particular form, related to the specific disease pattern engendered by this increased sugar consumption, and the constraints and opportunities offered in the rapidly mechanizing world of Victorian Europe. As a result the mind set of dentistry, which is encountered in training institutions, research programmes and international organizations, whether or not they are located in the developed or developing world, is that of the developed world (Hobdell and Sheiham, 1981). This is not to argue that there should be different principles on which the practice of clinical dentistry and research rest in developed and developing countries, but rather to suggest that these principles need to be translated into sustainable practice in ways appropriate to the circumstances prevailing in all countries, whether they are classified as developing or developed. And, therefore, that sustainable practice may look very different in one country to that in another. But if these practices embody the defined principles of good service then they are of equal merit, regardless of the practical differences.

Two approaches to the development of oral health care and services

Out of this history there have arisen two competing models on which the organization of oral health care has been based in developing countries: the rational and the traditional.

The *rational* development of services and practices is based on carefully gathered and analysed quantitative and qualitative data, which are then translated into strategic and operational plans (including patient treatment, education and research), based on scientifically sound principles and the availability of resources. The other is based on *tradition* and is usually found in the training institutions. It reflects the activities of dental practitioners (dental hygienists, therapists and dentists) which have been inherited from the past. It is pervasive and persistent and is to be found not only in developing but also in developed countries.

Sri Lanka–an example of the rational and traditional approaches

Sri Lanka was one of the first developing countries to begin the training of dental therapists, who were originally called school dental nurses. The school dental nurse programme was begun, in Sri Lanka, soon after the Second World War and modelled entirely on the teaching in New Zealand, to the extent that in 1980 they were still using the original teaching materials from New Zealand. By then it had become a good example of a traditionally based system. But that had not always been the case.

The reasons for starting the training of school dental nurses, for example, were rational and based on the scientific information available at that time. The pattern of oral disease and the requirements of the population were well-served by this approach. But, as time went on, there was little local input to the adaptation and development of the programmes. They became outdated. The school programme, for example, used an incremental care approach, so that in theory at least children on admission to the school were examined and given comprehensive care. Then the next year this group passed to maintenance care, and the new intake received the comprehensive care. Unfortunately after a while it was clear that not all children managed to receive comprehensive care in their first year at school, and even when they did, maintenance demands were high and were given priority over the provision of care for the new pupils. The result was that most of the dental nurses' time was spent on a small core of children, who after a while showed all the signs of overtreatment (Hobdell, 1981).

Since the early 1980s much has changed and the programmes, both in training and service, now better reflect the needs of the population. This is largely as a result of the influence of the Health Promotion Unit of the Ministry of Health, which has a strong oral health element. The rational approach has been used, replacing what had become the traditional approach. Maintaining the new approach will depend on monitoring and evaluation being used, and adjustments being made, on a regular basis. Failure to do this in the past resulted in the programme lapsing into one based on tradition.

Critical changes in economic approaches

In all this finance plays a vital part, particularly in relation to the availability of resources in developing countries. In those developing countries, which have in recent years changed their economic approach from that of a planned economy to that of the free market, there are major implications for the health sector and the health of their people (Green, 1989). The argument in favour of allowing free-market forces to operate in health care is as follows: providers of health care, that is paid for directly, by either patients or third parties, come under greater pressure to be accountable to patients and make their care work, than those in services which are free at the time of use, and who are salaried. In other words, the services are more efficient in economic terms particularly. Examples of the latter type of service are the centrally planned and operated services developed for ideological reasons by many newly independent countries. This consumer pressure, generated by the free market, reinforces the use of the rational rather than traditional approach to the organization of programmes and also individual treatment plans. Under such pressure even the most traditional establishments are now being forced to bring their programmes and activities into line with the economic reality. The down side of all this is that, in the free market, access to care is restricted to those who can afford it. In developing countries, like Mozambique, it is a very small percentage of the

population and far fewer than had access before external pressures forced the introduction of the free market. Indeed it was this very fact that prompted the newly independent countries to opt for the system they developed after independence, because of their commitment to social justice.

Oral health and disease characteristics of developing countries

Dental caries and periodontal diseases

Considerations of the prevalence of oral diseases can be found in Chapter 6. For developing countries, caries levels are still generally lower than in the majority of developed countries. However, data from several studies support the findings that levels of dental caries are increasing in urban areas of developing countries where people have greater access to sugar-containing products. In sugar-producing countries, there is widespread consumption of sugar cane and locally prepared sweets are being manufactured. The latter phenomenon has been reported in Nigeria and Tanzania.

Much of the data on disease prevalence has come from small-scale studies that have rarely been representative of the whole country. There has been a recent national survey in Nigeria and the results are described here as they have many features that will be common to other developing countries. At 12 years old, the mean DMFT was 0.8 and all of the caries experience was untreated decay; similarly, at 15, the DMFT was 1.3 with 1.2 DT. By 35–44, an average of 2.5 teeth had experienced caries and 1.4 were decayed with 1.1 extracted (Adegbembo et al., 1995). At 12, 30% of children had decayed teeth and for 5%, the teeth were so badly decayed they required extraction. There were regional differences in prevalence and there was evidence of an increased number of decayed teeth in the young (<20 years) and in those living in urban compared to rural areas. The authors projected from the survey figures that 7.3 million people needed dental extractions and 22.9 million needed restorations. In the same survey, periodontal status was assessed (Adegbembo and El-Nadeef, 1995). By 12 years old, 94% of children had calculus and this seemed to be the prevailing problem for the young and young adults. Calculus was present in virtually all sextants and the principal need the authors identified was for calculus removal and oral hygiene instruction. The majority of people used chewing sticks for oral hygiene. Chewing sticks, or *miswak,* have been shown to be as effective as a tooth-brush in removing plaque and some types have been shown to have antibacterial properties. The World Health Organization (1987b) has recommended and encouraged the use of chewing sticks as an effective oral hygiene tool, while acknowledging that community programmes may be needed to teach effective cleaning routines. In Nigeria, there is already a network of community health extension workers and the authors of this present survey suggested extending their role to carry out screening for oral diseases with a referral system (Adegbembo *et al.,* 1995), complemented by the use of operating auxiliaries.

Cancrum oris or noma

This condition is an important indicator of the level of development of a community; it is a disease of poverty. It occurred in many developed countries until the 1920s, where these populations were poorly housed and fed, and immunization against infectious diseases was limited. Malnutrition plays an important part in the establishment of this and other diseases which begin with oral ulceration because of its effect on the inflammatory response and immune system (Enwonwu, 1985, 1994). Unfortunately, few accurate data exist on this most serious and important of health problems in developing countries. World Health Organization has estimated that annually there are around half a million cases a year in children between the ages of 2 and 6 years. Ninety per cent of those who do not receive appropriate and timely care, die. The remainder who survive are grossly disfigured for life and frequently become outcasts from their families and communities (World Health Organization, 1994). It is believed that several hundred thousand of these cases occur in Africa each year and that in that continent the problem is growing in parallel with the growing numbers living in extreme poverty.

Dental hypoplasia and malnutrition

Some of the underlying reasons for the differences in disease patterns in developing and developed countries have already been discussed; however, most profound are the effects of extensive material deprivation. Poverty, marginalization, lack of well-developed transport systems, poor housing and water supplies, chronic undernourishment and overcrowding in periurban slums all contribute to the disease burden carried by many people in developing countries. Oral health is equally affected. Whilst the diet may contain–at least in the rural areas–for example, little sugar, attacks of infectious diseases, such as measles, and fever (frequently caused by malaria in the hotter regions), result in many teeth, particularly the primary dentition, being hypoplastic (Li *et al.,* 1995). These teeth are more susceptible to carious attack. In the urban areas where sugar is more available and frequently consumed, this hypoplasia plays an important part in the occurrence of the higher dental caries prevalence levels encountered amongst the malnourished population (Alvarez and Navia, 1989; Alvarez, 1995).

Trauma

The high trauma rates reflect a number of aspects of life in the developing world. The appalling living conditions of many in the developing world not only provoke alcohol abuse but, combined with domestic overcrowding, also feed interpersonal violence and accidents. Alcoholism, poor road conditions and vehicle safety increase the chances of serious road traffic accidents. A lack of safety controls in the home and workplace add further to the likelihood of trauma.

Oral cancer

The higher oral cancer rates in developing countries often reflect the habit of chewing tobacco. Where this is combined with the habit of betel leaf chewing the rates are particularly high, as is the case in India and Sri Lanka, where a third of all cancers are associated with the mouth and pharynx (Daftary *et al.,* 1991). Not only is the cause tobacco use but also the use of alcohol. Alcohol abuse, as already mentioned, is often high in socially deprived populations. The alcohol is often impure and drunk neat. This aggravates the effects of the tobacco in causing both oral cancer and periodontal diseases (World Health Organization, 1987a). Many of these factors, mentioned above, also influence the rate of spread of HIV infection in the population. It would not be surprising, therefore, to find a higher prevalence of oral mucosal lesions, associated with this infection, in the mouths of people in developing countries. Data are however at present too unreliable to make a more concrete statement. Oral cancer prevalence is described in further detail in Chapter 6.

Oral health care in developing countries– implications for the future

The purpose of an oral health care system is to influence the population's way of life so that oral health is promoted or maintained, and oral disease prevented; and to provide adequate treatment to those members of the population affected by oral disease so that disease is arrested at an early stage and loss of function is prevented (World Health Organization, 1987b). These two functions, in the context of the PHCA (see Chapter 2), apply no matter whether the service is in a developing or developed country. Using these functions as a basis, principles have been established to guide the development of oral health services or programmes in the Oral Health Alliance's Declaration of Berlin (Oral Health Alliance, 1992). These principles hold for developing and developed countries alike and provide a framework for rational consideration of the role of governments; reducing inequalities;

underdevelopment; dependence; empowerment; community involvement; partnerships; oral health promotion; preventive strategies; ethics; personnel preparation; rights of health workers and the scientific basis of oral health strategies. This framework allows the specification of the work of a community-based dentist (Table 17.9). In the oral health sector new optimism and determination exist, not to recapitulate the stages of oral health service development which developed countries have been through, but rather to adopt a rational scientifically based process.

This is summarized succinctly in the introduction to a paper written by oral health care workers in the Middle East (Al-Lafi and Ahabneh, 1995):

> Dental caries and periodontal disease determine the level of oral health status of a person. Unfortunately, such diseases are so common that essentially every adult in the world has one or other or both. Therefore, these two diseases can be considered a real public health problem. In general every country has, and should have, its own system to prevent and cure its nation from diseases according to its resources and culture. Dental health personnel trained in western scientific systems usually have views on the prevention of oral disease that differ basically from those of local communities. Instead of focusing on the real causes of these diseases (which are simply dirt and diet) and instead of directing all efforts to invent and encourage the use of effective tools to prevent and control these two diseases effectively, the profession has fallen in an endless, exhausting and costly routine of restorative treatment which consumes too much time, resources, effort and money.

All preventive avenues need to be explored, in particular those that can be sustained within the society and culture of the country, for whichever route is taken in organizing oral health care it is clear that even where the state accepts responsibility for funding (and in some cases also providing) oral health services there will only be a commitment of funds if the procedures and programmes are effective and efficiently run. The problem is that any funds available for the health sector are likely to be small and, for oral health, infinitesimal. This will be a test of the world's commitment to health as a fundamental human right (Hobdell, 1993) on an equal footing to that, say, of democracy, which has been so much promoted to bring about change in the developing world. It will also be the challenge to dentistry in the coming millennium.

Table 17.9 The work of a community-based dentist

Functions	Activities
Manager	Leader of primary oral health care team; monitor and control the oral health subsystem; organize/coordinate preventive, treatment and referral services; help data analysis research and information dissemination; help plan, supervise and evaluate the oral health activities
Agent of socioeconomic development	Development of community participation in oral health; liaison with the public, politicians and other sectors; participate in community meetings and development activities; participate in intersectoral projects (e.g. food and water); advocacy of better oral health; critical analysis of intersectoral plans for oral health and their implications; influence politicians to make healthful decisions; support appropriate development (e.g. local food production)
Dental officer	Complex treatment of patients; promotion of oral health at community, family and individual levels
Educator	Continuing education of colleagues; training of lower-level oral health workers; oral health education of families and communities

References

Adegbembo, A.O. and El-Nadeef, M.A.I. (1995) National survey of periodontal status and treatment need among Nigerians. *International Dental Journal* **45**:197–203.

Adegbembo, A.O., El-Nadeef, M.A.I. and Adeyinka, A. (1995) National survey of dental caries status and treatment needs in Nigeria. *International Dental Journal* **45**:35–44.

Ademuwagun, Z.A. (1969) The relevance of Yoruba Medicine men in public health practice in Nigeria. *Public Health Reports* **84**:1085–1091.

Akerele, D. (1987) Role of traditional medicine in health care delivery systems. *Tanzania Medical Journal* **4**:3–7.

Al-Lafi, T. and Ahabneh, H. (1995) The effect of the extract of the Miswak (chewing sticks) used in Jordan and the Middle East on oral bacteria.

Alvarez, J.O. (1995) Nutrition, tooth development and dental caries. *American Journal of Clinical Nutrition* **61**(2):410–416.

Alvarez, J.O. and Navia, J.M. (1989) Nutritional status, tooth eruption and dental caries. *American Journal of Clinical Nutrition* **49**:417–426.

Anh, N.t.N. and Tram, T.T. (1995) Integration of primary health care concepts in a children's hospital with limited resources. *Lancet* **346**:421–424.

Corbet, M.E. and Moore, W.J. (1976) Distribution of dental caries in ancient British populations, 4: the 19th Century. *Caries Research* **10**:401–414.

Daftary, D.K., Murti, P.R., Bhonsle, R.B. *et al.* (1991) Risk markers for oral cancer in high incidence areas of the world. In: *Risk Markers for Oral Diseases*, vol. 2. *Oral Cancer* (Johnson, N.W. *et al.*, eds), pp. 27–63. University of Cambridge Press, Cambridge.

Davey Smith, G., Shipley, M.J. and Rose, G. (1990) Magnitude and causes of socio-economic differentials in mortality: further evidence from the Whitehall study. *Journal of Epidemiology Community Health* **44**:265–270.

Davidson, H. (1980) *Black Mother–Africa and the Atlantic Slave Trade*. Penguin Books, Harmondsworth.

Denham, J. (1991) *The Debt Crisis–Origins and Overview*. Third World Now–Ireland and the Wider World, Comhlamh, Dublin, pp. 1–4.

Economist Intelligence Unit (1990) *Nigeria Country Profile 1990–91*. The Economist Intelligence Unit, London.

Enwonwu, C.O. (1985) Infectious oral necrosis in Nigerian children. A review. *Community Dental and Oral Epidemiology* **13**:190–194.

Enwonwu, C.O. (1994) Cellular and molecular effects of malnutrition and their relevance to periodental diseases. *Journal of Clinical and Periodontology* **21**:643–657.

Federal Office of Statistics (1985) *Digest of Statistics*. Federal Office of Statistics, Lagos.

Green, R.H. (1989) The broken pot: the social fabric, economic disaster and adjustment in Africa. In: *The IMF, The World Bank and The African Debt, Vol.2. The Social and Political Impact* (Onimode, B., ed.), pp. 31–35. Zed Books Ltd and the Institute for African Alternatives, London.

Hanlon, J. (1986) *Beggar your Neighbours–Apartheid Power in Southern Africa*. Catholic Institute for International Relations with James Currey, London.

Hanlon, J. (1991) *Mozambique–Who calls the Shots?* James Currey with Indiana University Press, London.

Hobdell, M.H. (1980) Dental health services in Mozambique. *British Dental Journal* **151**:161–162.

Hobdell, M.H. (1981) *Oral Health Services for School Children in Sri Lanka*. World Health Organization report. WHO, SEARO, New Delhi.

Hobdell, M.H. (1993) *The Magus in the Labyrinth or Medicine in a Muddle*. University of the Western Cape, Cape Town.

Hobdell, M.H. and Sheiham, A. (1981) Barriers to the promotion of dental health in developing countries. *Social Science and Medicine* **15A**:817–823.

Kale, R. (1995) Traditional healers in South Africa: a parallel health care system. *British Medical Journal* **310**:1182–1185.

Li, Y., Navia, J.M. and Bian, J.Y. (1995) Caries experience in the deciduous dentition in rural Chinese children 3 to 5 years old in relation to the presence or absence of enamel hypoplasia. *Community Dentistry and Oral Epidemiology* **23**(2):72–79.

Marthaler, T.M. (1990) Changes in the prevalence of dental caries: how much can be attributed to changes in diet? *Caries Research* **24** (suppl. 1):3–15.

Minter, W. (1994) *Apartheid's Contras: An Inquiry into the Roots of War in Angola and Mozambique*. Zed Press, London.

Mshiu, E.N. and Chhabra, S.C. (1982) Traditional healers and health care delivery in Tanzania. *Tropical Doctor* **12**:142–143.

Ngilisho, L.A.F., Mosha, H.J. and Poulsen, S.(1994) The role of traditional healers in the treatment of toothache in Tanza region, Tanzania. *Community Dental Health* **11**:240–242.

Olbrich, H. (1989) *Zucher–museum*. Zucher museum, Berlin.

Onoja, B.E. (1995) An appraisal of Nigeria's primary health care system. A personal view. *Journal of the Institute of Health Education* **33**:51–52.

Oral Health Alliance (1992) *The Berlin Declaration on Oral Health and Oral Health Services in Deprived Communities*, p. 24. Deutsch Stiftung für internationale Entwicklung, Berlin.

Stinson, W. (1984) Potential and limitation of community financing. *World Health Forum* **5**:123–125.

Subramian, M. (1995) The World Health report 1995: Bridging the gaps. *World Health* **2**:4–5.

WHO/UNICEF (1978) *Primary Health Care, Alma Ata 1978*. 'Health for All' series no. 1. Geneva, World Health Organization.

World Health Organization (1987a) *Oral Health in Community Health Programmes*. WHO, Geneva.

World Health Organization (1987b) *Alternative Systems of Oral Health Care Delivery*. Technical report series no. 750. WHO, Geneva.

World Health Organization (1994) *Noma, A Little-known Public Health Problem*. WHO 94.6. WHO, Geneva.

World Health Organization (1995) *The World Health Report 1995: Bridging the Gaps*. Office of World Health Reporting, WHO, Geneva.

Index